SPINOCEREBELLAR ATAXIA

Edited by **Jose Gazulla**

Spinocerebellar Ataxia
Edited by Jose Gazulla

Published by InTech
Janeza Trdine 9, 51000 Rijeka, Croatia

Publishing Process Manager Petra Nenadic

Technical Editor Teodora Smiljanic

Cover Designer InTech Design Team

Additional hard copies can be obtained from orders@intechopen.com

Spinocerebellar Ataxia, Edited by Jose Gazulla
p. cm.
ISBN 978-953-51-0542-8

For EU product safety concerns:
IN TECH d.o.o., Prolaz Marije Krucifikse Kozulić 3, 51000 Rijeka, Croatia,
info@intechopen.com or visit our website at intechopen.com.

Meet the editor

Born in 1957, Dr. José Gazulla performed his medical studies at the University of Navarra, and received training in Neurology at the Hospital Universitario Marqués de Valdecilla, in Santander (Spain). He worked at the Hospital General de Teruel and Hospital San Jorge, in Huesca, before joining the Service of Neurology of Hospital Universitario Miguel Servet, in Zaragoza (Spain). His deployment as a general neurologist has not impaired his interest in the degenerative diseases of the nervous system, especially of the cerebellum, spinal cord and peripheral nerves. Deeply interested in neurological semiology and pathophysiology, as well as in genetics, imaging and molecular biology of central and peripheral nervous system disorders, his interest in the field of degenerative ataxias became evident from early in his professional career. As a result of this, a number of reports concerning the clinical manifestations, imaging, neurochemistry and pharmacological treatment of the degenerative ataxias have been published, in collaboration with a small number of close collaborators.

Contents

Preface

The purpose of this book has been to depict as many biochemical, genetic and molecular advances as possible, in the vast field of the spinocerebellar ataxias. In addition, potential lines of pharmacological treatment in spinocerebellar ataxia type 3, enumerated by Professor Luis Pereira, are complemented by a chapter in which the pharmacological trials of the cerebellar ataxias have been reviewed in depth. Clinical manifestations of the spinocerebellar ataxias are also included in the text, like the description by Dr. Luis Velázquez-Pérez of those in spinocerebellar ataxia type 2, and the exhaustive review about eye movement abnormalities in cerebellar disease, written by Dr. Rodríguez-Labrada.

Dr. Jose Gazulla
Service of Neurology,
Hospital Universitario Miguel Servet,
Zaragoza,
Spain

1

Model Systems for Spinocerebellar Ataxias: Lessons Learned About the Pathogenesis

Thorsten Schmidt*#, Jana Schmidt* and Jeannette Hübener*
Eberhard-Karls-University Tuebingen, Medical Genetics
Germany

1. Introduction

Model systems are important tools for the investigation of pathogenic processes. Especially for diseases with a late onset of symptoms and slow progression, like most spinocerebellar ataxias (SCA), it is time-consuming or even impossible to analyze all aspects of the pathogenesis in humans. Due to the reduced lifespan of model organisms, it is possible to study disease progression in full within a reasonable timeframe and due to the shorter generation time of most model organisms more individuals can be generated and analyzed, thereby strengthening the reliability of data via an increased number of replicates. Detailed studies of the histopathology can only be performed as endpoint analyses in humans, but with the help of an animal model, multiple time points can be analyzed throughout the course of the disease. In addition, model systems allow not only for the reduction of time from idea to results but also reduce the complexity due to their smaller genome sizes, less genes, nonredundant pathways, and a simpler nervous system.

Before using a specific species to model a disease it is of interest to check whether the proteins affected in humans are conserved within the respective model organism in order to increase the probability that binding partners and other keyplayers, involved in the pathogenesis of this disease, are likewise conserved. For those SCA which are caused by polyglutamine (polyQ) expansions, the respective affected genes are conserved in most organisms used as models (Table 1). Especially the proteins affected in SCA2, SCA6 and SCA17 are conserved with high similarity down to even yeast. This is not surprising as the TATA-binding protein (affected in SCA17) or a subunit of a voltage-dependent calcium channel (affected in SCA6) are important proteins for cellular maintenance. Although polyQ repeats are comparatively frequent in drosophila (Alba et al., 2007), only the repeat region of the TATA-binding protein is conserved. For most other non-mammalian model organisms, the respective orthologues are smaller and the polyQ repeats itself or even including the whole surrounding domains are not conserved. For analyses of SCA, various model systems have been employed. From the worm (*Caenorhabditis elegans*) and the fly (*Drosophila melanogaster*) all the way to mammals, i.e. the mouse (*Mus musculus*), model systems have

---

* All three authors contributed equally to this work
# Corresponding author: Thorsten Schmidt, Ph.D.; University of Tuebingen; Medical Genetics; Tuebingen; Germany; Email: Thorsten.Schmidt@med.uni-tuebingen.de

made important contributions to the understanding of disease progression and will be important tools for the first line tests of potential treatment strategies.

This review aims to sum up the model systems used for the investigation of SCA and especially focuses on the lessons learned from these models about the pathogenesis of SCA. We also compare commons and differences in the results obtained using these animal models and highlight the species-specific advantages and possible problems associated with the use of this species as a model organism.

2. Lessons learned from non-mammalian models of SCA

2.1 Lessons learned from worm models

The nematode *Caenorhabditis elegans* is frequently used as a model organism, primarily because of its anatomic and biochemical simplicity as well as its genetic tractability. The worm genome encodes orthologues for about 65% of all known human disease genes. Moreover, it allows for easy and rapid establishment of transgenic lines, thus facilitating screening and characterization of human disease-causing mutations *in vivo*. Overall it is an often used model organism to analyze pathological features of neurodegenerative diseases (Huntington's disease, Parkinson's disease or Alzheimer's disease) (reviewed in Driscoll and Gerstbrein, 2003 and Brignull et al., 2006b). Except for ataxin-7, the worm contains orthologues for all SCA caused by polyQ expansion. Interestingly, for SCA *C. elegans* strains have only been generated and characterized for SCA2 and SCA3 (Ciosk et al., 2004; Khan et al., 2006; Kiehl et al., 2000; Rodrigues et al., 2007; Teixeira-Castro et al., 2011).

In the field of polyQ diseases (e.g. HD or SCA) the formation of aggregates, and therefore, the transition of polyQ proteins to their toxic forms is not well understood. Due to its transparency, *C. elegans* is especially suitable to address this question. PolyQ proteins can be attached to a fluorescent protein (e.g. GFP, YFP, CFP) and the dynamics of aggregate formation both within individual cells and over time can be examined throughout the worm lifespan. Transgenic lines can be rapidly generated by feeding *C. elegans* wildtype strains with genetically transformed bacteria or by microinjection of manipulated DNA into the germline. The worm's life-cycle of about 2 to 3 weeks under suitable living conditions is short. This allows studying the aggregate formation of many different constructs with various polyQ lengths, with or without flanking sequences of the endogenous protein and under control of a wide range of different promoters. When expressed in the body wall muscle of *C. elegans*, even short polyQ stretches (with less than 40 Qs) without any flanking sequences from endogenous proteins tend to aggregate in old worms indicating a balance of different factors including repeat length and changes in the cellular protein-folding environment over time (Morley et al., 2002). In neurons, however, the pathogenic threshold turned out to be about 35-40 repeats, which correlates well with the human disease. This means that in comparison with muscle cells, neuronal cells have a higher aggregation threshold (Brignull et al., 2006a). By way of contrast, the analysis of aggregation in the protein context of (full-length) ataxin-3 revealed that only a highly expanded polyQ stretch (Q130) was able to induce the formation of aggregates in the cytoplasm and nucleus of neuronal cells in transgenic *C. elegans* lines. Non-expanded (Q14, Q17) and even pathological expanded polyQ stretches (Q75, Q91) were diffusely distributed within neurons

	SCA1	SCA2	SCA3/MJD	SCA6	SCA7	SCA17
Human (***Homo sapiens***)	**ATXN1** **815 aa** **(6-39 Q)**	**ATXN2** **1313 aa** **(14-32 Q)**	**ATXN3** **361 aa** **(12-40 Q)**	**CACNA1A** **2512 aa** **(4-18 Q)**	**ATXN7** **945 aa** **(7-18 Q)**	**TBP** **339 aa** **(25-43 Q)**
Mouse (*Mus musculus*)	Atxn1 791 aa (2 Q) 89 %	Atxn2 1286 aa (1 Q) 91 %	Atxn3 355 aa (6 Q) 87 %	Cacna1a 2368 aa (no polyQ) 93 %	Atxn7 867 aa (5 Q) 87 %	Tbp 316 aa (13 Q) 95 %
Zebrafish (*Danio Rerio*)	atxn1a 781 aa (no polyQ) 52 %	si:dkey-165i4.1 1112 aa (no polyQ) 66 %	atxn3 266 aa (no polyQ) 71 %	cacna1ab 2338 aa (no polyQ) 79 %	LOC100001490 918 aa (1 Q) 55 %	tbp 302 aa (6 Q) 91 %
Fly (*Drosphila melanogaster*)	Atx-1 230 aa (no polyQ)	Atx2 1084 aa (no polyQ) 30 %	n. o.	cac 1850 aa (no polyQ) 63 %	n. o.	Tbp 353 aa (8 Q) 68 %
Worm (*Caenorhabditis elegans*)	K04F10.1 299 aa (no polyQ)	ATX2 959 aa (no polyQ)	atx-3 317 aa (no polyQ) 38 %	unc-2 2087 aa (no polyQ) 55 %	n. o.	tbp-1 340 aa (no polyQ) 59 %
Yeast (*Saccharomyces cerevisiae*)	n. o.	PBP1 722 aa (no polyQ)	n. o.	CCH1 2039 aa (no polyQ)	SGF73 657 aa (no polyQ)	SPT15 240 aa (no polyQ) 79 %

Table 1. Orthologues of the affected proteins in spinocerebellar ataxias caused by polyglutamine expansions. For each protein, its name, size in aa, number of polyglutamine repeats and % of sequence identity (if specified in HomoloGene) is listed. Sizes of human proteins depend on polyglutamine repeat number. Orthologues were selected according to Rubin et al. (2000), Ciosk et al. (2004), Khurana and Lindquist (2010) and Tsuda et al. (2005) as well as using HomoloGene (Sayers et al., 2011); Repeat numbers according to Schöls et al. (2004). n. o., no orthologue; no polyQ, the polyglutamine repeat expanded in humans is not conserved in the respective orthologue

without aggregation (Khan et al., 2006; Teixeira-Castro et al., 2011). In a truncated protein of ataxin-3, however, just 63Q are sufficient for aggregation mainly in the perinuclear region but rarely in the nucleus (Khan et al., 2006). These results are in line with observations made in mouse models, where a truncated form of the polyQ expanded protein induced more aggregates and a more progressive neurological phenotype than the full-length protein (Ikeda et al., 1996).

C. elegans is also a useful organism for studying the normal distribution and function of polyQ proteins both during development and throughout the full lifespan. For example, a SCA2 transgenic model, which expressed the *C. elegans* orthologue of the human ataxin-2 gene under the control of the endogenous promoter, revealed a strong expression of ataxin-2 in the central nervous system of adult worm, but also allowed the detection of ataxin-2 even in the early embryo, beginning around the 4-cell stage (Kiehl et al., 2000). Likewise, the expression of the worm orthologue of the human ataxin-3 was strongly detected during the late embryogenesis and during all stages of postnatal development. Interestingly, ataxin-3 was not only detected in the central nervous system (in the neuronal dorsal and ventral cord as well as in neurons of the head and tail) but was also observed in the spermatheca, vulval muscle, hypoderm, coelomocytes and body muscles (Rodrigues et al., 2007).

Using knock-out strains or knocking down expression of polyQ proteins with a siRNA loaded diet has provided another method for the study of polyQ distribution and function. The knockdown of ataxin-2 by siRNA results in reduced numbers of eggs and developmental arrest whereas the knock-out of this gene was embryonically lethal (Kiehl et al., 2000). In comparison, the knock-out of ataxin-3 results in viable animals, which show no obvious morphological abnormalities as well as normal lifespan and behaviour (Rodrigues et al., 2007) but a significantly increased resistance to stress (Rodrigues et al., 2011).

Aside from protein distribution *C. elegans* has been used to study synaptic function (Khan et al., 2006) and to perform genome-wide RNAi-based genetic screens to identify modifiers (Poole et al., 2011). Such a RNAi screen identified that the aggregation of pure polyQ repeats was enhanced by factors involved in RNA metabolism and protein synthesis (leading to an increased production of misfolded proteins) as well as factors involved in protein folding, transport and degradation (leading to decreased protein clearance) (Nollen et al., 2004).

Invertebrate models, like *C. elegans,* are also particularly useful models for first-line screenings of possible therapeutic compounds, especially in late-onset neurodegenerative diseases such as SCA. The useful nature of *C. elegans* in such screenings was demonstrated in 2007 when a first drug screening for Huntington's disease was published. Voisine et al. developed a so called food clearance assay by exploiting that *C. elegans* can easily be cultured in solution. For this assay, wildtype *C. elegans* were incubated in *E. coli* liquid culture to determine the optimal drug concentration. The optical density was used to measure the consumption of *E. coli* (food source) to indicate the growth or survival of *C. elegans*. Drugs in the established concentrations were then used to treat worms with a polyQ expanded huntingtin (Htn-Q150) and analyzed using a starvation assay (by measuring the presence or absence of GFP expression in neurons). In this assay, a HDAC inhibitor (Trichostatin, TSA) was able to suppress neurodegeneration and LiCl decreased polyQ-induced neurodegeneration, while NaCl had no effect (Voisine et al., 2007).

Although no single model organism is able to recapitulate all features of a human disease, *C. elegans* models have proven to be a very good starting point. Worm models allow answering research relevant questions *in vivo* in an easy to handle and "low-cost" organism, before generating a more complex and expensive, but also more comparable model to human diseases, like mouse models.

2.2 Lessons learned from fly models

A big advantage of disease models involving *Drosophila melanogaster* is the so called GAL4-UAS system (Brand and Perrimon, 1993; Fischer et al., 1988). A specific promoter controls the expression of the transcription factor GAL4 which binds the UAS (upstream activating sequence) in the responder construct containing the gene of interest. The use of different promoter GAL4-lines, thereby, allows controlling the expression strength and/or directing the expression of the disease-causing gene to different organs or cell types. A frequently chosen promoter is the mainly eye specific gmr-GAL4 driver (Freeman, 1996) directing the transgene to the flies eyes. *Drosophila* eyes are highly organized structures thereby allowing a macroscopic observation of the degeneration of (visual) neurons without the need of even preparing and staining brain sections. The high reproducibility, the simple breeding and the ease of analyzing neurodegeneration macroscopically make *Drosophila* models the ideal tool for the screening for and analysis of factors influencing neurodegenerative events in SCA. However, not all genes causing SCA are conserved in flies, e.g. there are no natural orthologues for ataxin-3 and ataxin-7 in *Drosophila melanogaster*. However, the *CACNA1A*, the affected gene in SCA6, as well as *ataxin-1* (Tsuda et al., 2005) and *ataxin-2* seem to be conserved albeit with only reduced homology (Rubin et al., 2000) as the CAG repeat is missing in these genes. This lack of endogenous genes excludes any knock-in or knock-out approaches and at first sight questions the chance of successful generation of transgenic models for these diseases as relevant binding partners for the affected proteins may also not be conserved. Interestingly, the sole overexpression of the *Drosophila* orthologue of ataxin-1 (*dAtx-1*) induced a similar phenotype than the overexpression of human ataxin-1 (*hATXN1*) although *dAtx-1* misses more than 60 % of *hATXN1* amino acids including the polyQ repeat (Tsuda et al., 2005). Not even a polyQ expansion is required as a high level of *hATXN1* with normal repeat length (30Q) caused neuronal degeneration (Fernandez-Funez et al., 2000). This data indicates that both *Drosophila* and human ataxin-1 are "intrinsically toxic at high levels" (Lu and Vogel, 2009). Likewise, the overexpression of *dAtx2*, the *Drosophila* orthologue of human ataxin-2, caused developmental defects and degeneration of tissues (Satterfield et al., 2002). As well the loss of dAtx2 had comparable effects, stressing the importance of maintaining normal ataxin-2 activity (Satterfield et al., 2002).

Analyses using *Drosophila* connected pathogenic mechanisms in SCA1, SCA2, and SCA3 and identified ataxin-2 as a potential key player both in SCA1 and SCA3 (Al-Ramahi et al., 2007; Lessing and Bonini, 2008): In both cases, the overexpression of *dAtx2* enhanced the neurodegeneration caused by ataxin-1 and ataxin-3, respectively, and downregulation of *dAtx2* had the opposite effect. Comparable observations were made even for a non-polyQ disease, amyotrophic lateral sclerosis (ALS) (Bonini and Gitler, 2011). This influence of *dAtx2* seems to be linked to the conserved PAM2 motif (PABP-interacting motif 2) within ataxin-2 which mediates the interaction of ataxin-2 with the Poly(A)-binding protein (PABP) (Lessing and Bonini, 2008) implicating ataxin-2 in the regulation of translation of specific mRNAs (Satterfield and Pallanck, 2006). The general importance of protein domains apart from the polyQ repeat were first addressed using pure polyQ repeats which proved to be toxic in *Drosophila* in expanded, but not in normal lengths (Marsh et al., 2000). However, adding as few as 26 additional amino acids (such as addition of a myc and a FLAG tag) and even more, adding the surrounding amino acids of a full protein is able to even neutralize the toxic effect of expanded polyQ repeats (Marsh et al., 2000).

Drosophila models were also used to assess the relevance of the intracellular localization of the affected protein: Ataxin-2 is normally a cytoplasmic protein and the occurrence of intranuclear aggregates in SCA2 patients is still controversial as both the presence and absence of nuclear aggregates have been described (Huynh et al., 2000; Koyano et al., 2000). However, the intracellular localization of dAtx2 strongly influences the phenotype in flies. While nuclear dAtx2 induces strong neurodegeneration, the phenotype of flies with cytoplasmic dAtx2 is much milder (Al-Ramahi et al., 2007).

As SCA are neurodegenerative disorders, with ubiquitous expression of the disease causing gene in humans, glial cells are usually not the main focus of interest. However the choice of different driver lines allows for the analysis of glial vs. neuronal expression of the disease-causing genes in *Drosophila*. Data suggest that the effect of glial expression of the transgene is more pronounced than of neuronal expression (Kretzschmar et al., 2005).

Another strong advantage of *Drosophila* as a model organism is the suitability for large-scale screens for modifying factors. Such screens for ataxin-1, ataxin-3 or even pure polyQ repeats identified somehow expected proteins involved in protein folding (like chaperones) and protein degradation (components of the ubiquitin-proteasome system and autophagy) (Bilen and Bonini, 2007; Fernandez-Funez et al., 2000; Kazemi-Esfarjani and Benzer, 2000; Latouche et al., 2007). In addition, these screens gave insight into further mechanisms relevant for polyQ disease pathogenesis like cellular detoxification, protein transport, transcriptional regulation and RNA and miRNA processing (Bilen and Bonini, 2007; Bilen et al., 2006; Fernandez-Funez et al., 2000; Latouche et al., 2007). The identification of *muscleblind* (*mbl*) as a modifier of an SCA3 fly model drew attention to the role of CAG repeat RNA in the pathogenesis of SCA3 (Li et al., 2008) and led to the conclusion that not only the expanded polyQ repeat but also the RNA coding for it has an effect on the pathogenesis of polyQ diseases at least in *Drosophila*. *Muscleblind* is known to be involved in Myotonic dystrophy caused by aberrant RNA containing massive CUG expansions (Jiang et al., 2004). The expression of an untranslated CAG repeat caused neurodegeneration in *Drosophila*. This toxicity was mitigated just by the interruption of the pure CAG repeat by replacing it with a CAACAG repeat (Li et al., 2008). These results were in line with previous data for a non-polyQ SCA, SCA8, also caused by non-coding RNA. Both a normal and an expanded CAG repeat led to neurodegeneration in a fly model of SCA8 (Mutsuddi et al., 2004). Interestingly, a screen for modifiers of this phenotype caused by non-coding RNA (containing expanded CAG repeats) pointed to several pathways which were also identified as modifiers of a phenotype caused by (translated RNA coding for) expanded polyQ repeats (Mutsuddi et al., 2004). Taken together, disease models in *Drosophila* facilitated both the identification and further analysis of multiple factors and mechanisms involved in the pathogenesis of SCA.

3. Lessons learned from mammalian models of SCA

In contrast to disease models in the worm or the fly, mouse models resemble pathogenic processes in humans much closer than their non-mammalian counterparts. For example the brain structure of mice is much closer to that of humans than those of flies or worms and mechanisms of special importance for late-onset diseases like SCA, e.g. gene expression changes during aging (Bishop et al., 2010), are better conserved. In particular, mouse models allow analyzing aspects of the disease which cannot be analyzed in simpler organisms. Although behavioural analyses are possible in *C. elegans* and *Drosophila* models, they are rather basic compared to more sophisticated behavioural tests possible with mouse models which even allow for e.g. fear and spatial learning analyses (Huynh et al., 2009).

3.1 Lessons learned from knock-out mouse models

In mouse models, it is possible to selectively inactivate a specific gene-of-interest via gene targeting. There is a large amount of insight to be gained from generating such knock-out models and a lot of information has been uncovered about the functional roles of specific genes in mammalian biology (Capecchi, 2005). To learn about the native function of genes affected in SCA knock-out mice were generated for SCA1, 2 and 3. All mice were viable, fertile and had a normal lifespan with no severe ataxic phenotype or neurodegeneration (SCA1: Matilla et al., 1998; SCA2: Kiehl et al., 2006; Lastres-Becker et al., 2008; SCA3: Schmitt et al., 2007; Switonski et al., 2011), providing evidence that loss-of-function is not the primary cause for ataxic symptoms in these disorders. However, these mice served to give indications for normal functions of the respective knock-out genes. For *ataxin-1*, the gene affected in SCA1, a role in learning and memory was identified (Matilla et al., 1998) and its function as a transcriptional co-regulator was elucidated (Goold et al., 2007). Knocking out the *ataxin-2* gene led to adult-onset obesity and reduced fertility (Kiehl et al., 2006; Lastres-Becker et al., 2008a) as well as hyperactivity and abnormal fear-related behaviour (Huynh et al., 2009). In *ataxin-3* knock-out mice increased levels of ubiquitinated proteins were detected reflecting its function as a deubiquitinating enzyme (Schmitt et al., 2007). However, in a second SCA3 knock-out model changes in the ubiquitination level were not observed. The authors suggested compensational effects as the cause for this opposing result (Switonski et al., 2011). Other analyses on SCA3 knock-out mice were able to show a protective function of ataxin-3 in the heat shock response pathway (Reina et al., 2010).

In contrast to only mild effects observed with the deletion of genes responsible for polyQ products, the knock-out of genes affected in non-polyQ SCA resulted in severe ataxic phenotypes. The deletion of the *Klhl1* gene which is mutated in SCA8 led to the loss of motor coordination due to degeneration of Purkinje cell function (He et al., 2006). The analysis of mice showing signs of a severe autosomal recessive movement disorder revealed a deletion in the inositol 1,4,5-triphosphate receptor (ITPR1 gene) as the cause of the observed symptoms. Knowing that the gene correlated to SCA15 in humans maps to the *ITPR1* genomical region, it was possible to identify a deletion in this gene as the cause of this autosomal dominant disorder (van de Leemput et al., 2007).

Taken together, the analyses of SCA knock-out mice demonstrated a toxic gain-of-function as the cause for SCA due to polyQ expansions, whereas for non-polyQ SCA loss-of-function seems to be the primary mechanism of pathogenesis.

3.2 Lessons learned from classical transgenic mouse models for SCA

Transgenic mouse models gave insight into various pathogenic mechanisms in SCA. Here, we review three examples: Lessons learned about the cell-type specificity of neurodegeneration, the aggregation and localization of the affected protein as well as transcriptional dysregulation caused by expanded polyQ proteins.

3.2.1 Lessons learned about the cell-type specificity of neurodegeneration

A classical transgenic mouse model is generated by using a specific promoter typically controlling the expression of a cDNA construct of the respective gene-of-interest. The effect of expressing different transgenes in a specific subgroup of neurons can be nicely compared among several proteins affected in SCA as the Purkinje-cell-specific promoter (Pcp2/L7 promoter) (Vandaele et al., 1991) was used for the generation of transgenic mice for SCA1 (Burright et al., 1995), SCA2 (Huynh et al., 2000), SCA3 (Ikeda et al., 1996), SCA7 (Yvert et al., 2000) and SCA17 (Chang et al., 2011), respectively. In the SCA1, SCA2 and SCA17 mouse models the expanded full-length transgene causes a strong degeneration of Purkinje cells (Burright et al., 1995; Chang et al., 2011; Huynh et al., 2000). By contrast, in the SCA7 mouse model, the sole expression of full-length *ataxin-7* with 90 Q induced a behavioural phenotype, but only mild degeneration of Purkinje cells in quite old mice (Yvert et al., 2000). Ironically, the expression of full-length *ataxin-7* (92 Q) in most neurons except for Purkinje cells (Garden et al., 2002; La Spada et al., 2001) or even just in Bergmann glia cells (Custer et al., 2006), led to a strong degeneration of Purkinje cells (Custer et al., 2006). Likewise, when a full-length ataxin-3 protein with 79 Q was expressed using the same promoter, no phenotype was induced. Only a fragment containing not more than a few amino acids surrounding the expanded polyQ repeat was able to induce a phenotype (Ikeda et al., 1996). These data demonstrate that Purkinje cells in transgenic mice seem to be more vulnerable by a repeat expansion within *ataxin-1*, *ataxin-2* and *ataxin-17*, than by an expansion within *ataxin-3* and *ataxin-7*, thereby –at first sight- nicely replicating the situation in humans where Purkinje cells are strongly affected in SCA1 (Cummings et al., 1999a), SCA2 (Lastres-Becker et al., 2008b) and SCA17 (Rolfs et al., 2003), but the loss of Purkinje cells can be observed but is not so prominent in SCA3 patients (Rüb et al., 2002a; Rüb et al., 2002b). In SCA7, however, Purkinje cells are typically affected (Holmberg et al., 1998), thereby possibly indicating that the pathogenic processes leading to Purkinje cell death in SCA7 differ from those in SCA1, SCA2 and SCA17.

3.2.2 Lessons learned about the aggregation of polyQ proteins and their localization

A common feature of polyQ as well as other neurodegenerative diseases is the accumulation of insoluble proteins in neurons, a feature recapitulated by most model systems of these disorders. Despite this fact the role of these so called neuronal nuclear inclusions (NIIs) in the pathological processes of polyQ diseases is still controversially discussed but it is known that these structures are associated with pathogenesis. Analysis of a *C. elegans* model of SCA3 directly linked the formation of aggregates to neuronal dysfunction (Teixeira-Castro et al., 2011), whereas several opposing results in mouse models exist. Observations in transgenic mouse models for SCA1, SCA2, SCA3 and SCA6 (Boy et al., 2010; Cummings et al., 1999b; Huynh et al., 2000; Klement et al., 1998; Silva-Fernandes et al., 2010; Watase et al., 2008) reveal that the development of a pathological phenotype is independent of the formation of inclusions excluding large aggregates as a primary cause for neuronal dysfunction. Even more, evidence exists for a protective role of inclusion bodies (Bowman et al., 2005). Inclusions in human SCA patients and respective mouse models stain positive for ubiquitin and other components of the ubiquitin-proteasome-system (UPS) (Bichelmeier et al., 2007; Cummings et al., 1998; Holmberg et al., 1998; Klement et al., 1998; Koyano et al., 1999; Paulson et al., 1997; Schmidt et al., 2002; Watase et al., 2002; Yvert et al., 2000) pointing to an involvement of this protein degradation system in the clearance of proteins with expanded CAG repeats. In *C. elegans* it was observed that expanded polyQ tracts impair the functions of UPS (Khan et al., 2006). In brains of SCA3 patients a marked misdistribution of proteasomal subunits was detected leaving only a subpopulation of neurons with the possibility to form functional proteasome complexes (Schmidt et al., 2002). Comparable results were obtained for SCA1 patients and transgenic mice (Cummings et al., 1998) and further studies revealed that an impairment or altered function of the ubiquitin and the proteasomal degradation system could contribute to the SCA1 pathogenesis (Cummings et al., 1999b; Hong et al., 2002). Data gained using a knock-in model, though, excluded an impairment of the ubiquitin-proteasome-system as a major neuropathological cause of SCA7 (Bowman et al., 2005).

The mechanism which leads to the formation of aggregates is not well understood. It has been proposed that proteolytic cleavage of polyQ-containing proteins is required for aggregate formation, because polyQ-containing fragments are predominantly found in NIIs. Another indication for the cleavage hypotheses is the detection of protein fragments in brains of mouse models for SCA3 (Goti et al., 2004), SCA7 (Garden et al., 2002) and SCA17 (Friedman et al., 2008) as well as human SCA patients (Garden et al., 2002; Goti et al., 2004). As possible protein cleavage enzymes, caspases or calpains are under controversial discussion. For ataxin-3, calpain (Haacke et al., 2007; Koch et al., 2011) and caspase cleavage was analyzed *in vitro* (Berke et al., 2004; Pozzi et al., 2008). It was shown that a C-terminal fragment of ataxin-3 containing the polyQ stretch leads to a more progressive phenotype (Ikeda et al., 1996), but also an N-terminal fragment without the CAG repeats can cause SCA3 symptoms (Hübener et al., 2011). In addition, mice expressing a fragment of the TATA-binding protein (affected in SCA17) exhibit a more severe phenotype (Friedman et al., 2008) than those expressing a full-length protein (Friedman et al., 2007). These studies suggest that cleavage of the affected protein is important for the pathogeneses of polyQ SCA. Although neuronal nuclear inclusions (NIIs) are a common feature of polyQ diseases, in some SCA the affected protein is normally localized in the cytoplasm. For this reason, the question arose whether the intracellular localization of the affected protein is of relevance for the pathogenesis of SCA. For an polyQ expansion within an ectopic protein context (Jackson et al., 2003), for ataxin-1 (Klement et al., 1998) and for ataxin-3 (Bichelmeier et al., 2007) it was demonstrated that the nuclear localization of the affected protein is a requirement for the manifestation of symptoms. Mice in which the respective protein was kept in the cytoplasm typically had less and smaller aggregates and milder or even almost no behavioural phenotype. For SCA1, Emamian et al. (2003) even went one step further demonstrating that although the nuclear localization of ataxin-1 is required, it is not sufficient to induce a phenotype. A serine residue close to the endogenous NLS within ataxin-1 (S776) was required additionally for the induction of a phenotype (Emamian et al., 2003).

3.2.3 Lessons learned about transcription dysregulation

Transcriptional dysregulation is a common feature of most polyQ diseases, but the underlying mechanisms which cause the differential regulation remain unknown. Many proteins affected in polyQ diseases are functioning as transcription factors/cofactors or at least interact with transcription factors: TBP (SCA17) is a general transcription factor, ataxin-7 is a part of a transcriptional co-activator complex and both ataxin-1 and ataxin-3 interact with various transcription factors (Helmlinger et al., 2006).

Especially for SCA1, the molecular basis of transcriptional dysregulation and therefore its influence on the pathogenesis is thoroughly studied. Transcriptional dysregulation mediated by ataxin-1 has been attributed to the interaction with the polyQ binding protein 1 (PQBP1). This interaction interferes with the cellular RNA polymerase-dependent transcription (Okazawa et al., 2002). Microarray analyses of SCA1 knock-in and knock-out mice revealed differential expression of proteins involved in calcium signaling (Crespo-Barreto et al., 2010). In SCA3 and SCA7, components of the NIIs are transcriptionally dysregulated, including subunits of the proteasome and heat shock proteins (Chou et al., 2010; Chou et al., 2008). Several other transcription factors such as CREB (cAMP response element binding protein) and HDAC proteins and therefore histone deacetylation is often differential regulated in polyQ diseases (McCampbell et al., 2000; McCullough and Grant, 2010). For this reason, treatment studies using HDAC inhibitors such as sodium butyrate were performed (Chou et al., 2011; McCampbell et al., 2001). In several studies, transcriptional dysregulation is associated with the degeneration of specific neurons: for SCA17, a downregulation of TrkA (nerve growth factor receptor) is linked to Purkinje cell degeneration (Shah et al., 2009), or for SCA1 an interaction of ataxin-1 and PQBP1 and therefore transcriptional dysregulation leads to selective neuronal loss in the cerebellum (Okazawa et al., 2002).

3.3 Lessons learned from YAC, BAC and knock-In mouse models

In the process of generating classical transgenic mice it is only possible to insert cDNA randomly into the animal genome, not allowing for controlling the expression of the pathogenic gene in the native genetic environment at endogenous levels or excluding alternative splicing events. Therefore, different techniques have been developed to overcome these limitations and to generate models which more closely resemble human disease conditions. One strategy was the use of a yeast artificial chromosome (YAC) containing a large fragment of the human *MJD1* locus for the generation of a model for SCA3 thus enabling the expression of a full-length *ataxin-3* gene with the endogenous regulatory elements needed for cell specificity and endogenous levels of expression (Cemal et al., 2002). Mice with expanded CAG tracts showed mild and slowly progressing cerebellar symptoms with nuclear inclusions and cell loss in specific brain regions closely resembling main features of the SCA3 disease in humans (Cemal et al., 2002). A likewise approach was used to generate a model for SCA8. Moseley *et al.* (2006) used a bacterial artificial chromosome (BAC) to control the expression of the SCA8 locus encoding a non-expressed transgene. If they would have used just a classical transgenic construct without 116 kb of flanking sequences they may not have observed that the construct is indeed expressed in both directions encoding both a non-translated RNA containing a CTG expansion as well as a polyQ containing protein expressed from the opposite strand (Moseley et al., 2006).

A different more widely used strategy in the generation of SCA mouse models is to take advantage of homologous recombination techniques leading to knock-in models. This allows for endogenous levels of expression in proper spatio-temporal patterns (Yoo et al.,

2003). The first knock-in model generated for SCA1 targeted an expanded CAG tract of 78 repeats to the endogenous *ataxin-1* mouse locus. These mice reflected genetic repeat instability observed in human SCA1 patients, but showed only mild behavioural changes in late life with no clear neuropathological changes (Lorenzetti et al., 2000). From this first attempt the conclusion was drawn that the short lifespan of mice seems to be a limiting factor and that the longer exposure of the mutant protein in humans might be necessary for the development of neuronal dysfunctions. This drawback can be overcome by either overexpression of mutant proteins or by the use of extremely long CAG tracts to produce neurodegeneration (Yoo et al., 2003; Zoghbi and Botas, 2002). Therefore, in the next knock-in model for SCA1, more CAG repeats (154 repeats) were used and this model then indeed resembled main features of the human SCA1 disease (Watase et al., 2002). Analyzing these mice it was also shown that there is no direct relationship between the degree of somatic instability and the selective neuronal toxicity (Watase et al., 2003), but that the selective neuropathology rather arises from alterations in the function of the ataxin-1 protein (Bowman et al., 2007). Furthermore, these mice served to demonstrate that a partial loss-of-function contributes to the SCA1 pathogenesis (Bowman et al., 2007; Crespo-Barreto et al., 2010; Lim et al., 2008). SCA6 knock-in mice with up to 84 (hyperexpanded) CAG repeats in the *CACNA1A* gene (encoding for a calcium channel subunit) gave evidence against the assumption that the SCA6 pathogenesis is caused by alterations of channel properties and rather indicated that it is due to the accumulation of mutant calcium channels (Saegusa et al., 2007; Watase et al., 2008). In infantile cases of SCA7 expansions of 200-460 CAG repeats were documented (Benton et al., 1998; van de Warrenburg et al., 2001) and knock-in mice with 266 CAG repeats indeed reproduced hallmark features of the infantile disease (Yoo et al., 2003). Using this knock-in model it was shown that polyQ nuclear inclusions seem to have a protective role against neuronal dysfunction, that an impairment of the ubiquitin-proteasome-system can be excluded as a major neuropathological cause (Bowman et al., 2005) and that SUMOylation influences the aggregation process of ataxin-7 (Janer et al., 2010). A most recent publication reported on the attempt to generate the first knock-in mouse model of SCA3, but due to unexpected splicing events ended up creating another SCA3 knock-out model (Switonski et al., 2011) showing some of the difficulties which may occur generating animal models.

3.4 Lessons learned from an alternative strategy to generate mouse models

An alternative approach for the generation of animal models is the use of viral injections. By using lentiviral vectors it was possible to overexpress wildtype or polyQ expanded ataxin-3 in brain regions of adult wildtype rats. An expression of polyQ-expanded ataxin-3 in the substantia nigra, an area affected in SCA3, led to the formation of ubiquitinated ataxin-3 positive aggregates, loss of dopaminergic markers and an apomorphine-induced turning behaviour. If polyQ expanded ataxin-3 is overexpressed in the striatum or cortex, regions previously not linked to SCA3 pathogenesis, by the lentiviral-based system it results in accumulation of misfolded ataxin-3 and loss of neuronal markers especially in the striatum (Alves et al., 2008b). Using the lentiviral vector system it is also possible to co-express ataxin-3 with knock-down vectors or other proteins and to analyze direct effects in specific brain regions. For example a co-expression of expanded ataxin-3 with beclin, an autophagic protein, led to stimulation of autophagic flux, clearance of mutant ataxin-3 and neuroprotective effects (Nascimento-Ferreira et al., 2011).

3.5 Treatment approaches using mouse models

At the moment, curative treatment for SCA is not possible. Only treatments directed towards alleviating symptoms are available (Duenas et al., 2006). Therefore, one or the most important goal in the research of SCA is the development of a cure.

The basic question of whether any treatment -if available- would be able to even reverse symptoms already manifested was addressed using conditional mouse models. With these models which allow to turn off the pathogenic trangene expression using the Tet-off system it was possible to demonstrate that already developed symptoms of SCA1 and SCA3 indeed can be reversed (Boy et al., 2009; Zu et al., 2004). Inhibiting or reducing the production of pathogenic proteins could therefore be a powerful tool in the therapy of dominant neurodegenerative diseases. Using the RNA interference (RNAi) technology (Mello and Conte, 2004) to inhibit the expression of mutant ataxin-1 in a mouse model of SCA1 led to improved motor coordination, restored cerebellar morphology as well as resolved ataxin-1 inclusions demonstrating the *in vivo* potential of this strategy (Xia et al., 2004). RNAi knockdown was also successfully used for a selective allele-specific silencing of mutant ataxin-3 showing to mitigate neuropathological abnormalities in a lentiviral-mediated model of SCA3 (Alves et al., 2008a; Alves et al., 2010) and may be a possible treatment approach. As protein misfolding and impaired protein degradation is implicated in the pathogenesis of polyQ SCA and other related diseases that present with intracellular inclusion bodies, supporting the correction of these alterations might be a therapeutic strategy. In this manner it was possible to show that crossbreeding of SCA1 transgenic mice with mice overexpressing a molecular chaperone leads to the mitigation of the SCA1 phenotype (Cummings et al., 2001).

In addition to genetic approaches, some of the published mouse models have already been used to test the effect of different compounds on the movement phenotype, neuronal loss and aggregate formation: Lithium carbonate enhanced the motor performances and improved spatial learning, but had neither an effect on the distribution and formation of aggregates nor did it improve the lifespan of the SCA1 knock-in mice (Watase et al., 2007). A treatment approach using lithium chloride in a *C. elegans* model for Huntington's disease, however, was beneficial (Voisine et al., 2007). A dietary supplementation with creatine improved survival and motor performance and delays neuronal atrophy in the R6/2 transgenic mouse model of Huntington's disease. In a SCA2 transgenic mouse model, however, creatine extended the Purkinje cell survival, but was not able to improve or delay ataxic symptoms (Kaemmerer et al., 2001). Two promising studies were performed using transgenic models for SCA3: The HDAC inhibitor sodium butyrate (SB) delayed the onset of ataxic symptoms and improved the survival rate by reversing polyQ induced histone hypoacetylation and transcriptional repression (Chou et al., 2011). In addition, a rapamycin ester (also called temsirolimus or CCI-779) which inhibits the mammalian target of rapamycin and upregulates the protein degradation by autophagy, reduced the number of aggregates and improved the motor performance (Menzies et al., 2010). In a study using a SCA2 mouse model, the Ca^{2+} stabilizer dantrolene was able both to alleviate motor symptoms and to reduce the loss of Purkinje cells in this model (Liu et al., 2009). Another group used a specific mouse model, the so called rolling mouse Nagoya, which has been suggested as an animal model for some human neurological diseases such as autosomal dominant cerebellar ataxia (SCA6). This model was treated with talrelin, a synthetic analogue of the thyrotropin-releasing hormone (TRH) which alters the metabolism of acetylcholine and dopamine and therefore activates the dopaminergic system. Talrelin significantly elevated the cerebellar dopamine and serotonin levels of mice and improved the locomotion phenotype (Nakamura et al., 2005).

Other therapeutical attempts are based on the functional restoration of affected cell populations. Expanded ataxin-1 causes the degeneration of Purkinje cells thereby also negatively effects the synthesis of the insulin-like growth factor–I (IGF-I) a factor promoting Purkinje cell development (Fukudome et al., 2003). Administering this factor to SCA1 transgenic mice (SCA1[82Q]) intranasally led to significant improvement of motor coordinative abilities as well as to partial restoration of Purkinje cell survival (Vig et al., 2006). Using the same SCA1 transgenic model, improved motor skills and a higher Purkinje cell survival rate was reached after grafting neural precursor cells into the cerebellar white matter (Chintawar et al., 2009). Although there is a long way from successful treatment approaches in animal models to clinical application, the recent results give hope that treatment of SCA will be possible in the future.

4. Commons and differences between SCA models in worms, flies and mice

It is self-evident that the data acquired in different model organisms especially those obtained in non-vertebrate compared with those from vertebrate models cannot be identical. However, if results obtained in a specific model are to be translated to the situation in humans one would expect that basic mechanisms in the pathogenesis of SCA are conserved among species. Previous studies revealed that many pathogenic mechanisms are indeed comparable among species, however, also indicated that there are some differences between model organisms (Table 2). Orthologues of ataxin-2 can be found all the way down to simple organisms and even in yeast (Table 1). However, the knock-out of ataxin-2 gave rise to contradictory results among model organisms: The knock-out of the endogenous SCA2 gene in the worm and the fly is embryonic lethal. In contrast to that, SCA2 knock-out mice are viable and showed no developmental defects. Further analyses of SCA2 knock-out worms demonstrated that ataxin-2 is functioning during development, since the knockdown by RNAi results in developmental arrest.

These results indicate that the function of homologous proteins as well as the interaction of different proteins in special pathways is not conserved in the species analyzed (Kiehl et al., 2006; Kiehl et al., 2000; Lastres-Becker et al., 2008a; Satterfield et al., 2002). Since in *C. elegans* the polyQ repeats in all orthologous genes are not conserved, one could assume that much shorter repeat expansions than e.g. in the mouse may already give rise to a phenotype. However, the exact opposite seems to be true: Within the full-length context of a protein, much higher polyQ repeat numbers are required to be toxic (Khan et al., 2006; Teixeira-Castro et al., 2011). Proteins with polyQ repeats are frequent in *Drosophila* (Alba et al., 2007), but these repeats are generally encoded by interrupted rather than pure CAG repeats and, therefore, more resistant to expansion (Alba et al., 2001). This could lead to the assumption that pure CAG repeats may behave unstable in *Drosophila* as observed in human SCA patients and mouse models (Boy et al., 2010; Kaytor et al., 1997; Lorenzetti et al., 2000). However, CAG repeats seem to be perfectly stable in *Drosophila* even within a challenging genomic context (Jackson et al., 2005) pointing to a specific protection mechanism against repeat expansion in *Drosophila*.

	Caenorhabditis elegans	*Drosophila melanogaster*	*Mus musculus*
knock-out	SCA2: lethal (1) SCA3: viable (2)	SCA2: lethal (3)	SCA1/2/3/8: viable (4-9)
overexpression of pure polyQ causes phenotype	yes (10; 11)	yes (12)	yes (13; 14)
truncated protein requires less repeats to induce phenotype	yes (15)	yes (16)	yes (13)
full-length protein causes phenotype	yes (≥ 130 Q) (15; 17)	wt: no or mild exp: strong (3; 18-22)	wt: no exp: mild to strong (23-26)
instability of repeats		no (27)	SCA1/3: yes (28-30) SCA2: no (24)
repeat numbers causing phenotype	≥ 130 Q (15; 17)	≥30 Q (18)	≥ 30 Q (18; 24; 26)
increasing repeat length intensifies phenotype	yes (15; 17)	yes (3; 18-22)	yes (23-26)
formation of aggregates	yes (15; 17)	yes (31)	yes (33; 25) no (24; 32) late (30; 34)
neurodegeneration/ neuronal loss		yes (18; 19; 35)	wt: no exp: mild to strong (13; 23; 24; 36)
switching-off led to reversal of symptom		yes (31)	yes (30; 37)
transgene leads to reduced lifespan	yes (17)	yes (31)	yes (25)

References: (1) Kiehl et al., 2000; (2) Rodrigues et al., 2007; (3) Satterfield et al., 2002; (4) Matilla et al., 1998; (5) Kiehl et al., 2006; (6) Lastres-Becker et al., 2008a; (7) Schmitt et al., 2007 ; (8) Switonski et al., 2011; (9) He et al., 2006; (10) Brignull et al., 2006a ; (11) Morley et al., 2002; (12) Marsh et al., 2000; (13) Ikeda et al., 1996; (14) Ordway et al., 1997; (15) Khan et al., 2006; (16) Lu and Vogel, 2009; (17) Teixeira-Castro et al., 2011); (18) Fernandez-Funez et al., 2000; (19) Al-Ramahi et al., 2007; (20) Warrick et al., 1998; (21) Warrick et al., 2005; (22) Moseley et al., 2006; (23) Burright et al., 1995; (24) Huynh et al., 2000; (25) Bichelmeier et al., 2007; (26) Friedman et al., 2007; (27) Jackson et al., 2005; (28) Kaytor et al., 1997; (29) Lorenzetti et al., 2000; (30) Boy et al., 2009; (31) Latouche et al., 2007; (32) Silva-Fernandes et al., 2010; (33) Cummings et al., 1999b ; (34) Watase et al., 2008; (35) Lessing and Bonini, 2008; (36) Aguiar et al., 2006; (37) Zu et al., 2004

Table 2. Exemplary phenotypical features of human SCA patients compared among model organisms. For clearness, only examples for the respective phenotypic features are listed. The table is not intended to be exhaustive. (wt, normal repeat; exp, expanded repeat).

5. Conclusion

Multiple successful attempts generating transgenic animal models for SCA were performed in different species. While each model organism has its own advantages and disadvantages, all animal models contributed to the knowledge about the pathogenesis of SCA. The transparency of *C.elegans* together with the simplicity to generate transgenic models as well as the option to study neurodegeneration even macroscopically by targeting the gene of interest to the *Drosophila* eye make smaller organisms like the worm or the fly especially suitable for the screening of compounds or genetic modifiers. Since many pathologic mechanisms in SCA are conserved in these models, there is a high probability that results obtained in worms and flies can be translated to mammals. Although unsuitable for large-scale (genetic and compound) screening approaches, mouse models are the ideal tools for verification of screening results in mammals. Viral injections now even allow a comparatively rapid analysis without the need of breeding or even generating transgenic mice. Especially to answer questions which require brain structures closer to humans or for analyses of ataxic movement or even emotional phenotypes, mammalian models are required. Taken together, model organisms are indispensable tools for the analysis of pathogenic mechanisms important for SCA *in vivo.*

6. Acknowledgment

We thank Anna S. Sowa for critical reading of the manuscript.

7. References

Aguiar, J.; Fernandez, J.; Aguilar, A.; Mendoza, Y.; Vazquez, M.; Suarez, J.; Berlanga, J.; Cruz, S.; Guillen, G.; Herrera, L.; Velazquez, L.; Santos, N. & Merino, N. (2006). Ubiquitous expression of human SCA2 gene under the regulation of the SCA2 self promoter cause specific Purkinje cell degeneration in transgenic mice. *Neurosci Lett*, Vol. 392, No. 3, pp. 202-6, ISSN 0304-3940

Al-Ramahi, I.; Perez, A. M.; Lim, J.; Zhang, M.; Sorensen, R.; de Haro, M.; Branco, J.; Pulst, S. M.; Zoghbi, H. Y. & Botas, J. (2007). dAtaxin-2 mediates expanded Ataxin-1-induced neurodegeneration in a Drosophila model of SCA1. *PLoS Genet*, Vol. 3, No. 12, pp. e234, ISSN 1553-7404

Alba, M. M.; Santibanez-Koref, M. F. & Hancock, J. M. (2001). The comparative genomics of polyglutamine repeats: extreme differences in the codon organization of repeat-encoding regions between mammals and Drosophila. *J Mol Evol*, Vol. 52, No. 3, pp. 249-59, ISSN 0022-2844

Alba, M. M.; Tompa, P. & Veitia, R. A. (2007). Amino acid repeats and the structure and evolution of proteins. *Genome Dyn*, Vol. 3, No. pp. 119-30, ISSN 1660-9263

Alves, S.; Nascimento-Ferreira, I.; Auregan, G.; Hassig, R.; Dufour, N.; Brouillet, E.; Pedroso de Lima, M. C.; Hantraye, P.; Pereira de Almeida, L. & Deglon, N. (2008a). Allele-specific RNA silencing of mutant ataxin-3 mediates neuroprotection in a rat model of Machado-Joseph disease. *PLoS One*, Vol. 3, No. 10, pp. e3341, ISSN 1932-6203

Alves, S.; Nascimento-Ferreira, I.; Dufour, N.; Hassig, R.; Auregan, G.; Nobrega, C.; Brouillet, E.; Hantraye, P.; Pedroso de Lima, M. C.; Deglon, N. & de Almeida, L. P. (2010). Silencing ataxin-3 mitigates degeneration in a rat model of Machado-Joseph disease: no role for wild-type ataxin-3? *Hum Mol Genet*, Vol. 19, No. 12, pp. 2380-94, ISSN 1460-2083

Alves, S.; Regulier, E.; Nascimento-Ferreira, I.; Hassig, R.; Dufour, N.; Koeppen, A.; Carvalho, A. L.; Simoes, S.; de Lima, M. C.; Brouillet, E.; Gould, V. C.; Deglon, N. & de Almeida, L. P. (2008b). Striatal and nigral pathology in a lentiviral rat model of Machado-Joseph disease. *Hum Mol Genet*, Vol. 17, No. 14, pp. 2071-83, ISSN 1460-2083

Benton, C. S.; de Silva, R.; Rutledge, S. L.; Bohlega, S.; Ashizawa, T. & Zoghbi, H. Y. (1998). Molecular and clinical studies in SCA-7 define a broad clinical spectrum and the infantile phenotype. *Neurology*, Vol. 51, No. 4, pp. 1081-6, ISSN 0028-3878

Berke, S. J.; Schmied, F. A.; Brunt, E. R.; Ellerby, L. M. & Paulson, H. L. (2004). Caspase-mediated proteolysis of the polyglutamine disease protein ataxin-3. *J Neurochem*, Vol. 89, No. 4, pp. 908-18, ISSN 0022-3042

Bichelmeier, U.; Schmidt, T.; Hubener, J.; Boy, J.; Ruttiger, L.; Habig, K.; Poths, S.; Bonin, M.; Knipper, M.; Schmidt, W. J.; Wilbertz, J.; Wolburg, H.; Laccone, F. & Riess, O. (2007). Nuclear localization of ataxin-3 is required for the manifestation of symptoms in SCA3: in vivo evidence. *J Neurosci*, Vol. 27, No. 28, pp. 7418-28, ISSN 1529-2401

Bilen, J. & Bonini, N. M. (2007). Genome-wide screen for modifiers of ataxin-3 neurodegeneration in Drosophila. *PLoS Genet*, Vol. 3, No. 10, pp. 1950-64, ISSN 1553-7404

Bilen, J.; Liu, N.; Burnett, B. G.; Pittman, R. N. & Bonini, N. M. (2006). MicroRNA pathways modulate polyglutamine-induced neurodegeneration. *Mol Cell*, Vol. 24, No. 1, pp. 157-63, ISSN 1097-2765

Bishop, N. A.; Lu, T. & Yankner, B. A. (2010). Neural mechanisms of ageing and cognitive decline. *Nature*, Vol. 464, No. 7288, pp. 529-35, ISSN 1476-4687

Bonini, N. M. & Gitler, A. D. (2011). Model Organisms Reveal Insight into Human Neurodegenerative Disease: Ataxin-2 Intermediate-Length Polyglutamine Expansions Are a Risk Factor for ALS. *J Mol Neurosci*, Vol., No., ISSN 1559-1166

Bowman, A. B.; Lam, Y. C.; Jafar-Nejad, P.; Chen, H. K.; Richman, R.; Samaco, R. C.; Fryer, J. D.; Kahle, J. J.; Orr, H. T. & Zoghbi, H. Y. (2007). Duplication of Atxn1l suppresses SCA1 neuropathology by decreasing incorporation of polyglutamine-expanded ataxin-1 into native complexes. *Nat Genet*, Vol. 39, No. 3, pp. 373-9, ISSN 1061-4036

Bowman, A. B.; Yoo, S. Y.; Dantuma, N. P. & Zoghbi, H. Y. (2005). Neuronal dysfunction in a polyglutamine disease model occurs in the absence of ubiquitin-proteasome system impairment and inversely correlates with the degree of nuclear inclusion formation. *Hum Mol Genet*, Vol. 14, No. 5, pp. 679-91, ISSN 0964-6906

Boy, J.; Schmidt, T.; Schumann, U.; Grasshoff, U.; Unser, S.; Holzmann, C.; Schmitt, I.; Karl, T.; Laccone, F.; Wolburg, H.; Ibrahim, S. & Riess, O. (2010). A transgenic mouse model of spinocerebellar ataxia type 3 resembling late disease onset and gender-specific instability of CAG repeats. *Neurobiol Dis*, Vol. 37, No. 2, pp. 284-93, ISSN 1095-953X

Boy, J.; Schmidt, T.; Wolburg, H.; Mack, A.; Nuber, S.; Bottcher, M.; Schmitt, I.; Holzmann, C.; Zimmermann, F.; Servadio, A. & Riess, O. (2009). Reversibility of symptoms in a conditional mouse model of spinocerebellar ataxia type 3. *Hum Mol Genet*, Vol. 18, No. 22, pp. 4282-95, ISSN 1460-2083

Brand, A. H. & Perrimon, N. (1993). Targeted gene expression as a means of altering cell fates and generating dominant phenotypes. *Development*, Vol. 118, No. 2, pp. 401-15, ISSN 0950-1991

Brignull, H. R.; Moore, F. E.; Tang, S. J. & Morimoto, R. I. (2006a). Polyglutamine proteins at the pathogenic threshold display neuron-specific aggregation in a pan-neuronal Caenorhabditis elegans model. *J Neurosci*, Vol. 26, No. 29, pp. 7597-606, ISSN 1529-2401

Brignull, H. R.; Morley, J. F.; Garcia, S. M. & Morimoto, R. I. (2006b). Modeling polyglutamine pathogenesis in C. elegans. *Methods Enzymol*, Vol. 412, No. pp. 256-82, ISSN 0076-6879

Burright, E. N.; Clark, H. B.; Servadio, A.; Matilla, T.; Feddersen, R. M.; Yunis, W. S.; Duvick, L. A.; Zoghbi, H. Y. & Orr, H. T. (1995). SCA1 transgenic mice: a model for neurodegeneration caused by an expanded CAG trinucleotide repeat. *Cell*, Vol. 82, No. 6, pp. 937-48, ISSN 0092-8674

Capecchi, M. R. (2005). Gene targeting in mice: functional analysis of the mammalian genome for the twenty-first century. *Nat Rev Genet*, Vol. 6, No. 6, pp. 507-12, ISSN 1471-0056

Cemal, C. K.; Carroll, C. J.; Lawrence, L.; Lowrie, M. B.; Ruddle, P.; Al-Mahdawi, S.; King, R. H.; Pook, M. A.; Huxley, C. & Chamberlain, S. (2002). YAC transgenic mice carrying pathological alleles of the MJD1 locus exhibit a mild and slowly progressive cerebellar deficit. *Hum Mol Genet*, Vol. 11, No. 9, pp. 1075-94, ISSN 0964-6906

Chang, Y. C.; Lin, C. Y.; Hsu, C. M.; Lin, H. C.; Chen, Y. H.; Lee-Chen, G. J.; Su, M. T.; Ro, L. S.; Chen, C. M. & Hsieh-Li, H. M. (2011). Neuroprotective effects of granulocyte-colony stimulating factor in a novel transgenic mouse model of SCA17. *J Neurochem*, Vol. 118, No. 2, pp. 288-303, ISSN 1471-4159

Chintawar, S.; Hourez, R.; Ravella, A.; Gall, D.; Orduz, D.; Rai, M.; Bishop, D. P.; Geuna, S.; Schiffmann, S. N. & Pandolfo, M. (2009). Grafting neural precursor cells promotes functional recovery in an SCA1 mouse model. *J Neurosci*, Vol. 29, No. 42, pp. 13126-35, ISSN 1529-2401

Chou, A. H.; Chen, C. Y.; Chen, S. Y.; Chen, W. J.; Chen, Y. L.; Weng, Y. S. & Wang, H. L. (2010). Polyglutamine-expanded ataxin-7 causes cerebellar dysfunction by inducing transcriptional dysregulation. *Neurochem Int*, Vol. 56, No. 2, pp. 329-39, ISSN 1872-9754

Chou, A. H.; Chen, S. Y.; Yeh, T. H.; Weng, Y. H. & Wang, H. L. (2011). HDAC inhibitor sodium butyrate reverses transcriptional downregulation and ameliorates ataxic symptoms in a transgenic mouse model of SCA3. *Neurobiol Dis*, Vol. 41, No. 2, pp. 481-8, ISSN 1095-953X

Chou, A. H.; Yeh, T. H.; Ouyang, P.; Chen, Y. L.; Chen, S. Y. & Wang, H. L. (2008). Polyglutamine-expanded ataxin-3 causes cerebellar dysfunction of SCA3 transgenic mice by inducing transcriptional dysregulation. *Neurobiol Dis*, Vol. 31, No. 1, pp. 89-101, ISSN 1095-953X

Ciosk, R.; DePalma, M. & Priess, J. R. (2004). ATX-2, the C. elegans ortholog of ataxin 2, functions in translational regulation in the germline. *Development*, Vol. 131, No. 19, pp. 4831-41, ISSN 0950-1991

Crespo-Barreto, J.; Fryer, J. D.; Shaw, C. A.; Orr, H. T. & Zoghbi, H. Y. (2010). Partial loss of ataxin-1 function contributes to transcriptional dysregulation in spinocerebellar ataxia type 1 pathogenesis. *PLoS Genet*, Vol. 6, No. 7, pp. e1001021, ISSN 1553-7404

Cummings, C. J.; Mancini, M. A.; Antalffy, B.; DeFranco, D. B.; Orr, H. T. & Zoghbi, H. Y. (1998). Chaperone suppression of aggregation and altered subcellular proteasome localization imply protein misfolding in SCA1. *Nat Genet*, Vol. 19, No. 2, pp. 148-54, ISSN 1061-4036

Cummings, C. J.; Orr, H. T. & Zoghbi, H. Y. (1999a). Progress in pathogenesis studies of spinocerebellar ataxia type 1. *Philos Trans R Soc Lond B Biol Sci*, Vol. 354, No. 1386, pp. 1079-81, ISSN 0962-8436

Cummings, C. J.; Reinstein, E.; Sun, Y.; Antalffy, B.; Jiang, Y.; Ciechanover, A.; Orr, H. T.; Beaudet, A. L. & Zoghbi, H. Y. (1999b). Mutation of the E6-AP ubiquitin ligase reduces nuclear inclusion frequency while accelerating polyglutamine-induced pathology in SCA1 mice. *Neuron*, Vol. 24, No. 4, pp. 879-92, ISSN 0896-6273

Cummings, C. J.; Sun, Y.; Opal, P.; Antalffy, B.; Mestril, R.; Orr, H. T.; Dillmann, W. H. & Zoghbi, H. Y. (2001). Over-expression of inducible HSP70 chaperone suppresses neuropathology and improves motor function in SCA1 mice. *Hum Mol Genet*, Vol. 10, No. 14, pp. 1511-8, ISSN 0964-6906

Custer, S. K.; Garden, G. A.; Gill, N.; Rueb, U.; Libby, R. T.; Schultz, C.; Guyenet, S. J.; Deller, T.; Westrum, L. E.; Sopher, B. L. & La Spada, A. R. (2006). Bergmann glia expression of polyglutamine-expanded ataxin-7 produces neurodegeneration by impairing glutamate transport. *Nat Neurosci*, Vol. 9, No. 10, pp. 1302-11, ISSN 1097-6256

Driscoll, M. & Gerstbrein, B. (2003). Dying for a cause: invertebrate genetics takes on human neurodegeneration. *Nat Rev Genet*, Vol. 4, No. 3, pp. 181-94, ISSN 1471-0056

Duenas, A. M.; Goold, R. & Giunti, P. (2006). Molecular pathogenesis of spinocerebellar ataxias. *Brain*, Vol. 129, No. Pt 6, pp. 1357-70, ISSN 1460-2156

Emamian, E. S.; Kaytor, M. D.; Duvick, L. A.; Zu, T.; Tousey, S. K.; Zoghbi, H. Y.; Clark, H. B. & Orr, H. T. (2003). Serine 776 of ataxin-1 is critical for polyglutamine-induced disease in SCA1 transgenic mice. *Neuron*, Vol. 38, No. 3, pp. 375-87, ISSN 0896-6273

Fernandez-Funez, P.; Nino-Rosales, M. L.; de Gouyon, B.; She, W. C.; Luchak, J. M.; Martinez, P.; Turiegano, E.; Benito, J.; Capovilla, M.; Skinner, P. J.; McCall, A.; Canal, I.; Orr, H. T.; Zoghbi, H. Y. & Botas, J. (2000). Identification of genes that modify ataxin-1-induced neurodegeneration. *Nature*, Vol. 408, No. 6808, pp. 101-6, ISSN 0028-0836

Fischer, J. A.; Giniger, E.; Maniatis, T. & Ptashne, M. (1988). GAL4 activates transcription in Drosophila. *Nature*, Vol. 332, No. 6167, pp. 853-6, ISSN 0028-0836

Freeman, M. (1996). Reiterative use of the EGF receptor triggers differentiation of all cell types in the Drosophila eye. *Cell*, Vol. 87, No. 4, pp. 651-60, ISSN 0092-8674

Friedman, M. J.; Shah, A. G.; Fang, Z. H.; Ward, E. G.; Warren, S. T.; Li, S. & Li, X. J. (2007). Polyglutamine domain modulates the TBP-TFIIB interaction: implications for its normal function and neurodegeneration. *Nat Neurosci*, Vol. 10, No. 12, pp. 1519-28, ISSN 1097-6256

Friedman, M. J.; Wang, C. E.; Li, X. J. & Li, S. (2008). Polyglutamine expansion reduces the association of TATA-binding protein with DNA and induces DNA binding-independent neurotoxicity. *J Biol Chem*, Vol. 283, No. 13, pp. 8283-90, ISSN 0021-9258

Fukudome, Y.; Tabata, T.; Miyoshi, T.; Haruki, S.; Araishi, K.; Sawada, S. & Kano, M. (2003). Insulin-like growth factor-I as a promoting factor for cerebellar Purkinje cell development. *Eur J Neurosci*, Vol. 17, No. 10, pp. 2006-16, ISSN 0953-816X

Garden, G. A.; Libby, R. T.; Fu, Y. H.; Kinoshita, Y.; Huang, J.; Possin, D. E.; Smith, A. C.; Martinez, R. A.; Fine, G. C.; Grote, S. K.; Ware, C. B.; Einum, D. D.; Morrison, R. S.; Ptacek, L. J.; Sopher, B. L. & La Spada, A. R. (2002). Polyglutamine-expanded ataxin-7 promotes non-cell-autonomous purkinje cell degeneration and displays proteolytic cleavage in ataxic transgenic mice. *J Neurosci*, Vol. 22, No. 12, pp. 4897-905, ISSN 1529-2401

Goold, R.; Hubank, M.; Hunt, A.; Holton, J.; Menon, R. P.; Revesz, T.; Pandolfo, M. & Matilla-Duenas, A. (2007). Down-regulation of the dopamine receptor D2 in mice lacking ataxin 1. *Hum Mol Genet*, Vol. 16, No. 17, pp. 2122-34, ISSN 0964-6906

Goti, D.; Katzen, S. M.; Mez, J.; Kurtis, N.; Kiluk, J.; Ben-Haiem, L.; Jenkins, N. A.; Copeland, N. G.; Kakizuka, A.; Sharp, A. H.; Ross, C. A.; Mouton, P. R. & Colomer, V. (2004). A mutant ataxin-3 putative-cleavage fragment in brains of Machado-Joseph disease patients and transgenic mice is cytotoxic above a critical concentration. *J Neurosci*, Vol. 24, No. 45, pp. 10266-79, ISSN 1529-2401

Haacke, A.; Hartl, F. U. & Breuer, P. (2007). Calpain inhibition is sufficient to suppress aggregation of polyglutamine-expanded ataxin-3. *J Biol Chem*, Vol. 282, No. 26, pp. 18851-6, ISSN 0021-9258

He, Y.; Zu, T.; Benzow, K. A.; Orr, H. T.; Clark, H. B. & Koob, M. D. (2006). Targeted deletion of a single Sca8 ataxia locus allele in mice causes abnormal gait, progressive loss of motor coordination, and Purkinje cell dendritic deficits. *J Neurosci*, Vol. 26, No. 39, pp. 9975-82, ISSN 1529-2401

Helmlinger, D.; Tora, L. & Devys, D. (2006). Transcriptional alterations and chromatin remodeling in polyglutamine diseases. *Trends Genet*, Vol. 22, No. 10, pp. 562-70, ISSN 0168-9525

Holmberg, M.; Duyckaerts, C.; Durr, A.; Cancel, G.; Gourfinkel-An, I.; Damier, P.; Faucheux, B.; Trottier, Y.; Hirsch, E. C.; Agid, Y. & Brice, A. (1998). Spinocerebellar ataxia type 7 (SCA7): a neurodegenerative disorder with neuronal intranuclear inclusions. *Hum Mol Genet*, Vol. 7, No. 5, pp. 913-8, ISSN 0964-6906

Hong, S.; Kim, S. J.; Ka, S.; Choi, I. & Kang, S. (2002). USP7, a ubiquitin-specific protease, interacts with ataxin-1, the SCA1 gene product. *Mol Cell Neurosci*, Vol. 20, No. 2, pp. 298-306, ISSN 1044-7431

Hübener, J.; Vauti, F.; Funke, C.; Wolburg, H.; Ye, Y.; Schmidt, T.; Wolburg-Buchholz, K.; Schmitt, I.; Gardyan, A.; Driessen, S.; Arnold, H. H.; Nguyen, H. P. & Riess, O. (2011). N-terminal ataxin-3 causes neurological symptoms with inclusions, endoplasmic reticulum stress and ribosomal dislocation. *Brain*, Vol. 134, No. Pt 7, pp. 1925-1942, ISSN 1460-2156

Huynh, D. P.; Figueroa, K.; Hoang, N. & Pulst, S. M. (2000). Nuclear localization or inclusion body formation of ataxin-2 are not necessary for SCA2 pathogenesis in mouse or human. *Nat Genet*, Vol. 26, No. 1, pp. 44-50, ISSN 1061-4036

Huynh, D. P.; Maalouf, M.; Silva, A. J.; Schweizer, F. E. & Pulst, S. M. (2009). Dissociated fear and spatial learning in mice with deficiency of ataxin-2. *PLoS One*, Vol. 4, No. 7, pp. e6235, ISSN 1932-6203

Ikeda, H.; Yamaguchi, M.; Sugai, S.; Aze, Y.; Narumiya, S. & Kakizuka, A. (1996). Expanded polyglutamine in the Machado-Joseph disease protein induces cell death in vitro and in vivo. *Nat Genet*, Vol. 13, No. 2, pp. 196-202, ISSN 1061-4036

Jackson, S. M.; Whitworth, A. J.; Greene, J. C.; Libby, R. T.; Baccam, S. L.; Pallanck, L. J. & La Spada, A. R. (2005). A SCA7 CAG/CTG repeat expansion is stable in Drosophila melanogaster despite modulation of genomic context and gene dosage. *Gene*, Vol. 347, No. 1, pp. 35-41, ISSN 0378-1119

Jackson, W. S.; Tallaksen-Greene, S. J.; Albin, R. L. & Detloff, P. J. (2003). Nucleocytoplasmic transport signals affect the age at onset of abnormalities in knock-in mice expressing polyglutamine within an ectopic protein context. *Hum Mol Genet*, Vol. 12, No. 13, pp. 1621-9, ISSN 0964-6906

Janer, A.; Werner, A.; Takahashi-Fujigasaki, J.; Daret, A.; Fujigasaki, H.; Takada, K.; Duyckaerts, C.; Brice, A.; Dejean, A. & Sittler, A. (2010). SUMOylation attenuates the aggregation propensity and cellular toxicity of the polyglutamine expanded ataxin-7. *Hum Mol Genet*, Vol. 19, No. 1, pp. 181-95, ISSN 1460-2083

Jiang, H.; Mankodi, A.; Swanson, M. S.; Moxley, R. T. & Thornton, C. A. (2004). Myotonic dystrophy type 1 is associated with nuclear foci of mutant RNA, sequestration of muscleblind proteins and deregulated alternative splicing in neurons. *Hum Mol Genet*, Vol. 13, No. 24, pp. 3079-88, ISSN 0964-6906

Kaemmerer, W. F.; Rodrigues, C. M.; Steer, C. J. & Low, W. C. (2001). Creatine-supplemented diet extends Purkinje cell survival in spinocerebellar ataxia type 1 transgenic mice but does not prevent the ataxic phenotype. *Neuroscience*, Vol. 103, No. 3, pp. 713-24, ISSN 0306-4522

Kaytor, M. D.; Burright, E. N.; Duvick, L. A.; Zoghbi, H. Y. & Orr, H. T. (1997). Increased trinucleotide repeat instability with advanced maternal age. *Hum Mol Genet*, Vol. 6, No. 12, pp. 2135-9, ISSN 0964-6906

Kazemi-Esfarjani, P. & Benzer, S. (2000). Genetic suppression of polyglutamine toxicity in Drosophila. *Science*, Vol. 287, No. 5459, pp. 1837-40, ISSN 0036-8075

Khan, L. A.; Bauer, P. O.; Miyazaki, H.; Lindenberg, K. S.; Landwehrmeyer, B. G. & Nukina, N. (2006). Expanded polyglutamines impair synaptic transmission and ubiquitin-proteasome system in Caenorhabditis elegans. *J Neurochem*, Vol. 98, No. 2, pp. 576-87, ISSN 0022-3042

Khurana, V. & Lindquist, S. (2010). Modelling neurodegeneration in Saccharomyces cerevisiae: why cook with baker's yeast? *Nat Rev Neurosci*, Vol. 11, No. 6, pp. 436-49, ISSN 1471-0048

Kiehl, T. R.; Nechiporuk, A.; Figueroa, K. P.; Keating, M. T.; Huynh, D. P. & Pulst, S. M. (2006). Generation and characterization of Sca2 (ataxin-2) knockout mice. *Biochem Biophys Res Commun*, Vol. 339, No. 1, pp. 17-24, ISSN 0006-291X

Kiehl, T. R.; Shibata, H. & Pulst, S. M. (2000). The ortholog of human ataxin-2 is essential for early embryonic patterning in C. elegans. *J Mol Neurosci*, Vol. 15, No. 3, pp. 231-41, ISSN 0895-8696

Klement, I. A.; Skinner, P. J.; Kaytor, M. D.; Yi, H.; Hersch, S. M.; Clark, H. B.; Zoghbi, H. Y. & Orr, H. T. (1998). Ataxin-1 nuclear localization and aggregation: role in polyglutamine-induced disease in SCA1 transgenic mice. *Cell*, Vol. 95, No. 1, pp. 41-53, ISSN 0092-8674

Koch, P.; Breuer, P.; Peitz, M.; Jungverdorben, J.; Kesavan, J.; Poppe, D.; Doerr, J.; Ladewig, J.; Mertens, J.; Tüting, T.; Hoffmann, P.; Klockgether, T.; Evert, B. O.; Wüllner, U.; Brüstle, O. (2011). Excitation-induced ataxin-3 aggregation in neurons from patients with Machado-Joseph disease. *Nature*, Epub ahead of print, ISSN 1476-4687

Koyano, S.; Uchihara, T.; Fujigasaki, H.; Nakamura, A.; Yagishita, S. & Iwabuchi, K. (1999). Neuronal intranuclear inclusions in spinocerebellar ataxia type 2: triple-labeling immunofluorescent study. *Neurosci Lett*, Vol. 273, No. 2, pp. 117-20, ISSN 0304-3940

Koyano, S.; Uchihara, T.; Fujigasaki, H.; Nakamura, A.; Yagishita, S. & Iwabuchi, K. (2000). Neuronal intranuclear inclusions in spinocerebellar ataxia type 2. *Ann Neurol*, Vol. 47, No. 4, pp. 550, ISSN 0364-5134

Kretzschmar, D.; Tschape, J.; Bettencourt Da Cruz, A.; Asan, E.; Poeck, B.; Strauss, R. & Pflugfelder, G. O. (2005). Glial and neuronal expression of polyglutamine proteins induce behavioral changes and aggregate formation in Drosophila. *Glia*, Vol. 49, No. 1, pp. 59-72, ISSN 0894-1491

La Spada, A. R.; Fu, Y. H.; Sopher, B. L.; Libby, R. T.; Wang, X.; Li, L. Y.; Einum, D. D.; Huang, J.; Possin, D. E.; Smith, A. C.; Martinez, R. A.; Koszdin, K. L.; Treuting, P. M.; Ware, C. B.; Hurley, J. B.; Ptacek, L. J. & Chen, S. (2001). Polyglutamine-expanded ataxin-7 antagonizes CRX function and induces cone-rod dystrophy in a mouse model of SCA7. *Neuron*, Vol. 31, No. 6, pp. 913-27, ISSN 0896-6273

Lastres-Becker, I.; Brodesser, S.; Lutjohann, D.; Azizov, M.; Buchmann, J.; Hintermann, E.; Sandhoff, K.; Schurmann, A.; Nowock, J. & Auburger, G. (2008a). Insulin receptor and lipid metabolism pathology in ataxin-2 knock-out mice. *Hum Mol Genet*, Vol. 17, No. 10, pp. 1465-81, ISSN 1460-2083

Lastres-Becker, I.; Rub, U. & Auburger, G. (2008b). Spinocerebellar ataxia 2 (SCA2). *Cerebellum*, Vol. 7, No. 2, pp. 115-24, ISSN 1473-4230

Latouche, M.; Lasbleiz, C.; Martin, E.; Monnier, V.; Debeir, T.; Mouatt-Prigent, A.; Muriel, M. P.; Morel, L.; Ruberg, M.; Brice, A.; Stevanin, G. & Tricoire, H. (2007). A conditional pan-neuronal Drosophila model of spinocerebellar ataxia 7 with a reversible adult phenotype suitable for identifying modifier genes. *J Neurosci*, Vol. 27, No. 10, pp. 2483-92, ISSN 1529-2401

Lessing, D. & Bonini, N. M. (2008). Polyglutamine genes interact to modulate the severity and progression of neurodegeneration in Drosophila. *PLoS Biol*, Vol. 6, No. 2, pp. e29, ISSN 1545-7885

Li, L. B.; Yu, Z.; Teng, X. & Bonini, N. M. (2008). RNA toxicity is a component of ataxin-3 degeneration in Drosophila. *Nature*, Vol. 453, No. 7198, pp. 1107-11, ISSN 1476-4687

Lim, J.; Crespo-Barreto, J.; Jafar-Nejad, P.; Bowman, A. B.; Richman, R.; Hill, D. E.; Orr, H. T. & Zoghbi, H. Y. (2008). Opposing effects of polyglutamine expansion on native protein complexes contribute to SCA1. *Nature*, Vol. 452, No. 7188, pp. 713-8, ISSN 1476-4687

Liu, J.; Tang, T. S.; Tu, H.; Nelson, O.; Herndon, E.; Huynh, D. P.; Pulst, S. M. & Bezprozvanny, I. (2009). Deranged calcium signaling and neurodegeneration in spinocerebellar ataxia type 2. *J Neurosci*, Vol. 29, No. 29, pp. 9148-62, ISSN 1529-2401

Lorenzetti, D.; Watase, K.; Xu, B.; Matzuk, M. M.; Orr, H. T. & Zoghbi, H. Y. (2000). Repeat instability and motor incoordination in mice with a targeted expanded CAG repeat in the Sca1 locus. *Hum Mol Genet*, Vol. 9, No. 5, pp. 779-85, ISSN 0964-6906

Lu, B. & Vogel, H. (2009). Drosophila models of neurodegenerative diseases. *Annu Rev Pathol*, Vol. 4, No. pp. 315-42, ISSN 1553-4014

Marsh, J. L.; Walker, H.; Theisen, H.; Zhu, Y. Z.; Fielder, T.; Purcell, J. & Thompson, L. M. (2000). Expanded polyglutamine peptides alone are intrinsically cytotoxic and cause neurodegeneration in Drosophila. *Hum Mol Genet*, Vol. 9, No. 1, pp. 13-25, ISSN 0964-6906

Matilla, A.; Roberson, E. D.; Banfi, S.; Morales, J.; Armstrong, D. L.; Burright, E. N.; Orr, H. T.; Sweatt, J. D.; Zoghbi, H. Y. & Matzuk, M. M. (1998). Mice lacking ataxin-1 display learning deficits and decreased hippocampal paired-pulse facilitation. *J Neurosci*, Vol. 18, No. 14, pp. 5508-16, ISSN 0270-6474

McCampbell, A.; Taye, A. A.; Whitty, L.; Penney, E.; Steffan, J. S. & Fischbeck, K. H. (2001). Histone deacetylase inhibitors reduce polyglutamine toxicity. *Proc Natl Acad Sci U S A*, Vol. 98, No. 26, pp. 15179-84, ISSN 0027-8424

McCampbell, A.; Taylor, J. P.; Taye, A. A.; Robitschek, J.; Li, M.; Walcott, J.; Merry, D.; Chai, Y.; Paulson, H.; Sobue, G. & Fischbeck, K. H. (2000). CREB-binding protein sequestration by expanded polyglutamine. *Hum Mol Genet*, Vol. 9, No. 14, pp. 2197-202, ISSN 0964-6906

McCullough, S. D. & Grant, P. A. (2010). Histone acetylation, acetyltransferases, and ataxia--alteration of histone acetylation and chromatin dynamics is implicated in the pathogenesis of polyglutamine-expansion disorders. *Adv Protein Chem Struct Biol*, Vol. 79, No. pp. 165-203, ISSN 1876-1631

Mello, C. C. & Conte, D., Jr. (2004). Revealing the world of RNA interference. *Nature*, Vol. 431, No. 7006, pp. 338-42, ISSN 1476-4687

Menzies, F. M.; Huebener, J.; Renna, M.; Bonin, M.; Riess, O. & Rubinsztein, D. C. (2010). Autophagy induction reduces mutant ataxin-3 levels and toxicity in a mouse model of spinocerebellar ataxia type 3. *Brain*, Vol. 133, No. Pt 1, pp. 93-104, ISSN 1460-2156

Morley, J. F.; Brignull, H. R.; Weyers, J. J. & Morimoto, R. I. (2002). The threshold for polyglutamine-expansion protein aggregation and cellular toxicity is dynamic and influenced by aging in Caenorhabditis elegans. *Proc Natl Acad Sci U S A*, Vol. 99, No. 16, pp. 10417-22, ISSN 0027-8424

Moseley, M. L.; Zu, T.; Ikeda, Y.; Gao, W.; Mosemiller, A. K.; Daughters, R. S.; Chen, G.; Weatherspoon, M. R.; Clark, H. B.; Ebner, T. J.; Day, J. W. & Ranum, L. P. (2006). Bidirectional expression of CUG and CAG expansion transcripts and intranuclear polyglutamine inclusions in spinocerebellar ataxia type 8. *Nat Genet*, Vol. 38, No. 7, pp. 758-69, ISSN 1061-4036

Mutsuddi, M.; Marshall, C. M.; Benzow, K. A.; Koob, M. D. & Rebay, I. (2004). The spinocerebellar ataxia 8 noncoding RNA causes neurodegeneration and associates with staufen in Drosophila. *Curr Biol*, Vol. 14, No. 4, pp. 302-8, ISSN 0960-9822

Nakamura, T.; Honda, M.; Kimura, S.; Tanabe, M.; Oda, S. & Ono, H. (2005). Taltirelin improves motor ataxia independently of monoamine levels in rolling mouse nagoya, a model of spinocerebellar atrophy. *Biol Pharm Bull*, Vol. 28, No. 12, pp. 2244-7, ISSN 0918-6158

Nascimento-Ferreira, I.; Santos-Ferreira, T.; Sousa-Ferreira, L.; Auregan, G.; Onofre, I.; Alves, S.; Dufour, N.; Colomer Gould, V. F.; Koeppen, A.; Deglon, N. & Pereira de Almeida, L. (2011). Overexpression of the autophagic beclin-1 protein clears mutant ataxin-3 and alleviates Machado-Joseph disease. *Brain*, Vol. 134, No. Pt 5, pp. 1400-15, ISSN 1460-2156

Nollen, E. A.; Garcia, S. M.; van Haaften, G.; Kim, S.; Chavez, A.; Morimoto, R. I. & Plasterk, R. H. (2004). Genome-wide RNA interference screen identifies previously undescribed regulators of polyglutamine aggregation. *Proc Natl Acad Sci U S A*, Vol. 101, No. 17, pp. 6403-8, ISSN 0027-8424

Okazawa, H.; Rich, T.; Chang, A.; Lin, X.; Waragai, M.; Kajikawa, M.; Enokido, Y.; Komuro, A.; Kato, S.; Shibata, M.; Hatanaka, H.; Mouradian, M. M.; Sudol, M. & Kanazawa, I. (2002). Interaction between mutant ataxin-1 and PQBP-1 affects transcription and cell death. *Neuron*, Vol. 34, No. 5, pp. 701-13, ISSN 0896-6273

Ordway, J. M.; Tallaksen-Greene, S.; Gutekunst, C. A.; Bernstein, E. M.; Cearley, J. A.; Wiener, H. W.; Dure, L. S. t.; Lindsey, R.; Hersch, S. M.; Jope, R. S.; Albin, R. L. & Detloff, P. J. (1997). Ectopically expressed CAG repeats cause intranuclear inclusions and a progressive late onset neurological phenotype in the mouse. *Cell*, Vol. 91, No. 6, pp. 753-63, ISSN 0092-8674

Paulson, H. L.; Perez, M. K.; Trottier, Y.; Trojanowski, J. Q.; Subramony, S. H.; Das, S. S.; Vig, P.; Mandel, J. L.; Fischbeck, K. H. & Pittman, R. N. (1997). Intranuclear inclusions of expanded polyglutamine protein in spinocerebellar ataxia type 3. *Neuron*, Vol. 19, No. 2, pp. 333-44, ISSN 0896-6273

Poole, R. J.; Bashllari, E.; Cochella, L.; Flowers, E. B. & Hobert, O. (2011). A Genome-Wide RNAi Screen for Factors Involved in Neuronal Specification in Caenorhabditis elegans. *PLoS Genet*, Vol. 7, No. 6, pp. e1002109, ISSN 1553-7404

Pozzi, C.; Valtorta, M.; Tedeschi, G.; Galbusera, E.; Pastori, V.; Bigi, A.; Nonnis, S.; Grassi, E. & Fusi, P. (2008). Study of subcellular localization and proteolysis of ataxin-3. *Neurobiol Dis*, Vol. 30, No. 2, pp. 190-200, ISSN 1095-953X

Reina, C. P.; Zhong, X. & Pittman, R. N. (2010). Proteotoxic stress increases nuclear localization of ataxin-3. *Hum Mol Genet*, Vol. 19, No. 2, pp. 235-49, ISSN 1460-2083

Rodrigues, A. J.; Coppola, G.; Santos, C.; Costa Mdo, C.; Ailion, M.; Sequeiros, J.; Geschwind, D. H. & Maciel, P. (2007). Functional genomics and biochemical characterization of the C. elegans orthologue of the Machado-Joseph disease protein ataxin-3. *Faseb J*, Vol. 21, No. 4, pp. 1126-36, ISSN 1530-6860

Rodrigues, A. J.; Neves-Carvalho, A.; Teixeira-Castro, A.; Rokka, A.; Corthals, G.; Logarinho, E. & Maciel, P. (2011). Absence of ataxin-3 leads to enhanced stress response in C. elegans. *PLoS One*, Vol. 6, No. 4, pp. e18512, ISSN 1932-6203

Rolfs, A.; Koeppen, A. H.; Bauer, I.; Bauer, P.; Buhlmann, S.; Topka, H.; Schols, L. & Riess, O. (2003). Clinical features and neuropathology of autosomal dominant spinocerebellar ataxia (SCA17). *Ann Neurol*, Vol. 54, No. 3, pp. 367-75, ISSN 0364-5134

Rüb, U.; de Vos, R. A.; Brunt, E. R.; Schultz, C.; Paulson, H.; Del Tredici, K. & Braak, H. (2002a). Degeneration of the external cuneate nucleus in spinocerebellar ataxia type 3 (Machado-Joseph disease). *Brain Res*, Vol. 953, No. 1-2, pp. 126-34, ISSN 0006-8993

Rüb, U.; de Vos, R. A.; Schultz, C.; Brunt, E. R.; Paulson, H. & Braak, H. (2002b). Spinocerebellar ataxia type 3 (Machado-Joseph disease): severe destruction of the lateral reticular nucleus. *Brain*, Vol. 125, No. Pt 9, pp. 2115-24, ISSN 0006-8950

Rubin, G. M.; Yandell, M. D.; Wortman, J. R.; Gabor Miklos, G. L.; Nelson, C. R.; Hariharan, I. K.; Fortini, M. E.; Li, P. W.; Apweiler, R.; Fleischmann, W.; Cherry, J. M.; Henikoff, S.; Skupski, M. P.; Misra, S.; Ashburner, M.; Birney, E.; Boguski, M. S.; Brody, T.; Brokstein, P.; Celniker, S. E.; Chervitz, S. A.; Coates, D.; Cravchik, A.; Gabrielian, A.; Galle, R. F.; Gelbart, W. M.; George, R. A.; Goldstein, L. S.; Gong, F.; Guan, P.; Harris, N. L.; Hay, B. A.; Hoskins, R. A.; Li, J.; Li, Z.; Hynes, R. O.; Jones, S. J.; Kuehl, P. M.; Lemaitre, B.; Littleton, J. T.; Morrison, D. K.; Mungall, C.; O'Farrell, P. H.; Pickeral, O. K.; Shue, C.; Vosshall, L. B.; Zhang, J.; Zhao, Q.; Zheng, X. H. & Lewis, S. (2000). Comparative genomics of the eukaryotes. *Science*, Vol. 287, No. 5461, pp. 2204-15, ISSN 0036-8075

Saegusa, H.; Wakamori, M.; Matsuda, Y.; Wang, J.; Mori, Y.; Zong, S. & Tanabe, T. (2007). Properties of human Cav2.1 channel with a spinocerebellar ataxia type 6 mutation expressed in Purkinje cells. *Mol Cell Neurosci*, Vol. 34, No. 2, pp. 261-70, ISSN 1044-7431

Satterfield, T. F.; Jackson, S. M. & Pallanck, L. J. (2002). A Drosophila homolog of the polyglutamine disease gene SCA2 is a dosage-sensitive regulator of actin filament formation. *Genetics*, Vol. 162, No. 4, pp. 1687-702, ISSN 0016-6731

Satterfield, T. F. & Pallanck, L. J. (2006). Ataxin-2 and its Drosophila homolog, ATX2, physically assemble with polyribosomes. *Hum Mol Genet*, Vol. 15, No. 16, pp. 2523-32, ISSN 0964-6906

Sayers, E. W.; Barrett, T.; Benson, D. A.; Bolton, E.; Bryant, S. H.; Canese, K.; Chetvernin, V.; Church, D. M.; DiCuccio, M.; Federhen, S.; Feolo, M.; Fingerman, I. M.; Geer, L. Y.; Helmberg, W.; Kapustin, Y.; Landsman, D.; Lipman, D. J.; Lu, Z.; Madden, T. L.; Madej, T.; Maglott, D. R.; Marchler-Bauer, A.; Miller, V.; Mizrachi, I.; Ostell, J.; Panchenko, A.; Phan, L.; Pruitt, K. D.; Schuler, G. D.; Sequeira, E.; Sherry, S. T.; Shumway, M.; Sirotkin, K.; Slotta, D.; Souvorov, A.; Starchenko, G.; Tatusova, T. A.; Wagner, L.; Wang, Y.; Wilbur, W. J.; Yaschenko, E. & Ye, J. (2011). Database resources of the National Center for Biotechnology Information. *Nucleic Acids Res*, Vol. 39, No. Database issue, pp. D38-51, ISSN 1362-4962

Schmidt, T.; Lindenberg, K. S.; Krebs, A.; Schöls, L.; Laccone, F.; Herms, J.; Rechsteiner, M.; Riess, O. & Landwehrmeyer, G. B. (2002). Protein surveillance machinery in brains with spinocerebellar ataxia type 3: redistribution and differential recruitment of 26S proteasome subunits and chaperones to neuronal intranuclear inclusions. *Ann Neurol*, Vol. 51, No. 3, pp. 302-10, ISSN 0364-5134

Schmitt, I.; Linden, M.; Khazneh, H.; Evert, B. O.; Breuer, P.; Klockgether, T. & Wuellner, U. (2007). Inactivation of the mouse Atxn3 (ataxin-3) gene increases protein ubiquitination. *Biochem Biophys Res Commun*, Vol. 362, No. 3, pp. 734-9, ISSN 0006-291X

Schöls, L.; Bauer, P.; Schmidt, T.; Schulte, T. & Riess, O. (2004). Autosomal dominant cerebellar ataxias: clinical features, genetics, and pathogenesis. *Lancet Neurol*, Vol. 3, No. 5, pp. 291-304, ISSN 1474-4422

Shah, A. G.; Friedman, M. J.; Huang, S.; Roberts, M.; Li, X. J. & Li, S. (2009). Transcriptional dysregulation of TrkA associates with neurodegeneration in spinocerebellar ataxia type 17. *Hum Mol Genet*, Vol. 18, No. 21, pp. 4141-52, ISSN 1460-2083

Silva-Fernandes, A.; Costa Mdo, C.; Duarte-Silva, S.; Oliveira, P.; Botelho, C. M.; Martins, L.; Mariz, J. A.; Ferreira, T.; Ribeiro, F.; Correia-Neves, M.; Costa, C. & Maciel, P. (2010). Motor uncoordination and neuropathology in a transgenic mouse model of Machado-Joseph disease lacking intranuclear inclusions and ataxin-3 cleavage products. *Neurobiol Dis*, Vol. 40, No. 1, pp. 163-76, ISSN 1095-953X

Switonski, P. M.; Fiszer, A.; Kazmierska, K.; Kurpisz, M.; Krzyzosiak, W. J. & Figiel, M. (2011). Mouse ataxin-3 functional knock-out model. *Neuromolecular Med*, Vol. 13, No. 1, pp. 54-65, ISSN 1559-1174

Teixeira-Castro, A.; Ailion, M.; Jalles, A.; Brignull, H. R.; Vilaca, J. L.; Dias, N.; Rodrigues, P.; Oliveira, J. F.; Neves-Carvalho, A.; Morimoto, R. I. & Maciel, P. (2011). Neuron-specific proteotoxicity of mutant ataxin-3 in C. elegans: rescue by the DAF-16 and HSF-1 pathways. *Hum Mol Genet*, Vol. 20, No. 15, pp. 2996-3009, ISSN 1460-2083

Tsuda, H.; Jafar-Nejad, H.; Patel, A. J.; Sun, Y.; Chen, H. K.; Rose, M. F.; Venken, K. J.; Botas, J.; Orr, H. T.; Bellen, H. J. & Zoghbi, H. Y. (2005). The AXH domain of Ataxin-1 mediates neurodegeneration through its interaction with Gfi-1/Senseless proteins. *Cell*, Vol. 122, No. 4, pp. 633-44, ISSN 0092-8674

van de Leemput, J.; Chandran, J.; Knight, M. A.; Holtzclaw, L. A.; Scholz, S.; Cookson, M. R.; Houlden, H.; Gwinn-Hardy, K.; Fung, H. C.; Lin, X.; Hernandez, D.; Simon-Sanchez, J.; Wood, N. W.; Giunti, P.; Rafferty, I.; Hardy, J.; Storey, E.; Gardner, R. J.; Forrest, S. M.; Fisher, E. M.; Russell, J. T.; Cai, H. & Singleton, A. B. (2007). Deletion at ITPR1 underlies ataxia in mice and spinocerebellar ataxia 15 in humans. *PLoS Genet*, Vol. 3, No. 6, pp. e108, ISSN 1553-7404

van de Warrenburg, B. P.; Frenken, C. W.; Ausems, M. G.; Kleefstra, T.; Sinke, R. J.; Knoers, N. V. & Kremer, H. P. (2001). Striking anticipation in spinocerebellar ataxia type 7: the infantile phenotype. *J Neurol*, Vol. 248, No. 10, pp. 911-4, ISSN 0340-5354

Vandaele, S.; Nordquist, D. T.; Feddersen, R. M.; Tretjakoff, I.; Peterson, A. C. & Orr, H. T. (1991). Purkinje cell protein-2 regulatory regions and transgene expression in cerebellar compartments. *Genes Dev*, Vol. 5, No. 7, pp. 1136-48, ISSN 0890-9369

Vig, P. J.; Subramony, S. H.; D'Souza, D. R.; Wei, J. & Lopez, M. E. (2006). Intranasal administration of IGF-I improves behavior and Purkinje cell pathology in SCA1 mice. *Brain Res Bull*, Vol. 69, No. 5, pp. 573-9, ISSN 0361-9230

Voisine, C.; Varma, H.; Walker, N.; Bates, E. A.; Stockwell, B. R. & Hart, A. C. (2007). Identification of potential therapeutic drugs for huntington's disease using Caenorhabditis elegans. *PLoS One*, Vol. 2, No. 6, pp. e504, ISSN 1932-6203

Warrick, J. M.; Morabito, L. M.; Bilen, J.; Gordesky-Gold, B.; Faust, L. Z.; Paulson, H. L. & Bonini, N. M. (2005). Ataxin-3 suppresses polyglutamine neurodegeneration in Drosophila by a ubiquitin-associated mechanism. *Mol Cell*, Vol. 18, No. 1, pp. 37-48, ISSN 1097-2765

Warrick, J. M.; Paulson, H. L.; Gray-Board, G. L.; Bui, Q. T.; Fischbeck, K. H.; Pittman, R. N. & Bonini, N. M. (1998). Expanded polyglutamine protein forms nuclear inclusions and causes neural degeneration in Drosophila. *Cell*, Vol. 93, No. 6, pp. 939-49, ISSN 0092-8674

Watase, K.; Barrett, C. F.; Miyazaki, T.; Ishiguro, T.; Ishikawa, K.; Hu, Y.; Unno, T.; Sun, Y.; Kasai, S.; Watanabe, M.; Gomez, C. M.; Mizusawa, H.; Tsien, R. W. & Zoghbi, H. Y. (2008). Spinocerebellar ataxia type 6 knockin mice develop a progressive neuronal dysfunction with age-dependent accumulation of mutant CaV2.1 channels. *Proc Natl Acad Sci U S A*, Vol. 105, No. 33, pp. 11987-92, ISSN 1091-6490

Watase, K.; Gatchel, J. R.; Sun, Y.; Emamian, E.; Atkinson, R.; Richman, R.; Mizusawa, H.; Orr, H. T.; Shaw, C. & Zoghbi, H. Y. (2007). Lithium therapy improves neurological function and hippocampal dendritic arborization in a spinocerebellar ataxia type 1 mouse model. *PLoS Med*, Vol. 4, No. 5, pp. e182, ISSN 1549-1676

Watase, K.; Venken, K. J.; Sun, Y.; Orr, H. T. & Zoghbi, H. Y. (2003). Regional differences of somatic CAG repeat instability do not account for selective neuronal vulnerability in a knock-in mouse model of SCA1. *Hum Mol Genet*, Vol. 12, No. 21, pp. 2789-95, ISSN 0964-6906

Watase, K.; Weeber, E. J.; Xu, B.; Antalffy, B.; Yuva-Paylor, L.; Hashimoto, K.; Kano, M.; Atkinson, R.; Sun, Y.; Armstrong, D. L.; Sweatt, J. D.; Orr, H. T.; Paylor, R. & Zoghbi, H. Y. (2002). A long CAG repeat in the mouse Sca1 locus replicates SCA1 features and reveals the impact of protein solubility on selective neurodegeneration. *Neuron*, Vol. 34, No. 6, pp. 905-19, ISSN 0896-6273

Xia, H.; Mao, Q.; Eliason, S. L.; Harper, S. Q.; Martins, I. H.; Orr, H. T.; Paulson, H. L.; Yang, L.; Kotin, R. M. & Davidson, B. L. (2004). RNAi suppresses polyglutamine-induced neurodegeneration in a model of spinocerebellar ataxia. *Nat Med*, Vol. 10, No. 8, pp. 816-20, ISSN 1078-8956

Yoo, S. Y.; Pennesi, M. E.; Weeber, E. J.; Xu, B.; Atkinson, R.; Chen, S.; Armstrong, D. L.; Wu, S. M.; Sweatt, J. D. & Zoghbi, H. Y. (2003). SCA7 knockin mice model human SCA7 and reveal gradual accumulation of mutant ataxin-7 in neurons and abnormalities in short-term plasticity. *Neuron*, Vol. 37, No. 3, pp. 383-401, ISSN 0896-6273

Yvert, G.; Lindenberg, K. S.; Picaud, S.; Landwehrmeyer, G. B.; Sahel, J. A. & Mandel, J. L. (2000). Expanded polyglutamines induce neurodegeneration and trans-neuronal alterations in cerebellum and retina of SCA7 transgenic mice. *Hum Mol Genet*, Vol. 9, No. 17, pp. 2491-506, ISSN 0964-6906

Zoghbi, H. Y. & Botas, J. (2002). Mouse and fly models of neurodegeneration. *Trends Genet*, Vol. 18, No. 9, pp. 463-71, ISSN 0168-9525

Zu, T.; Duvick, L. A.; Kaytor, M. D.; Berlinger, M. S.; Zoghbi, H. Y.; Clark, H. B. & Orr, H. T. (2004). Recovery from polyglutamine-induced neurodegeneration in conditional SCA1 transgenic mice. *J Neurosci*, Vol. 24, No. 40, pp. 8853-61, ISSN 1529-2401

2

Non-Mendelian Genetic Aspects in Spinocerebellar Ataxias (SCAS): The Case of Machado-Joseph Disease (MJD)

Manuela Lima[1,2], Jácome Bruges-Armas[1,3] and Conceição Bettencourt[1,2,4]

[1]*Genetic and Arthritis Research Group, Institute for Molecular and Cell Biology (IBMC), University of Porto, Porto*

[2]*Center of Research in Natural Resources (CIRN) and Department of Biology, University of the Azores, Ponta Delgada*

[3]*Serviço Especializado de Epidemiologia e Biologia Molecular, Hospital de Santo Espírito de Angra do Heroísmo*

[4]*Laboratorio de Biología Molecular, Instituto de Enfermedades Neurológicas, Fundación Socio-Sanitaria de Castilla-La Mancha, Guadalajara*

[1,2,3]*Portugal*

[4]*Spain*

1. Introduction

Monogenic disorders of Mendelian nature, defined as those resulting of mutation at a single locus, and in which the observed alteration is both necessary and sufficient for phenotypic manifestation (Gropman & Adams, 2007), constituted, until recently, the main target of gene-finding studies. Mendelian or otherwise "simple" phenotypes are frequently referred in the scientific literature in opposition to the "complex" ones; the designation of "Mendelian", therefore, should reflect the occurrence of such diseases in accordance with simple, predictable family patterns, with a single locus determining its manifestation. It has, however, become very evident that even in the case of individual causative genes, the associated phenotypes can display attributes which result in non-Mendelian patterns of the trait or disease whose expression is being considered (Gropman & Adams, 2007; Sherman, 1997). In practical terms, this implies that the number of diseases for which the respective phenotypes can be explained by the effect of mutations at a single locus is dramatically diminishing (Gropman & Adams, 2007). Several diseases, initially characterized as monogenic, are now known to be modulated by a yet undetermined number of loci. Incomplete genotype-phenotype correlations observed in a large number of diseases have, therefore, forced the widening of the monogenic model, to allow the accommodation of the remaining factors, which can potentially explain the spectrum of the phenotypic variability (Badano & Katsanis, 2002). The incompleteness of the genotype-phenotype correlations seen in such situations confirms that the product of the primary mutation is imbedded in a highly complex system, in which polymorphic variation, mutations at other loci as well as environmental variables modulate the differences observed amongst individuals (Van Heyningen & Yeyati, 2004).

Factors that produce atypical or irregular patterns of inheritance are frequently referred as "complicating factors". The understanding of the mechanisms on the basis of such patterns is pertinent not only at a theoretical level, but also due to implications in terms of diagnosis and genetic risk assessment, conditioning, furthermore, the ability to predict the initiation and course of disease (Haines & Pericak-Vance, 2006; Van Heyningen & Yeyati, 2004). On the other hand, in the context of research related with the identification of deleterious genes, such irregularities can imply, amongst other aspects, severe obstacles in the interpretation of pedigrees, as well as difficulties in the selection of families (*e.g.*, in the context of linkage studies). Several of such complicating factors are frequently cited, namely clinical variability, expressivity, pleiotropism, anticipation, incomplete penetrance, age-dependent penetrance and meiotic drive. Underlying these observations are mechanisms such as allelic and locus heterogeneity, presence of modifier genes, intergenerational instability, somatic instability, genomic imprinting and *de novo* mutations (Gilchrist et al., 2000).

Amongst the several diseases with a known causative mutation but which, nevertheless, display complicating features are those associated with triplet repeat expansions. Four classes of triplet repeat disorders are usually considered, based on the location of the repeat motif in 5´or 3´untranslated regions, in introns or in coding regions (revised in Bettencourt et al., 2007). Polyglutamine (Poly-Q) disorders are part of this "expansion disorders" group, being caused by a CAG repeat expansion in the coding region of the respective causative genes; enclosed within this group are several spinocerebellar ataxias (SCAs), namely SCA1, SCA2, SCA3, SCA6, SCA7, SCA17 as well as dentato-rubro-pallido-luysian atrophy (DRPLA). Poly-Q diseases exhibit atypical features, difficult to integrate in the classic mendelian expectations (Tsuji, 1997). Machado-Joseph disease (MJD/SCA3) is considered the most frequent SCA worldwide (Cagnoli et al., 2006; Paulson, 2007; Schöls et al., 2004); using MJD as a paradigm, this review aims to explore complicating, non-Mendelian aspects of Poly-Q SCAs, from a perspective that synthesizes the current knowledge concerning such complicating factors as well as their implications at several levels, namely at the level of genetic counseling (GC).

2. Machado-Joseph disease: general perspective

Machado-Joseph disease, also known as spinocerebellar ataxia type 3 (MJD/SCA3 - MIM 109150) is an autosomal dominant neurodegenerative disorder. Described as a disorder of adulthood, with an average age at onset rounding 40 years (Coutinho, 1992), this disease has, nevertheless, reported onset extremes of 4 (Carvalho et al., 2008) and 70 years (Coutinho, 1992). Average survival time is of 21 years (Coutinho, 1992; Kieling et al., 2007). MJD is characterized by a complex and pleiotropic phenotype, involving the cerebellar, oculomotor, pyramidal, extra-pyramidal and peripheral systems. The high clinical variability observed in this disorder has led to its systematization into three clinical types, which can occasionally be present in a single family (Coutinho & Andrade, 1978).

MJD was originally described in North American patients of Azorean ancestry, residing in the United States (Nakano et al., 1972; Rosenberg et al., 1976; Woods & Schaumburg, 1972). The history of its initial description, as three distinct clinical entities, clearly reflects the high phenotypic variability that characterizes this disorder, whose unification was dependent of the identification, in a single family, of the different clinical forms that were described in the original reports (Coutinho & Andrade, 1978). The common ancestry of the three families that were described between 1972 and 1976 (known as Machado, Thomas and Joseph), has largely conditioned the interpretations about the origin of the disease, initially considered as Azorean, and designated as "Azorean disease of the nervous system" (Romanul et al., 1977). The molecular screening of MJD's causative mutation allowed, afterwards, the differential diagnosis, which has led to an epidemiological profile clearly distinct from the one obtained on the basis of clinical criteria alone (Lopes-Cendes et al., 1996). In Portugal, MJD represents about 58% of the families with dominant ataxias (Vale et al., 2009). In the Azores, more precisely in the small island of Flores, the disease achieves the highest values of prevalence reported worldwide (Bettencourt et al., 2008a; Lima et al., 1997).

Two main studies have addressed the issue of the worldwide origin of the MJD mutation. Gaspar et al. (2001), using flanking and intragenic markers, have identified two main haplotypes in 94% of the families studied. In the Azores, these two haplotypes were present, and were related with the islands of higher prevalence (Flores and São Miguel), indicating that two mutational events were responsible for the presence of MJD in the families of Azorean origin, a result previously disclosed by genealogical analysis (Lima et al., 1998). Aiming to determine the origin, age and dispersion of these two main mutational events, Martins et al. (2007) have conducted a more extensive haplotype analysis, which revealed that the TTACAC lineage, the most frequently found in the expanded alleles of patients from all over the world, achieved its highest variability in Asia (specifically in the Japanese population). A "Short Tandem Repeat" (STR) based haplotype was identified in this population and an approximate age of 5774±1116 years was suggested.

The MJD locus was mapped to 14q24.3-q32 in 1993 (Takiyama et al., 1993). In the following year, Kawaguchi and colleagues (Kawaguchi et al., 1994) isolated and characterized a cDNA clone, designated as MJD1a, identifying MJD's causative mutation as an expansion of a CAG motif in the coding region of the *ATXN3* gene. Initially described as containing 11 exons, *ATXN3* spans a genomic region of around 48 kb, with the CAG tract located in exon 10, at 5' (Ichikawa et al., 2001). Two novel exons were identified recently, in a study that used information from cDNA clones of Azorean MJD patients and controls (Bettencourt et al., 2010a). In the MJD locus, normal chromosomes have from 12 to 44 CAG repeats, whereas in patients, usually heterozygous, the number of repeats in the mutated allele consensually ranges between 61 and 87 (Maciel et al., 2001). Intermediate alleles are rare and, as a result, their behavior is poorly understood. For example, in a family described by Maciel and colleagues (Maciel et al., 2001), an allele with 51 repeats apparently was not associated with the disease. On the other hand, alleles of intermediate size have been associated with the MJD phenotype (*e.g.*, Padiath et al., 2005; Van Alfen et al., 2001); in the study of Van Alfen et al. (2001), four symptomatic family members presented CAG tract sizes between 53 and 54 repeats. Although rare, the cases of intermediate alleles imply that the distinction, initially very clear, between normal and mutated alleles has become much more difficult to establish. Alleles with around 50 repeats seem, in certain cases, to act as fully penetrant, a scenario that remains, nevertheless, rare (Paulson, 2007). In Portugal, and despite the high prevalence of the disease, a study of nearly 2000 chromosomes from the general population, representing all Portuguese districts, failed to detect the presence of intermediate alleles (Lima et al., 2005). Normal and pathogenic repeat size ranges are not definitive, and gathering of up-dated information should be a concern of laboratories offering molecular testing.

The *ATXN3* gene is ubiquously expressed in neuronal and non-neuronal tissues; it encodes for ataxin-3, a protein with an approximate molecular weight of 42kD, in its native form. In the neurons, ataxin-3 is found essentially in the cytoplasm (Paulson et al., 1997). Five products of the *ATXN3* gene, referring to transcripts of different sizes, were described by Ichikawa and colleagues (Ichikawa et al., 2001). More recently, the sequence of 56 distinct transcripts, generated by alternative splicing, was described, and the high transcriptional variability of MJD's causative gene has been demonstrated (Bettencourt et al., 2010a). Ataxin-3 belongs to the family of cysteine-proteases; structurally it is composed by 339 aa, to which a variable number of glutamines is added (Poly-Q tract) (Kawaguchi et al., 1994). This protein is composed by a Josephine domain (JD), located in its N-terminal portion, containing, at its C-terminal, two or three ubiquitin-interacting motifs (UIMs) and the Poly-Q tract. It has been proposed that the native form of the protein acts as a deubiquitinating enzyme in the ubiquitin-proteossome pathway (revised in Bettencourt & Lima, 2011). Therefore, evidence concerning the proprieties of ataxin-3 suggests that this protein participates in cellular pathways related to quality control of proteins (see, amongst others, Schmitt et al., 2007). The involvement of the normal form of the protein in the regulation of transcription has also been suggested (Chou et al., 2008).

In the MJD locus, the presence of an expanded allele leads to a protein enriched in glutamines. The Poly-Q tract expansion should lead to a gain of neurotoxic function of the corresponding protein and, as a consequence, to neuronal death, by a process which remains, nevertheless, incompletely understood. Models of pathogenesis include the formation of toxic oligomers of ataxin-3, as well as aberrant protein-protein interactions, which disrupt normal cellular functions; revisions on the aspects of MJD's pathogenesis can be found, amongst others, in Paulson (2007) and Katsuno et al. (2008).

Notwithstanding the fact that MJD constitutes a relatively well defined clinical entity, its clinical diagnosis can, in many situations, be difficult to establish. Such is the case, when the disease is at its initial stage and minor, but more specific signs are absent. Moreover, in apparently isolated cases, or in cases that appear associated to a less common geographic distribution, a clinical diagnosis can also be hard to establish with certainty (Lopes-Cendes et al., 1996). Therefore, in the differential diagnosis of MJD, molecular testing, available after the identification of the causative mutation, has become of major importance (Maciel et al., 2001). Furthermore, predictive testing (PT), as well as prenatal diagnosis (PND) became available (Sequeiros et al., 1998). More recently, pre-implantation genetic diagnosis (PGD) is also feasible (Drüsedau et al., 2004). The program of PT and GC, available for MJD in Portugal since the end of 1995, was based on the previous experience with Huntington's disease (HD) (Sequeiros, 1996). This program is ongoing in the Azores since 1996, and its impact in patients and families is periodically revised (Gonzalez et al., 2004; Lima et al., 2001).

Presently there is no effective pharmacological approach for SCAs. Specific drugs have been prescribed to minimize some of the symptoms, such as ataxia or dystonia (reviewed in Bettencourt & Lima, 2011). Cell and animal models have also been fundamental in the understanding of the pathogenesis and gene therapy search (*e.g.*, Gould, 2005); the use of interference RNA and the administration of antisense oligonucleotides showed promising results according to Alves et al. (2008; 2010) and Hu et al. (2009), respectively.

3. Complicating factors in MJD

Several aspects of non-compliance with the Mendelian expectations can be readily recognized for MJD. Variation in the age at onset, variability in clinical presentation, presence of anticipation as well as repeat instability (somatic and germ line), have been described as the main complicating factors in MJD (Tsuji, 1997). Other factors, which will be referred, are also noteworthy.

3.1 Clinical variability

As previously referred, MJD is characterized by a complex phenotype, which is highly variable amongst patients. The recognition of its high degree of clinical variability has led to the proposal of Coutinho & Andrade (1978), in which patients could be classified into three clinical types. According to Coutinho (1992), type 1 has an early onset (average of 24 years) and a more rapid progression of symptoms, being characterized by pyramidal signs and dystonia. Type 2 is the most frequent, and occurs around 40 years of age, being dominated by ataxia and ophtalmoplegia, with or without pyramidal signs. Type 3 has a latter onset (average of 47 years) and progresses slowly, with amyothrophies. The three clinical types can, occasionally, be present in the same family. A fourth type, a rare presentation that associates parkinsonism to cerebellar signs (Suite et al., 1986), and a fifth type, associated with spastic paraplegia (Sakai & Kawakami, 1996), have also been proposed. Notwithstanding the fact that some clinical features, if present, can help in the differential diagnosis of MJD (*e.g.*, ophthalmoplegia, bulging eyes or face and tongue fasciculations), phenotypic overlapping with other SCAs has implications for GC and PT. Therefore, at-risk individuals entering the PT program must have an affected close relative with a definitive molecular diagnosis - "mutation-positive" familial control (Sequeiros et al., 2010).

Variation in age at onset, evidenced by its reported extremes (4 and 70 years) described by Carvalho et al. (2008) and Coutinho (1992), constitutes a particular aspect of the clinical variability of this disorder. A significant, but partial, negative correlation between the size of the expanded allele (and thus, the extension of the Poly-Q tract) and the age of appearance of symptoms explains between nearly 50 to 75% of the variation in the age at onset, depending on the analyzed series of patients (*e.g.*, Maciel et al., 1995; Maruyama et al., 1995). The size of the mutated allele also correlates with the frequency of particular clinical signs, such as pyramidal signs, which are more frequent in patients with larger repeats (Takiyama et al., 1995). In the Azorean series of patients, for example, the number of CAG repeats, determined in genomic DNA and in mRNA, explains 68% and 67% of variation in the age at onset, respectively (Bettencourt et al., 2010b). The incompleteness of the correlation observed between the size of the CAG tract and the age at onset implies that such information cannot be used for counseling purposes; whether allele sizes should be disclosed in the molecular test report is still being debated (Sequeiros et al., 2010).

The reported incompleteness of the genotype-phenotype correlation, observed in MJD as well as in other SCAs, confirms the involvement of non-CAG factors in the explanation of the phenotype, that can either be genetic or environmental (van de Warrenburg et al., 2005). For MJD, the hypothesis that an important fraction of the residual of the disease onset (after accounting for the CAG repeat size) is of genetic nature has been reinforced (DeStefano et al., 1996; van de Warrenburg et al., 2005). The few studies that attempted to identify MJD modifiers have used candidate gene approaches; Jardim et al. (2003), in a study that considers the effect of the CAG tract at several expansion loci (namely SCA2, SCA6 and DRPLA), only found a correlation between the severity of fasciculations and the size of the CAG tract at the SCA2 locus. Recently, Bettencourt and colleagues (2011) found a significant association between the presence of the *APOE* ε2 allele and an earlier onset in MJD.

3.2 Gene dosage effect

The reduced number of homozygous patients described for MJD makes any generalization, concerning the impact of gene dosage on clinical presentation, hard to perform. The few cases described in the literature, nevertheless, reinforce the fact that the phenotype is more severe and the onset is earlier in homozygous carriers of the mutated allele (*e.g.*, Carvalho et al., 2008; Lerer et al., 1996). This indicates that gene dosage is an important determinant of the onset. The increased severity observed in homozygous is common in dominant diseases, which do not follow the Mendelian expectation of phenotypic overlapping between homo and heterozygous. In specific populations, known to have a particularly high prevalence of MJD, such as the Azorean island of Flores, the possibility of mating between carriers of the MJD mutation must be taken into consideration when planning GC sessions.

3.3 Incomplete and age-dependent pattern of penetrance

In MJD pedigrees, skipped generations are rarely observed. Coutinho (1992) refers that the majority of such cases can be explained by a premature death of the obligate carrier, in relation to the average onset of the disease. Other factors, such as migration, can further prevent the confirmation of the disease status in the obligate carrier. With an estimated value of 98%, the MJD gene penetrance presents an age-dependent pattern, which implies that the *a posteriori*, or residual risk, differs considerably depending on the age of the individual. Residual risk tables constitute, in this context, important tools for GC (Bettencourt et al., 2008a), since they allow the geneticist to estimate the probability that an asymptomatic at-risk individual has to develop the disease at a certain age.

3.4 Intergenerational instability of the CAG tract

Within the Poly-Q disorders, anticipation is more marked for DRPLA, SCA2, SCA7 and HD (Paulson, 2007; Takiyama et al., 1999). In MJD, however, the aggravation of symptoms, and the decrease in the age at onset in successive generations, is also observed. On the basis of anticipation in MJD is the instability of the *ATXN3* gene region containing the expanded CAG tract, which, during cellular division, can lead to alterations in the size of the repeat tract, resulting in expansions or, more rarely, in contractions. Although the decrease in the age at onset is highly related with the increase in the size of the CAG tract, families with a higher degree of anticipation than it would be expected for each repeat unit increase were identified (Takiyama et al., 1998).

Germline mosaicism has been consistently described for MJD (*e.g.*, Cancel et al., 1995). The tendency for the increase of the repeat size is more marked in male than in female meiosis; processes specific to sperm or oocyte development should be involved in such differences.

Maciel et al. (1995) reported that the size of the repeat tract varies in 55% of transmissions; from these, 78% correspond to expansions and 22% to contractions.

Several factors have been implicated as modulating the intergenerational instability in MJD, such as the sex of the transmitting parent as well as the intragenic environment (see, amongst others, Igarashi et al., 1996; Maciel et al., 1999). The results obtained by Takiyama et al. (1997) suggests the presence of an inter-allelic association involved in the instability of the CAG tract, trough yet poorly known mechanisms. Other inter-allelic and *cis* factors have also been studied by Martins et al. (2008); these authors have concluded that distinct origins of the mutation (established on the basis of haplotypes constructed using intragenic SNPs) present different behaviors on what concerns repeat instability. Evidences gathered so far support the presence of a mechanism associated to DNA repair, rather than associated with replication, on the basis of meiotic instability observed in this locus (Martins et al., 2008).

Little is known about the mutational process that leads to the emergence of repeats within the pathological size. It has been postulated that a mutational bias, in favor of expansions, exists in trinucleotide repeat loci, suggesting that the upper end of the normal allele distribution would provide a "reservoir" from which expanded alleles would be generated (Rubinsztein et al., 1994). The hypothesis that normal alleles of larger size could constitute such a reservoir was not supported by a study of nearly 2000 chromosomes of a representative sample of the general Portuguese population (Lima et al., 2005). On the contrary, the report from Lima and colleagues (2005), shows that the allelic distribution was skewed towards smaller size alleles. In a subsequent study, Martins et al. (2006) have integrated not only the analysis of the CAG repeat, but also information on haplotypes built using intragenic and flanking markers; the conclusions indicate that a multistep mechanism is on the basis of the evolution of the CAG repeats in MJD, originated either by gene conversion or DNA slippage.

3.5 Somatic mosaicism

The instability of the expanded polyglutamine-coding (CAG)n tracts during mitotic cell division can lead to changes in repeat length, either contractions or more frequently expansions, resulting in certain populations of cells carrying different repeat sizes. For MJD, the somatic mosaicism has been described by several authors (see, amongst others, Cancel et al., 1995; Lopes-Cendes et al., 1996; Maciel et al., 1997).

In the central nervous system (CNS), the pattern of mosaicism for mutated alleles is similar in the several structures, with the exception of the cerebellar cortex, which presents slightly reduced tracts (Cancel et al., 1998; Hashida et al., 1997). In non-neuronal tissues, the instability is lower in muscle (Tanaka et al., 1999). The studies conducted have consistently failed to demonstrate a correlation between the degree of mosaicism and the selective neuronal vulnerability (Cancel et al., 1998; Ito et al., 1998). The pattern of mosaicism in genomic DNA is maintained in mRNA, and the variation in the size of the CAG repeat in mRNA is also not relatable with the severity of the pathological involvement of the several tissues (Ito et al., 1998).

Somatic mosaicism contributes to the limitations in the precision of sizing the MJD repeat motif, since it originates differences in (CAG)n length among subpopulations of lymphocytes as well as between lymphocytes (where length is usually measured) and CNS cells (revised in Lima et al., 2006). Thus an error of ±1 CAG repeat is considered as acceptable (Maciel et al., 2001; Sequeiros et al., 2010).

3.6 Segregation distortion

Alterations to the Mendelian proportions in the segregation of the *ATXN3* alleles were firstly highlighted by Ikeuchi and colleagues, in 1996. These authors suggested the occurrence of "meiotic drive" to justify the observation of an excess of affected descendents of MJD patients, a fact hardly explainable by the Mendelian principle of random segregation of alleles (Ikeuchi et al., 1996). Their results pointed to the existence of segregation distortion, in the male meiosis. This issue, however, is far from consensual. A single-sperm typing performed in Japanese patients, by Takiyama et al. (1997) indicated a preferential transmission of mutated alleles. On the other hand, a similar study by Grewal et al. (1999), which used sperm samples from patients of French origin, failed to report the presence of segregation distortion. Using a methodology based on the analysis of pedigrees of patients belonging to Azorean MJD families, Bettencourt et al. (2008a) also investigated the presence of segregation distortion in the transmission of mutated *ATXN3* alleles. According to that study, segregation is done in agreement with the expected Mendelian proportions.

The behavior postulated for the wild-type and the mutated *ATXN3* alleles is not necessarily comparable. Nevertheless, studies with normal individuals have also been conducted, aiming to contribute to the understanding of this issue (Bettencourt et al., 2008b; MacMillan et al., 1999; Rubinsztein & Leggo, 1997). Rubinsztein and Leggo (1997), in a segregation study of MJD alleles in normal heterozygous individuals, reported the presence of segregation distortion only when the transmitting parent was a female, with the smaller allele being preferably transmitted. Results from another study, by Bettencourt et al. (2008b), followed the same trend, with a preference for the transmission of the smaller allele. These last authors also reinforced the importance of the genotypic constitution of the sample being analyzed, which may act as a confounding factor in the detection of segregation distortion.

4. Conclusion

Poly-Q diseases occur as a result of a mutation at the respective causative genes, representing, from that perspective, simple, monogenic diseases. Several aspects of complexity are, nevertheless, present in this group of disorders. Many of the complicating factors present are displayed by MJD and were approached here; the majority of them have implications for patients management and, therefore, its understanding is of major importance.

5. Acknowledgements

C.B. is a postdoctoral fellow of "Fundação para a Ciência e a Tecnologia" - FCT [SFRH/BPD/63121/2009].

6. References

Alves, S.; Nascimento-Ferreira, I.; Auregan, G.; et al. (2008). Allele-specific RNA silencing of mutant ataxin-3 mediates neuroprotection in a rat model of Machado-Joseph disease. *PLoS One*, 3: e3341.

Alves, S.; Nascimento-Ferreira, I.; Dufour, N.; et al. (2010) Silencing ataxin-3 mitigates degeneration in a rat model of Machado-Joseph disease: no role for wild-type ataxin-3? *Human Molecular Genetics*, 19(12): 2380-94.

Badano, J. L. & Katsanis, N. (2002). Beyond Mendel: an evolving view of human genetic disease transmission. *Nature Reviews-Genetics*, 3: 779-789.

Bettencourt, C.; Silva-Fernandes, A.; Montiel, R.; et al. (2007). Triplet Repeats: Features, Dynamics and Evolutionary Mechanisms. *In*: Santos, C. & Lima, M. (Eds.), *Recent Advances in Molecular Biology and Evolution: Applications to Biological Anthropology*, pp. 83-114. Kerala Research Signpost, India.

Bettencourt, C.; Santos, C.; Kay, T.; et al. (2008a). Analysis of Segregation Patterns in Machado-Joseph Disease Pedigrees. *Journal of Human Genetics*, 53(10): 920-923.

Bettencourt, C.; Fialho, R. N.; Santos, C.; et al. (2008b). Segregation distortion of wild-type alleles at the Machado-Joseph disease locus: a study in normal families from the Azores islands (Portugal). *Journal of Human Genetics*, 53: 333-39.

Bettencourt, C.; Santos, C.; Montiel, R.; et al. (2010a). Increased transcript diversity: novel splicing variants of Machado-Joseph Disease gene (ATXN3). *Neurogenetics*, 11(2): 193-202.

Bettencourt, C.; Santos, C.; Montiel, R.; et al. (2010b). The $(CAG)_n$ tract of Machado-Joseph Disease gene (*ATXN3*): a comparison between DNA and mRNA in patients and controls. *European Journal of Human Genetics*, 18(5): 621-3.

Bettencourt, C. & Lima, M. (2011). Machado-Joseph Disease: from first descriptions to new perspectives. *Orphanet Journal of Rare Diseases*, 6(1): 35.

Bettencourt, C.; Raposo, M.; Kazachkova, N.; et al. (2011). The ε2 allele of *APOE* increases the risk of earlier age-at-onset in Machado-Joseph Disease (MJD/SCA3). *Archives of Neurology*. 68(12):1580-3

Cagnoli, C.; Mariotti, C.; Taroni, F.; et al. (2006). SCA28, a novel form of autosomal dominant cerebellar ataxia on chromosome 18p11.22-q11.2. *Brain*, 129: 235-42.

Cancel, G.; Abbas, N.; Stevanin, G.; et al. (1995). Marked phenotypic heterogeneity associated with expansion of a CAG repeat sequence at the spinocerebellar ataxia 3/Machado-Joseph disease locus. *American Journal of Human Genetics*, 57(4): 809-16.

Cancel, G.; Gourfinkel-An, I.; Stevanin, G.; et al. (1998). Somatic mosaicism of the CAG repeat expansion in spinocerebellar ataxia type 3/Machado-Joseph disease. *Human Mutation*, 11(1): 23-7.

Carvalho, D. R.; La Rocque-Ferreira, A.; Rizzo, I. M.; et al. (2008). Homozygosity enhances severity in spinocerebellar ataxia type 3. *Pediatric Neurology*, 38: 296-299.

Chou, A. H.; Yeh, T. H.; Ouyand, P. *et al.* (2008). Polyglutamine-expanded ataxin-3 causes cerebellar dysfunction of SCA3 transgenic mice by inducing transcriptional dysregulation. *Neurobiology of Disease*, 31(1): 89-101.

Coutinho, P. & Andrade, C. (1978). Autosomal dominant system degeneration in Portuguese families of the Azores Islands. A new genetic disorder involving cerebellar, pyramidal, extrapyramidal and spinal cord motor functions. *Neurology*, 28(7): 703-9.

Coutinho, P. (1992). *Doença de Machado-Joseph: Tentativa de definição*, 247pp. Dissertação de Doutoramento, Instituto de Ciências Biomédicas Abel Salazar, Universidade do Porto, Porto.

DeStefano, A. L.; Cupples, L. A.; Maciel, P.; et al. (1996). A familial factor independent of CAG repeat length influences age at onset of Machado-Joseph disease. *American Journal of Human Genetics*, 59(1): 119-27.

Drüsedau, M.; Dreesen, J. C.; De Die-Smulders, C.; et al. (2004). Preimplantation genetic diagnosis of spinocerebellar ataxia 3 by (CAG)(n) repeat detection. *Molecular Human Reproduction*, 10(1): 71-5.

Gaspar, C.; Lopes-Cendes, I.; Hayes, S.; et al. (2001). Ancestral Origins of the Machado-Joseph Disease Mutation: A Worldwide Haplotype Study. *American Journal of Human Genetics*, 68: 523-528.

Gilchrist, D.; Glerum, D. M. & Wevrick, R. (2000). Deconstructing Mendel: new paradigms in genetic mechanisms. *Clinical and Investigative Medicine*, 23(3): 188-98.

Gonzalez, C.; Lima, M.; Kay, T.; et al. (2004). Short-Term impact of predictive testing for the Machado-Joseph disease: Depression and Anxiety levels in individuals at risk from the Azores (Portugal). *Community Genetics*, 7(4): 196-201.

Gould, V. F. C. (2005). Mouse models of Machado-Joseph disease and other polyglutamine spinocerebellar ataxias. *NeuroRx: the journal of the American Society for Experimental NeuroTherapeutics*, 2(3): 480-3.

Grewal, R. P.; Cancel, G.; Leeflang, E. P.; et al. (1999). French Machado-Joseph disease patients do not exhibit gametic segregation distortion: a sperm typing analysis. *Human Molecular Genetics*, 8(9): 1779-84.

Gropman, A. L. & Adams, D. R. (2007). Atypical Patterns of Inheritance. *Seminars in Pediatric Neurology*, 14: 34-45.

Haines, J. L. & Pericak-Vance, M. A. (2006). *Genetic analysis of complex disease*. 485pp. Wiley-Liss, New Jersey, USA.

Hashida, H.; Goto, J.; Kurisaki, H.; et al. (1997). Brain regional differences in the expansion of a CAG repeat in the spinocerebellar ataxias: dentatorubral-pallidoluysian atrophy, Machado-Joseph disease, and spinocerebellar ataxia type 1. *Annals of Neurology*, 41(4): 505-11.

Hu J.; Matsui M.; Gagnon, K.T.; et al. (2009). Allele-specific silencing of mutant huntingtin and ataxin-3 genes by targeting expanded CAG repeats in mRNAs. *Nature Biotechnology*, 27(5):478-84.

Ichikawa, Y.; Goto, J.; Hattori, M.; et al. (2001). The genomic structure and expression of MJD, the Machado-Joseph disease gene. *Journal Human Genetics*, 46: 413-22.

Igarashi, S.; Takiyama, Y.; Cancel, G.; et al. (1996). Intergenerational instability of the CAG repeat of the gene for Machado-Joseph disease (MJD1) is affected by the genotype of the normal chromosome: implications for the molecular mechanisms of the instability of the CAG repeat. *Human Molecular Genetics*, 5(7): 923-32.

Ikeuchi, T.; Igarashi, S.; Takiyama, Y.; et al. (1996). Non-Mendelian transmission in dentatorubral-pallidoluysian atrophy and Machado-Joseph disease: the mutant allele is preferentially transmitted in male meiosis. *American Journal of Human Genetics*, 58(4): 730-3.

Ito, Y.; Tanaka, F.; Yamamoto, M.; et al. (1998). Somatic mosaicism of the expanded CAG trinucleotide repeat in mRNAs for the responsible gene of Machado-Joseph disease

(MJD), dentatorubral pallidoluysian atrophy (DRPLA), and spinal and bulbar muscular atrophy (SBMA). *Neurochemical Research*, 23(1): 25-32.

Jardim, L.; Silveira, I.; Pereira, M. L.; et al. (2003). Searching for modulating effects of SCA2, SCA6 and DRPLA CAG tracts on the Machado-Joseph disease (SCA3) phenotype. *Acta Neurologica Scandinavica*, 107(3): 211-4.

Kawaguchi, Y.; Okamoto, T.; Taniwaki, M.; et al. (1994). CAG expansions in a novel gene for Machado-Joseph disease at chromosome 14q32.1. *Nature Genetics*, 8: 221-228.

Katsuno, M.; Banno, H.; Suzuki, K.; et al. (2008). Molecular genetics and biomarkers of polyglutamine diseases. *Current Molecular Medicine*, 8(3): 221-34.

Kieling, C.; Prestes, P. R.; Saraiva-Pereira, M. L.; et al. (2007). Survival estimates for patients with Machado-Joseph disease (SCA3). *Clinical Genetics*, 72(6): 543-5.

Lerer, I.; Merims, D.; Abeliovich, D.; et al. (1996). Machado-Joseph disease: correlation between the clinical features, the CAG repeat length and homozygosity for the mutation. *European Journal of Human Genetics*, 4(1): 3-7.

Lima, M.; Mayer, F. M.; Coutinho, P.; et al. (1997). Prevalence, geographical distribution and genealogical investigation of Machado-Joseph disease in the islands of the Azores (Portugal). *Human Biology*, 69(3): 383-391.

Lima, M.; Mayer, F. M.; Coutinho, P.; et al. (1998). Origins of a mutation: Population Genetics of Machado-Joseph disease in the Azores (Portugal). *Human Biology*, 70(6): 1011-1023.

Lima, M.; Kay, T.; Vasconcelos, J.; et al. (2001). Disease knowledge and attitudes toward Predictive Testing and Prenatal Diagnosis in families with Machado-Joseph disease from the Azores Islands (Portugal). *Community Genetics*, 4(1): 36-42.

Lima, M.; Costa, M. C.; Montiel, R.; et al. (2005). Population genetics of wild-type CAG repeats in the Machado-Joseph disease gene in Portugal. *Human Heredity*, 60(3): 156-63.

Lima, M.; Santos, C.; Bettencourt, C.; et al. (2006). Genetic testing for late-onset disorders: the experience of Machado-Joseph disease in the Azores Islands. *In*: KLAUSEN P. R. (Ed.), *Trends in Birth Defects Research*, pp 83-94. Nova Science Publishers, Inc., New York.

Lopes-Cendes, I.; Silveira, I.; Maciel, P.; et al. (1996). Limits of clinical assessment in the accurate diagnosis of Machado-Joseph disease. *Archives of Neurology*, 53(11): 1168-74.

Maciel, P.; Gaspar, C.; DeStefano, A. L.; et al. (1995). Correlation between CAG repeat length and clinical features in Machado-Joseph disease. *American Journal of Human Genetics*, 57(1): 54-61.

Maciel, P.; Lopes-Cendes, I.; Kish, S.; et al. (1997). Mosaicism of the CAG repeat in CNS tissue in relation to age at death in spinocerebellar ataxia type 1 and Machado-Joseph disease patients. *American Journal of Human Genetics*, 60(4): 993-6.

Maciel, P.; Gaspar, C.; Guimarães, L.; et al. (1999). Study of three intragenic polymorphisms in the Machado-Joseph disease gene (MJD1) in relation to genetic instability of the (CAG)n tract. *European Journal of Human Genetics*, 7(2): 147-56.

Maciel, P.; Costa, M. C.; Ferro, A.; et al. (2001). Improvement in the molecular diagnosis of Machado-Joseph disease. *Archives of Neurology*, 58: 1821-7.

MacMillan, J.C.; Voisey, J.; Healey, S. C.; et al. (1999). Mendelian segregation of normal CAG trinucleotide repeat alleles at three autosomal loci. *Journal of Medical Genetics*, 36(3): 258-9.

Martins, S.; Calafell, F.; Wong, V. C.; et al. (2006). A multistep mutation mechanism drives the evolution of the CAG repeat at MJD/SCA3 locus. *European Journal of Human Genetics*, 14(8): 932-40.

Martins, S.; Calafell, F.; Gaspar, C.; et al. (2007). Asian origin for the worldwide-spread mutational event in Machado-Joseph disease. *Archives of Neurology*, 64(10): 1502-8.

Martins, S.; Coutinho, P.; Silveira, I.; et al. (2008). Cis-acting factors promoting the CAG intergenerational instability in Machado-Joseph disease. *American Journal of Medical Genetics, B Neuropsychiatric Genetics*, 147B(4): 439-46.

Maruyama, H.; Nakamura, S.; Matsuyama, Z.; et al. (1995). Molecular features of the CAG repeats and clinical manifestation of Machado-Joseph disease. *Human Molecular Genetics*, 4: 807-12.

Nakano, K. K.; Dawson, D. M. & Spence, A. (1972). Machado disease. A hereditary ataxia in Portuguese emigrants to Massachusetts. *Neurology*, 22(1): 49-55.

Padiath, Q. S.; Srivastava, A. K.; Roy, S.; et al. (2005). Identification of a novel 45 repeat unstable allele associated with a disease phenotype at the MJD1/SCA3 locus. *American Journal of Medical Genetics- B Neuropsychiatric Genetics*, 133B (1): 124-6.

Paulson, H. L.; Das, S. S.; Crino, P. B.; et al. (1997). Machado-Joseph disease gene product is a cytoplasmic protein widely expressed in brain. *Annals of Neurology*, 41(4): 453-62.

Paulson, H. L. (2007). Dominantly inherited ataxias: lessons learned from Machado-Joseph disease/spinocerebellar ataxia type 3. *Seminars in Neurology*, 27(2): 133-42.

Romanul, F. C.; Fowler, H. L.; Radvany, J.; et al. (1977). Azorean disease of the nervous system. *New England Journal of Medicine*, 296(26): 1505-8.

Rosenberg, R. N.; Nyhan, W. L.; Bay, C.; et al. (1976). Autosomal dominant striatonigral degeneration. A clinical, pathologic, and biochemical study of a new genetic disorder. *Neurology*, 26(8): 703-14.

Rubinsztein, D. C.; Amos, W; Leggo J.; et al. (1994). Mutational bias provides a model for the evolution of Huntington's disease and predicts a general increase in disease prevalence. *Nature Genetics*, 7(4): 525-30.

Rubinsztein, D. C. & Leggo, J. (1997). Non-Mendelian transmission at the Machado-Joseph disease locus in normal females: preferential transmission of alleles with smaller CAG repeats. *Journal of Medical Genetics*, 34(3): 234-6.

Sakai T.; Kawakami, H. (1996). Machado-Joseph disease: A proposal of spastic paraplegic subtype. *Neurology*, 46(3): 846-7.

Schmitt, I.; Linden, M.; Khazneh, H.; et al. (2007). Inactivation of the mouse Atxn3 (Ataxin-3) gene increases protein ubiquitination. *Biochemichal and Biophysical Research Communications*, 362(3): 734-739.

Schöls, L.; Bauer, P.; Schmidt, T.; et al. (2004). Autosomal dominant cerebellar ataxias: clinical features, genetics, and pathogenesis. *Lancet Neurology*, 3(5): 291-304.

Sequeiros, J. (1996). Genética Clássica e Genética Molecular na Doença de Machado-Joseph. *In*: Sequeiros, J. (Ed.), *O teste preditivo da doença de Machado-Joseph*, pp. 33-48. UnIGENe, Porto.

Sequeiros, J.; Maciel, P.; Taborda, F.; et al. (1998). Prenatal diagnosis of Machado-Joseph disease by direct mutation analysis. *Prenatal Diagnosis*, 18(6): 611-7.

Sequeiros J.; Seneca S.; Martindale J. (2010). Consensus and controversies in best practices for molecular genetic testing of spinocerebellar ataxias. *European Journal of Human Genetics*, 18(11): 1188-95.

Sherman, S. L. (1997). Evolving Methods in Genetic Epidemiology. IV. Approaches to Non-Mendelian Inheritance. *Epidemiologic Reviews*, 19(1): 44-51.

Suite, N. D; Sequeiros, J. & McKhann, G. M. (1986). Machado-Joseph disease in a Sicilian-American family. *Journal of Neurogenetics*, 3(3): 177-82.

Takiyama, Y.; Nishizawa, M.; Tanaka, H.; et al. (1993). The gene for Machado-Joseph disease maps to human chromosome 14q. *Nature Genetics*, 4(3): 300-4.

Takiyama, Y.; Igarashi, S.; Rogaeva, E. A.; et al. (1995). Evidence for inter-generational instability in the CAG repeat in the MJD1 gene and for conserved haplotypes at flanking markers amongst Japanese and Caucasian subjects with Machado-Joseph disease. *Human Molecular Genetics*, 4(7): 1137-46.

Takiyama Y.; Sakoe, K.; Amaike, M.; et al. (1997). Single sperm analysis of the CAG repeats in the gene for Machado-Joseph disease (*MJD1*): evidence for non-Mendelian transmission of the MJD1 gene and for the effect of the intragenic CGG/GGG polymorphism on the intergenerational instability. *Human Molecular Genetics*, 6(7): 1063-8.

Takiyama, Y.; Shimazaki, H.; Morita, M.; et al. (1998). Maternal anticipation in Machado-Joseph disease (MJD): some maternal factors independent of the number of CAG repeat units may play a role in genetic anticipation in a Japanese MJD family. *Journal of Neurological Sciences*, 155(2): 141-5.

Takiyama, Y.; Sakoe, K.; Amaike, M.; et al. (1999). Single sperm analysis of the CAG repeats in the gene for dentatorubral-pallidoluysian atrophy (DRPLA): the instability of the CAG repeats in the DRPLA gene is prominent among the CAG repeat diseases. *Human Molecular Genetics*, 8(3): 453-7.

Tanaka, F.; Ito, Y. & Sobue, G. (1999). Somatic mosaicism of expanded CAG trinucleotide repeat in the neural and nonneural tissues of Machado-Joseph disease (MJD). *Nippon Rinsho*, 57(4): 838-42.

Tsuji, S. (1997). Molecular Genetics of Triplet Repeats: Unstable expansion of triplet repeats as a new mechanism for neurodegenerative diseases. *Internal Medicine*, 36:1: 3-8.

Vale, J.; Bugalho, P.; Silveira, I.; et al. (2009). Autosomal dominant cerebellar ataxia: frequency analysis and clinical characterization of 45 families from Portugal. *European Journal of Neurology*, 17(1):124-8.

Van Alfen, N.; Sinke, R. J.; Zwarts, M. J.; et al. (2001). Intermediate CAG repeat lengths (53, 54) for MJD/SCA3 are associated with an abnormal phenotype. *Annals of Neurology*, 49(6): 805-7.

Van Heyningen, V. & Yeyati, P. L. (2004). Mechanisms of non-Mendelian inheritance in genetic disease. *Human Molecular Genetics*, 13(2): R225-R233.

Van de Warrenburg, B. P.; Hendriks, H.; Dürr, A.; et al. (2005). Age at onset variance analysis in spinocerebellar ataxias: a study in a Dutch-French cohort. *Annals of Neurology*, 7(4): 505-12.

Woods, B. T. & Schaumburg, H. H. (1972). Nigro-spino-dentatal degeneration with nuclear ophthalmoplegia. A unique and partially treatable clinico-pathological entity. *Journal of Neurological Sciences*, 17(2): 149-66.

3

Spinocerebellar Ataxia with Axonal Neuropathy (SCAN1): A Disorder of Nuclear and Mitochondrial DNA Repair

Hok Khim Fam, Miraj K. Chowdhury and Cornelius F. Boerkoel
University of British Columbia
Canada

1. Introduction

Spinocerebellar ataxias (SCAs) are a group of progressive and irreversible neurological diseases affecting gait and movement coordination. Many result from cerebellar degeneration or the impairment of a portion of the neuroaxis that contributes to cerebellar inflow or outflow (Embirucu et al., 2009). In the cerebellum, the dysfunction and death of Purkinje cells, granule cells or interneurons can cause SCA. Molecular mechanisms for this pathology include polyglutamine tract expansion (SCA1, SCA2, SCA3), flawed basal transcription (SCA17) and defective DNA repair (ataxia telangiectasia, spinocerebellar ataxia with axonal neuropathy (SCAN1) and ataxia with oculomotor apraxia type 1) (Hire et al., 2010).

The mechanism by which defective DNA repair causes neuronal dysfunction and death is not yet fully understood, but damage to the nuclear and mitochondrial genomes underlie each potential explanation. Dysfunction of nuclear DNA repair enzymes results in nuclear DNA damage that impedes transcription and also induces programmed neuronal death (Fishel et al., 2007). Dysfunction of mitochondrial DNA repair enzymes leads to mitochondrial DNA damage that impairs mitochondrial gene expression causing mitochondrial dysfunction, oxidative stress and subsequently programmed neuronal death (Bender et al., 2006). Accumulation of DNA breaks within the neuronal nuclear genome has also been proposed to initiate expression of cell-cycle activators as a cellular response to repair genomic damage through replication-dependent mechanisms; however, these neurons are frequently unable to establish a new G0 quiescent state and this in turn activates neuronal death mechanisms (Kruman et al., 2004). Lastly, besides direct affects on the neurons, defective DNA repair also indirectly induces neuronal death by causing dysfunction of glia, which have trophic interactions with neurons and modulate neurotransmitter levels at synapses (Barzilai, 2011; Lobsiger and Cleveland, 2007).

For the purposes of this review, we focus on SCAN1, an autosomal recessive DNA repair disorder caused by the p.His493Arg active site mutation in tyrosyl-DNA phosphodiesterase 1 (Tdp1), an enzyme that enables DNA repair by processing blocked 3′ DNA termini. This mutation impairs this activity and also predisposes to the formation of Tdp1-DNA adducts.

Since the loss of Tdp1 activity predisposes to both nuclear and mitochondrial DNA damage, this review focuses on understanding SCAN1 etiology from the perspectives of DNA repair and mitochondrial dynamics.

2. Spinocerebellar ataxia with axonal neuropathy (SCAN1)

The only reported SCAN1 patients are from an extended Saudi Arabian family having nine affected individuals (Takashima et al., 2002). SCAN1 is characterized by normal intelligence and a late-childhood onset progressive cerebellar ataxia and peripheral neuropathy. Initial features include ataxic gait, gaze nystagmus and cerebellar dysarthria. As the disease advances, the affected individuals develop impaired pain, vibration and touch sensation in the hands and legs and eventually a steppage gait and pes cavus. With further progression of their cerebellar, motor and sensory symptoms, affected individuals become wheelchair-dependent in early adulthood (Hirano et al., 1993). Magnetic resonance imaging studies show cerebellar atrophy, especially of the vermis (Takashima et al., 2002). Nerve conduction studies show decreased amplitudes characteristic of axonal neuropathy. These clinical findings suggest a disease of large, terminally differentiated, post-mitotic neurons, especially those of the cerebellum, dentate nuclei, anterior spinal horn and dorsal root ganglia.

Currently, there are only symptomatic treatments for SCAN1. Physical therapy is recommended for maintaining activity. Prostheses, walking aids and wheelchairs are recommended for improving mobility. In addition, based on studies of cells from SCAN1 patients and animal models, SCAN1 patients should avoid exposure to genotoxic agents such as camptothecin, irinotecan, topotecan, bleomycin and radiation (Hirano et al., 2007).

Clinically, SCAN1 can be considered in the differential diagnosis for individuals who have 1) a slowly progressive cerebellar ataxia with onset in late-childhood or adolescence, 2) peripheral axonal neuropathy, 3) no signs of oculomotor apraxia and 4) no evidence of extraneurologic features such as telangiectasias, cancers or immunodeficiency. Supportive findings include increased serum cholesterol and decreased serum albumin (Takashima et al., 2002). The only known genetic defect causing SCAN1 is the c.1478A>G mutation in *TDP1*. This missense mutation, which encodes the p.His493Arg amino acid alteration, can be detected by DNA sequencing or by digestion of the PCR product with *Bsa*AI (Hirano et al., 2007; Takashima et al., 2002).

3. DNA repair mechanisms and progressive neurodegeneration

As exemplified by SCAN1, many DNA repair defects cause progressive neurodegenerative disease (Table 1) (Barekati et al., 2010; Sahin and Depinho, 2010). Neurons are particularly vulnerable to the accumulation of unrepaired DNA lesions because they are long-lived, post-mitotic and not readily replaced.

DNA lesions arise as a consequence of endogenous or exogenous genotoxic insults. However, the seclusion of central neurons, which are frequently more severely affected than peripheral neurons, by the blood-brain barrier suggests that the DNA lesions arise predominantly from endogenous genotoxic insults, particularly the oxidative damage arising from mitochondrial dysfunction (Harman, 1972, 1981)

Repair of DNA lesions is mediated by four major DNA repair pathways: double-strand break repair (DSBR), mismatch repair (MMR), nucleotide excision repair (NER), and base excision repair (BER). DSBR corrects double-strand breaks (DSB) in the DNA backbone; MMR corrects mismatches of normal bases; NER repairs bulky helix distorting DNA lesions, and BER repairs damage to a single nucleotide and handles single-strand DNA breaks (SSB). Dysfunction of each of these DNA repair processes causes or has been associated with progressive neurodegenerative disease (Table 1) (Jeppesen et al., 2011).

Gene(s)	DNA Repair Defect	Clinical Syndrome	Main Symptoms
SETX	Defective DSBR	Ataxia with oculomotor apraxia type 2	Cerebellar atrophy Axonal sensorimotor neuropathy Oculomotor apraxia Elevated serum concentration of alpha-fetoprotein
ATM	Defective DSBR	Ataxia telangiectasia	Progressive ataxia Defective muscle coordination Dilation of blood vessels in skin and eyes Immune deficiency Predisposition to cancer
MRE11	Defective DSBR	Ataxia telangiectasia-like	Slowly progressive cerebellar ataxia Ionizing radiation hypersensitivity
XPA, XPF, XPG, POLH, ERCC1-4, DDB2	Defective NER	Xeroderma pigmentosum	Sensitivity to sunlight Slow neurodegeneration Skin cancer
ERCC6, ERCC8	Defective NER and TC-NER	Cockayne's Syndrome	Sensitivity to sunlight Growth retardation Neurological impairment Progeria
ERCC2, ERCC3, GTF2H5	Defective NER	Trichothiodystrophy	Sensitivity to sunlight Dystrophy Short brittle hair with low sulfur content, Neurological and psychomotoric defects
TDP1	Defective BER	Spinocerebellar ataxia with axonal neuropathy 1	Progressive degeneration of post-mitotic neurons
APTX	Defective BER	Ataxia with oculomotor apraxia type 1	Slowly progressive cerebellar ataxia, followed by oculomotor apraxia Severe primary motor peripheral axonal motor neuropathy
ALS2, SETX, SOD1, VAPB	Defective BER	Amyotrophic lateral sclerosis	Progressive degeneration of motor neurons Muscle weakness and atrophy
C10orf2	Defective mitochondrial DNA repair	Infantile-onset spinocerebellar ataxia	Muscle hypotonia Loss of deep-tendon reflexes Athetosis

Table 1. DNA repair enzymes with mutations causing neurodegenerative disease. NER: Nucleotide excision repair, TC-NER: Transcription-coupled nucleotide excision repair, MMR: Mismatch repair, BER: Base excision repair, DSBR: Double-strand break repair, (Embirucu et al., 2009; Katyal and McKinnon, 2007; Subba Rao, 2007)

3.1 Double-strand break repair

DSBR corrects DNA double-strand breaks (DSBs) induced by exogenous sources such as ionizing radiation and genotoxic compounds or by endogenous sources such as reactive oxygen species, replication fork collapse, and errors of meiotic recombination (Ciccia and Elledge, 2010). The two major DSBR pathways in mammalian cells are homologous recombination (HR) and non-homologous end-joining (NHEJ). HR allows high fidelity repair of DSBs during DNA replication by using the intact sister chromatid as a template, whereas NHEJ allows for the error-prone repair of DSBs by modifying and ligating the two DNA termini of a DSB without using an undamaged template. HR is restricted to the late S to G2/M phase of the cell cycle when a sister chromatid is available in proliferating cells, whereas NHEJ operates throughout the cell cycle and can repair DSBs in differentiated cells. Therefore, since the mature nervous system is predominately post-mitotic cells, NHEJ is the major DSBR pathway in the postnatal brain.

Two NHEJ disorders with progressive neurodegeneration of the postnatal brain are ataxia telangiectasia and ataxia telangiectasia-like disorder. The neurological symptoms of ataxia telangiectasia are an early childhood onset of ataxia that generally leads to wheel chair dependence before adolescence. The neurological symptoms of ataxia telangiectasia-like disorder are similar to those of ataxia telangiectasia but of later onset and slower progression. For both disorders, the neurodegeneration is characterized by the loss of cerebellar granule and Purkinje cells.

3.2 Mismatch repair

MMR removes base-base mismatches and insertion-deletion loops that arise during DNA replication and recombination. Base-base mismatches are created when errors escape DNA polymerase proofreading, and insertion-deletion loops arise when the primer and template strand in a microsatellite or repetitive sequence dissociate and re-anneal incorrectly causing the number of microsatellite-repeat units in the template and in the newly synthesized strand to differ. Interestingly, expression of MMR components is not limited to replicating cells but is also observed in non-replicating postnatal neurons suggesting that this pathway plays a role in maintaining the genomic integrity of differentiated cells too (Ciccia and Elledge, 2010).

Consistent with a function in differentiated cells, studies of the Huntington trinucleotide repeat (CAG) in mice have shown somatic age-dependent repeat expansion that is suppressed by deficiency of some MMR components and is triggered by DNA glycosylases of the BER pathway (Kovtun et al., 2007; Owen et al., 2005). The relevance of the MMR pathway to trinucleotide repeat expansions of the human neurological disorders remains undefined however.

3.3 Nucleotide excision repair

In human cells, recognition of bulky helix distorting DNA lesions leads to the removal of a short single-stranded DNA segment surrounding and including the lesion. This creates a single-strand gap in the DNA that is subsequently filled during repair synthesis by a DNA polymerase using the undamaged strand as a template. NER can be divided into two sub-pathways, global genomic NER (GG-NER) and transcription-coupled NER (TC-NER). GG-NER and TC-NER differ in the recognition of the DNA lesion but subsequently use the same excision mechanism. GG-NER recognizes and repairs DNA lesions anywhere in the genome, whereas TC-NER only resolves lesions in the actively transcribed DNA strand (de Laat et al., 1999).

Two NER-associated disorders, xeroderma pigmentosum and Cockayne syndrome, feature progressive neurodegeneration (Kraemer et al., 1987). About 30% of xeroderma pigmentosum patients have neurological symptoms that include abnormal motor control, ataxia, peripheral neuropathy, dementia, brain and spinal cord atrophy, microcephaly and sensorineural deafness. In contrast, nearly all Cockayne syndrome patients have progressive neurological disease characterized by demyelination in the cerebral and cerebellar cortex, calcification in the basal ganglia and cerebral cortex, neuronal loss, sensorineural hearing loss and decreased nerve conduction (Nance and Berry, 1992). The progressive neurodegeneration in both xeroderma pigmentosum and Cockayne syndrome are attributable to apoptotic cell death (Lehmann, 2003).

3.4 Base excision repair

BER corrects the most common forms of DNA damage by recognizing, excising and replacing a broad spectrum of specific forms of DNA modifications including those arising from deamination, oxidation and alkylation. It is initiated by a distinct lesion-specific mono- or bi-functional DNA glycosylase and completed by either of two sub-pathways: short-patch BER (SP-BER) that replaces one nucleotide or long-patch BER (LP-BER) that replaces 2–13 nucleotides (Frosina et al., 1996).

The BER proteins are also responsible for repairing DNA SSBs. SSBs are some of the most common lesions found in chromosomal DNA and arise via enzymatic cleavage of the phosphodiester backbone or from oxidative damage or ionizing radiation. Examples of enzymatic cleavage causing SSBs include those arising during BER (Connelly and Leach, 2004) and during DNA topoisomerase I (Topo I) activity (Pommier et al., 2003).

Ataxia with oculomotor apraxia type 1 and SCAN1 are both associated with defects in the repair of SSBs, specifically the processing of obstructive termini (Table 1). The neurodegenerative features of ataxia with oculomotor apraxia type 1 include progressive cerebellar atrophy, late axonal peripheral motor neuropathy, ataxia and oculomotor apraxia. The features of SCAN1, which is caused by a mutation of *TDP1*, have been described above.

4. Tdp1 function

TDP1 encodes tyrosyl-DNA phosphodiesterase 1 (Tdp1), a 608 amino acid enzyme that contains a bipartite nuclear localization sequence and two conserved HxKx4Dx6G (G/S) HKD (histidine-lysine-arginine) signature motifs. The two HKD motifs form a single symmetrical active site characteristic of the phospholipase D superfamily and catalyze a phosphoryl transfer that is common to enzymes in this superfamily (Interthal et al., 2001). The HKD motifs are very important for the catalytic function of Tdp1. Tdp1 enables SSBR and DSBR by removing obstructing compounds linked by a phosphodiester bond to DNA 3′ termini and complements the 5′-phosphodiesterase function of TTRAP (Tdp2) (Cortes Ledesma et al., 2009; el-Khamisy and Caldecott, 2007; Zhou et al., 2009). Tdp1 endogenous substrates include 3′ tyrosine-DNA phosphodiester moieties, phosphoglycolates, mononulceosides and tetrahydrofurans, and exogenous substrates include 4-methylphenol, 4-nitrophenol and 4-methylumbelliferone (Figure 1) (Dexheimer et al., 2008; Interthal et al., 2005a). Tdp1 has the highest affinity for the 3′ tyrosine-DNA phosphodiester moieties, which are characteristic of Topo I-DNA intermediates (Dexheimer et al., 2010).

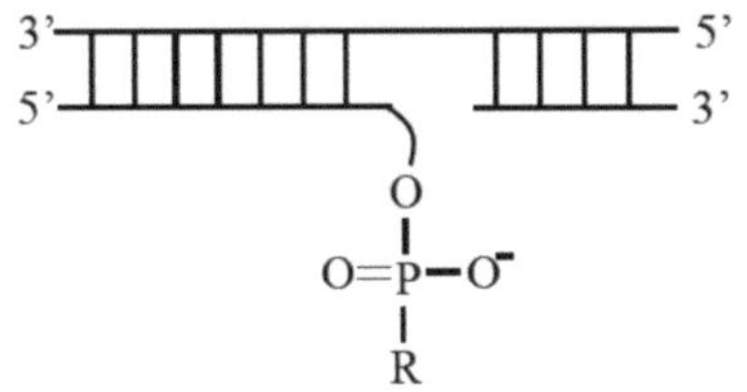

Physiologic R
Proteolysed Topo I, Tyrosine, Glycolate, Tdp1, Tetrahydrofuran and Mononucleoside
Non-physiologic R
4-methylphenol, 4-nitrophenol and 4-methylumbelliferone

Fig. 1. Substrates of Tdp1. Tdp1 can remove both physiologic substrates and non-physiologic substrates. R = Substrates.

During repair, replication, transcription, recombination and chromatin remodeling, Topo I relaxes superhelical tension by nicking DNA to allow controlled rotation of the broken DNA strand around the intact strand. After DNA relaxation has occurred, a nucleophilic attack by the DNA 5′ hydroxyl group on the phosphotyrosyl linkage between Topo I and the 3′ end of the DNA at the nick usually religates the DNA, and the Topo I dissociates. However, DNA damage such as abasic sites, nicks, and mismatched base pairs frequently impede removal of Topo I from the DNA by causing a misalignment of the 5′ hydroxyl end of the DNA that prevents it from acting as a nucleophile. (Pommier et al., 1998; Pommier et al., 2003; Pourquier and Pommier, 2001) Additionally, the 3′-Topo I-DNA intermediate can become unduly long-lived if Topo I binds oxidative base lesions (Interthal et al., 2005b). These trapped or long-lived Topo I-DNA covalent intermediates can then be converted to irreversible DNA breaks when the DNA replication machinery or RNA polymerase collides with the Topo I-DNA complex (Hsiang et al., 1989; Tsao et al., 1993; Wu and Liu, 1997)

Clearance of the trapped or stalled 3′-Topo I-DNA intermediates occurs via SSBR or DSBR if the SSB is converted to a DSB by collision of the DNA replication machinery with the trapped or stalled 3′-Topo I-DNA intermediate. Following recognition of the break, the trapped or stalled Topo I is proteolytically cleaved leaving a peptide bound to the 3′ end of the DNA by the phosphodiester bond formed between the DNA and the Topo I active site tyrosine (Tyr723). Tdp1 then acts on the phosphodiester bond and removes the obstructing Topo I peptide from the 3′ terminus (Debethune et al., 2002; Liu et al., 2002). The Tdp1 reaction removes the peptide from the DNA by an S_N2 nucleophilic attack of His263, which resides in the first HKD motif, on the phosphodiester bond; Tdp1 is then released from the DNA by the catalytic activity of His493, which resides in the second HKD motif (Figure 2).

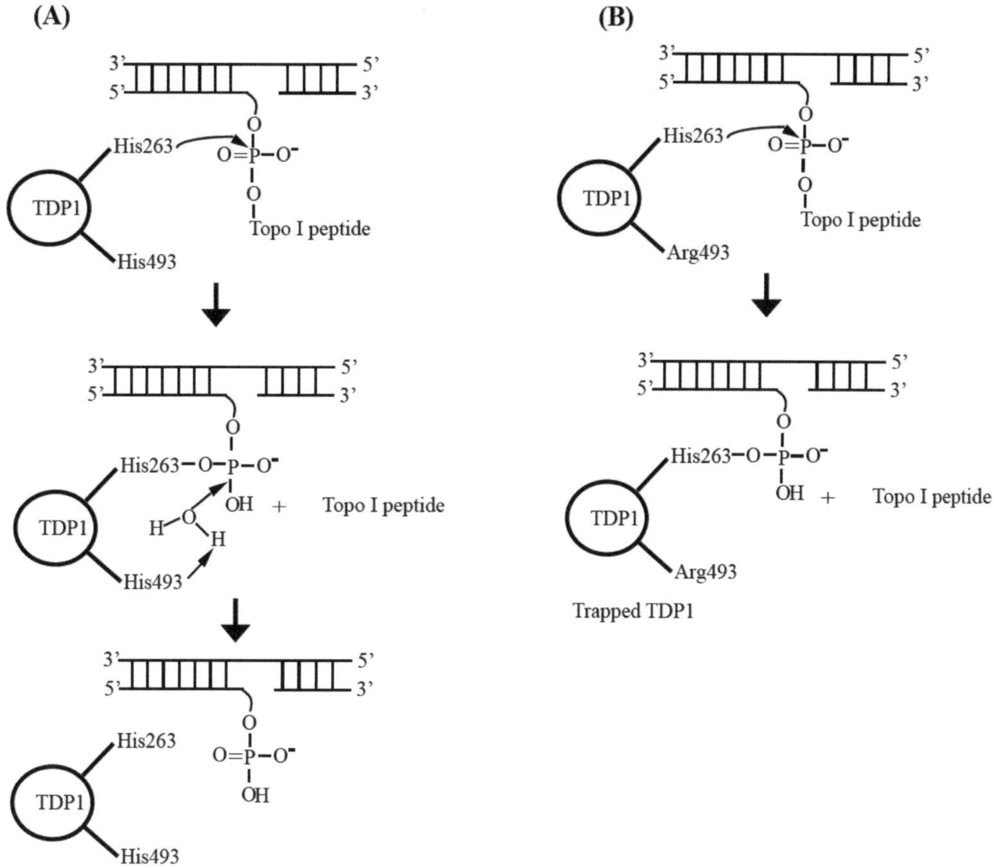

Fig. 2. Mechanism of Tdp1 catalytic activity. (A) Wild type Tdp1 removes proteolysed Topo I and forms a covalent intermediate with DNA before His493 of the second HKD motif excises Tdp1 from DNA through a nucleophilic substitution. (B) In SCAN1, the mutated Tdp1 (p.His493Arg) removes proteolysed Topo I but remains trapped on DNA and leads to accumulation of Tdp1-DNA adducts.

4.1 Tdp1 and nuclear DNA repair

Within the nucleus, Tdp1 is a component of the SSB multi-protein repair complex containing PARP1, LIG3α, XRCC1 and PNKP (Das et al., 2009). This repair complex is activated after proteasomal degradation of stalled Topo I (Zhang et al., 2004). PARP1 is an important regulator of the SSBR/BER pathway as it enhances the recruitment of DNA repair proteins. PARP1 hydrolyzes NAD^+ to catalyze the synthesis of ADP-ribose units onto glutamate

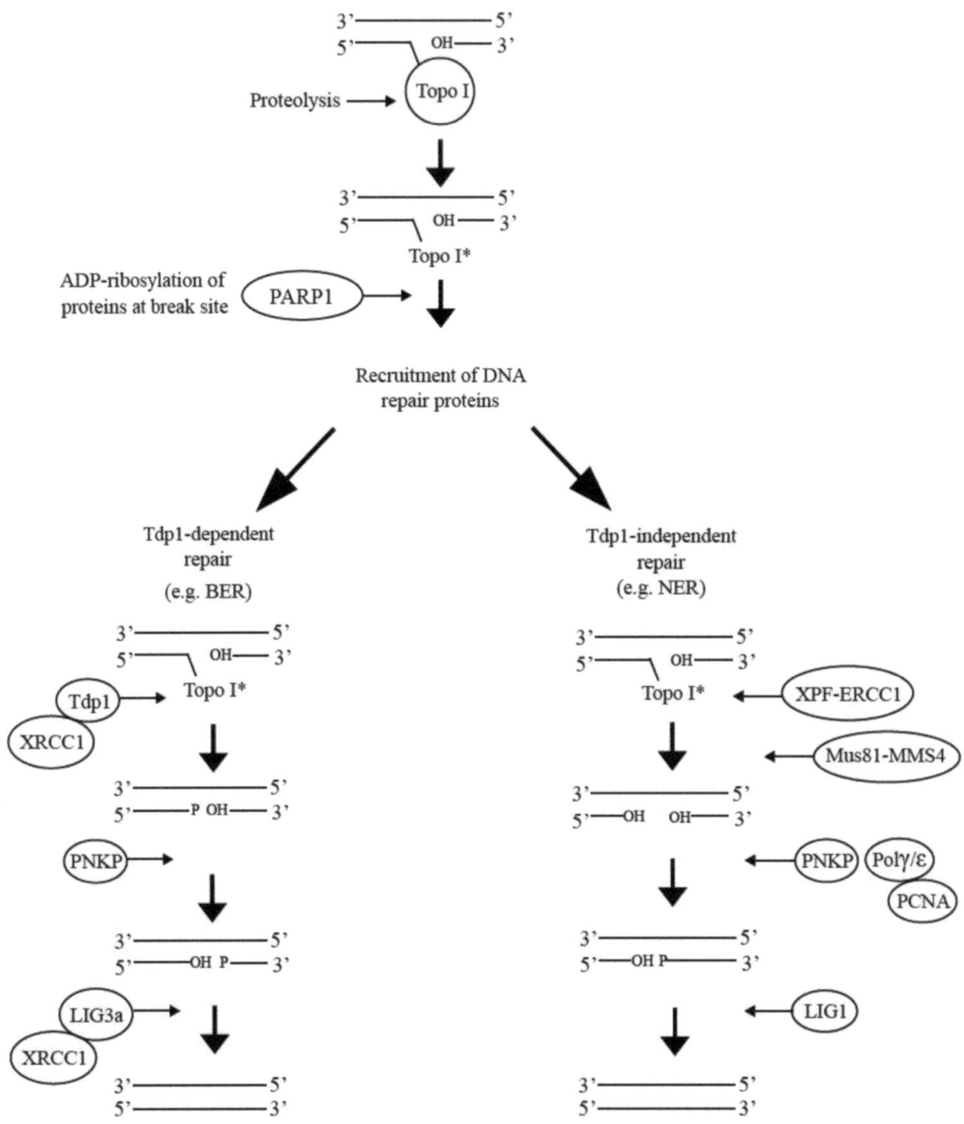

Fig. 3. Tdp1-dependent and Tdp1-independent pathways for the removal of Topo I-DNA covalent complexes. After Topo I is trapped on the DNA, proteolysis of Topo I occurs. The remaining Topo I peptide can be removed by either Tdp1-dependent pathway or Tdp1-independent pathways. Topo I* = Topo I peptide.

molecules of acceptor proteins. The addition of poly-ADP ribosyl (PAR) polymers onto histones promotes the relaxation of chromatin, while SSBR proteins such as XRCC1 and Lig3a are electrostatically attracted to PAR and are thus recruited to the site of DNA damage (El-Khamisy et al., 2003; Krishnakumar and Kraus, 2010). It is thought that XRCC1 acts as a molecular scaffold for the binding of Tdp1 and Lig3a and stabilizes the enzyme complex in the processing of Topo I derived SSBs. Processing of the 3′ tyrosine-DNA phosphodiester moieties by Tdp1 leaves a 3′-P terminus that is converted to 3′-OH by the phosphatase action of PNKP. The kinase activity of PNKP phosphorylates the 5′-OH terminus, allowing gap filling by DNA polymerase β (Polß), and finally the DNA nick is sealed by lig3a with the aid of the XRCC1 scaffold (Figure 3).

How Tdp1 processes obstructing 3′ overhangs on DNA DSBs has not been fully defined. The dependence of Tdp1 processing of DSB termini on the autophosphorylation activity of the NHEJ component DNA-PK suggests that Tdp1 contributes within the NHEJ pathway and that DNA-PK modulates the accessibility of DNA ends enabling Tdp1 to accomplish the processing necessary for eventual end-joining (Zhou et al., 2009).

One redundant DNA repair activity for Tdp1 is the nucleolytic removal of several DNA bases beginning upstream of the stalled Topo I. This is mediated by 3'-flap endonuclease complexes in the nucleus such as Mus81-MMS4 and XPF-ERCC1 that cleave at the 3'-flap created by stalled Topo I to enable short-patch gap filling. In comparison to Tdp1 processing, however, this mechanism is error-prone and less efficient.

4.2 Tdp1 and mitochondrial DNA repair

Besides its role in the repair of nuclear DNA, Tdp1 also plays a role in mitochondrial DNA (mtDNA) repair (Das et al., 2010). Mitochondria are membrane-enclosed organelles that generate most of the ATP via the electron transport chain at the inner mitochondrial membrane. This process leads to the generation of reactive oxygen species, and while mitochondria have various antioxidant enzymes to deactivate these highly reactive molecules, they do not constitute a perfect defense. This inevitably exposes the mtDNA to high levels of oxidative stress, particularly since the mtDNA is located in close proximity to the inner mitochondrial membrane and lacks protective histones (Ames et al., 1993). Consequently, the levels of oxidative base damage in mitochondrial DNA are 2–3 fold higher compared to nuclear DNA (Hudson et al., 1998), and the damage is more extensive and persistent than in nuclear DNA (Yakes and Van Houten, 1997).

Several DNA repair activities and pathways that function in the nucleus have also been identified and characterized in mammalian mitochondria. These include BER, MMR, and some components of DSBR (Larsen et al., 2005). Given the prevalence of small lesions generated by oxidative stress in the mitochondria, BER is the predominant mtDNA repair pathway. Mitochondrial BER proteins are not encoded by the mitochondrial genome; rather they are mitochondrial versions of nuclear-encoded proteins (Larsen et al., 2005). Among these is Tdp1, which could participate in the repair of oxidative mitochondrial DNA damage via resolution of 3′-phosphoglycolate obstructive termini and processing the apurinic/apyrimidinic (AP) sites arising from the DNA glycosylase removal of DNA lesions such as 7,8-dihydro-8-oxoguanine (8-oxoG). These two abilities of Tdp1 are also shared by APE1, although the relative contribution of each protein to either process is unclear.

Additionally, as there is a mitochondrial Topo I (mtTopo I) that has 71% identity and 87% similarity with the nuclear Topo I (Zhang et al., 2001), we hypothesize that the high level of mtDNA lesions predisposes to generation of long lived or trapped mtTopo I-DNA complexes similar to those in the nucleus and that the removal of mtTopo I peptides from mtDNA is also a function of mitochondrial Tdp1.

5. The molecular basis of SCAN1

In SCAN1, the p.His493Arg mutation in the second HKD motif of Tdp1 affects the active site of the protein and reduces its catalytic activity by 25-fold (Interthal et al., 2005b; Takashima et al., 2002). This alteration both decreases the processing of Topo I-DNA adducts and impairs the intermolecular reaction that would ordinarily release Tdp1. These Tdp1-DNA adducts can only be removed by wild-type Tdp1 (Figure 2) (Interthal et al., 2005b). This finding suggests that SCAN1 might arise, at least in part, from accumulation of the Tdp1-DNA adducts and the inability of the cell to remove $Tdp1^{H493R}$ in a timely manner (Dexheimer et al., 2008; Hirano et al., 2007).

Currently, the molecular basis of SCAN1 and the reason that mice deficient for Tdp1 do not develop ataxia are incompletely understood. Although there are no prominent tissue differences in gene expression nor evidence of positive selection of the Tdp1 protein (as reported in the Selectome database) between human and mouse (Proux et al., 2009), two observations suggest possible explanations for SCAN1 pathogenesis and the lack of ataxia in Tdp1-deficient mice. First, human Tdp1 is predominantly expressed in the cytoplasm of the neurons predicted to be affected in SCAN1, whereas mouse Tdp1 is predominantly expressed in the nucleus of the analogous neurons. Second, *in vitro* and cell culture experiments show that the p.His493Arg Tdp1 forms long lived Tdp1-DNA adducts (Hirano et al., 2007; Interthal et al., 2005b); therefore, development of SCAN1 may be dependent on this "mutagenic" property of p.His493Arg Tdp1.

5.1 Mitochondrial dysfunction model

The prominent cytoplasmic expression of Tdp1 in human Purkinje, dentate nucleus, anterior horn, and dorsal ganglion neurons suggests a cytoplasmic function for Tdp1. Given the mitochondrial localization of cytoplasmic Tdp1, this suggests 1) that the majority of Tdp1 in these neurons functions in the mitochondria and 2) that SCAN1 may be arising from mitochondrial dysfunction secondary to loss of mtDNA integrity. In contrast, the low expression of Tdp1 in the cytoplasm of these neurons in mice would suggest that Tdp1 plays a minor role in maintenance of the mouse mitochondrial genome or that the analogous neurons have less mtDNA damage in mice than in humans.

The human cerebellum contains post-mitotic neurons with a large mitochondrial population. Despite the non-proliferative nature of cerebellar neurons, the biogenesis of mitochondria and the maintenance of mitochondrial integrity are of central importance for survival of these neurons (Chen and Chan, 2009). The closed circular mitochondrial genome predisposes it to helical tension during mitochondrial replication, which is resolved by mtTopo I. In the nucleus, binding of Topo I to 8-oxoG rearranges the active site of Topo I and stabilizes it in an inactive conformation (Lesher et al., 2002). If the same occurs in mitochondria with mtTopo I, which encounters a much higher level of 8-oxoG, then Tdp1 will be critical for resolution of these lesions in mtDNA. Hypothetically, a repair process analogous to that in the nucleus would resolve these long-lived complexes: 1) protease cleavage of mtTopo I, 2) Tdp1 mediated cleavage and release of the mtTopo I peptide to leave an 8-oxoG 5'overhang and a 3'-phosphate, and 3) SP-BER. SP-BER would proceed by PNKP removal of the 3'-phosphate and OGG1 removal of the 5' 8-oxoG lesion, followed by mitochondrial polymerase-ϒ filling in the missing nucleotides and Lig3a ligating the DNA strand (Figure 4a).

Based on these observations, we hypothesize that the processing of trapped or long-lived mtTopo I-DNA intermediates is hindered in cells from SCAN1 patients by the reduced catalytic activity of p.His493Arg Tdp1. Additionally, we hypothesize that mitochondria lack DNA repair pathways redundant for the activity of Tdp1 since 3'end processing flap endonucleases that could resolve mtTopo I-DNA adducts have not been detected in mitochondria (Liu et al., 2002). In this model, trapped or long-lived mtTopo I-DNA intermediates interfere with mitochondrial transcription and contribute to mtDNA damage. In turn, both transcriptional dysfunction and genomic instability cause mitochondrial dysfunction and thereby poor cellular health. Relative to other brain neurons, cerebellar neurons may be highly sensitive to this mitochondrial damage since they have a lower tolerance for mitochondrial dysfunction (Chen et al., 2007; Hakonen et al., 2008) (Figure 4b).

In summary, therefore, the dysfunction of mitochondrial Tdp1 may contribute to the pathogenesis of SCAN1. Also, the absence of ataxia in Tdp1 deficient mice may arise because mouse cerebellar and spinal cord neurons have a lower requirement for Tdp1 processing of damaged mtDNA (Hirano et al., 2007).

5.2 Tdp1 neomorph model

The formation and accumulation of Tdp1-DNA adducts by the mutant p.His493Arg Tdp1 causes increased DNA breaks in cells expressing this mutant Tdp1 (Hirano et al., 2007) and thus suggests that p.His493Arg Tdp1 acts as a mutagen. *In vitro*, wild type Tdp1 is the only identified enzyme that can remove the mutant Tdp1 from the DNA (Interthal et al., 2005a). However, *in vivo* it is possible that nuclear Tdp1-DNA adducts are processed by a DNA repair mechanism such as HR that is present in proliferating unaffected cells but not in affected quiescent neurons. Alternatively, there may not be an alternative repair pathway but simply replacement of cells that die from accumulated Tdp1-DNA adducts in proliferating tissues and a failure of replacement for non-proliferating neurons.

As an extension of this hypothesis, one might consider that both mitochondrial dysfunction and the neomorphic properties of p.His493Arg Tdp1 contribute to the pathogenesis of SCAN1. The repair of damaged DNA is costly, and if the costs exceed cellular energy resources (ATP/NADH), then cell death results (Zong and Thompson, 2006). In this context, a mechanism that could lead to cell death is the depletion of NAD^+ and ATP reserves by the over-activation of PARP1 due to accumulating SSBs created by $Tdp1^{His493Arg}$-DNA adducts in the nucleus and mitochondria. In the context of compromised mitochondria, such depletion of cellular energy reserves, which triggers permeabilization of the outer mitochondrial membrane and the release of cytochrome c and apoptosis-inducing factor

(AIF) (Wang et al., 2009), would occur at a lower threshold in affected versus unaffected cells of SCAN1 patients (Wang et al., 2011) (Chen and Chan, 2009). In this model, the neurons with the least energy reserves would be most sensitive and, unlike proliferating cells, difficult to replace (Figure 4c).

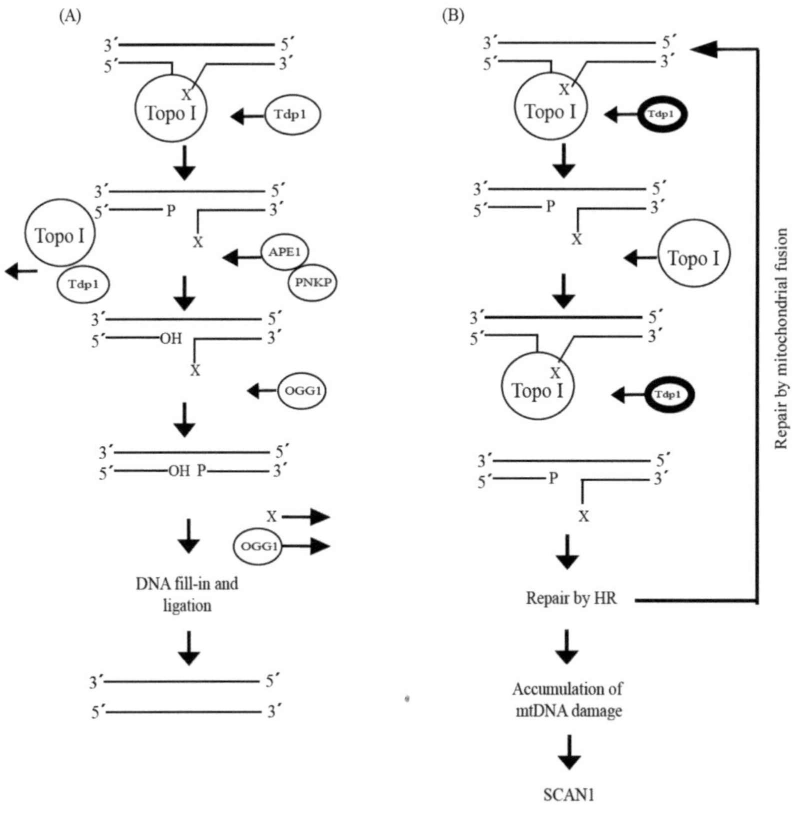

Fig. 4. A and B.

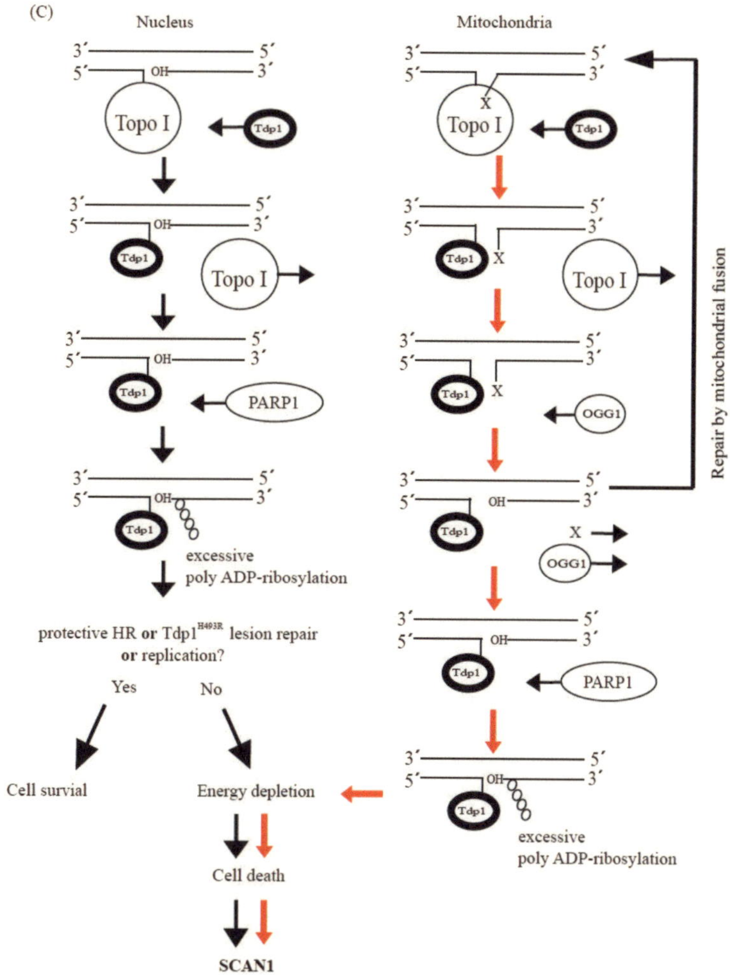

Fig. 4. Models for the pathobiology of SCAN1. (A) Putative Tdp1 function in the mitochondria. Wild type Tdp1 removes the residual peptide from stalled mtTopo I complexes. Interfering DNA lesions are processed by OGG1 and by PNKP or APE1. Religation synthesis would then proceed by mitochondrial short patch-BER. (B) The mitochondrial dysfunction model. In SCAN1, p.His493Arg Tdp1 (in bold) removes peptides derived from Topo I-DNA complexes at a severely compromised rate. This sluggish repair leads to a higher steady-state level of mtDNA SSBs and DSBs. To bypass the lack of Tdp1, error-prone repair may generate mtDNA deletions which impair mitochondrial function leading to cell death and SCAN1. (C) The Tdp1 neomorph model. Mutagenic p.His493Arg Tdp1 is trapped on DNA, and since wild type Tdp1 most efficiently repairs p.His493Arg Tdp1-DNA adducts, the unresolved p.His493Arg Tdp1-DNA adducts in cells from SCAN1 patients will lead to much higher steady state levels of nuclear and mitochondrial DNA SSBs. This could cause neuron death both by SSB-induced programmed cell death and by cellular energy depletion secondary to mitochondrial dysfunction. The energy depletion would be accentuated by the increased energy requirement for DNA repair as exemplified by PARP1 mediated poly ADP-ribosylation. X = interfering lesion.

6. Future directions

The discovery of Tdp1 in mitochondria places the pathobiology of SCAN1 in a new light although whether specific mitochondrial pathology is relevant to the pathogenesis of SCAN1 remains to be elucidated. To that end, the generation of $Tdp1^{His493Arg}$ mice will enable a thorough investigation of the physical and molecular characteristics of SCAN1.

Equally important is the precise elucidation of Tdp1 function in DNA processing. Research in mice and yeast has deciphered much about Tdp1 function but much remains to be discovered. Tdp1 orthologues have been described in 29 organisms, most recently in the plants *Arabidopsis sp.* and *Medicago sp.*, where Tdp1 repair of Topo I-induced damage is consistent with its role in mammalian cells (Lee et al., 2010; Macovei et al., 2010). As the time and cost of DNA sequencing continues to decline and techniques for probing the genome become more accessible to biologists, the study of emerging model organisms will provide valuable insights into the evolutionary conservation of Tdp1. This approach would allow more detailed evaluation of Tdp1 from an evolutionary perspective and enhance our mechanistic understanding. For example, this might enlighten us as to why the *Drosophila melanogaster* homologue *glaikit* appears to have a function distinct from that of the mammalian and plant Tdp1 homologues (Dunlop et al., 2000; Dunlop et al., 2004)

The study of SCAN1 has also defined Tdp1 as a reasonable drug target for other diseases. The absence of neurological disease in Tdp1 deficient mice and the adolescent onset of SCAN1 in humans suggest that Tdp1 could be inhibited briefly without severe adverse consequences. Since Tdp1 increases resistance to the Topo I poisons used as anticancer agents, these findings suggest that a combination therapy of Topo I poisons with Tdp1 inhibitors might enhance the efficacy of the Topo I poisons as anticancer drugs (Marchand et al., 2009).

7. Conclusion

Mitochondrial dysfunction is not yet the *sine qua non* of SCAs, but it is increasingly reported in neurodegenerative diseases. Besides the SCAs, mitochondrial dysfunction has been reported as contributing to the pathobiology of aging, Alzheimer disease, Parkinson disease, Huntington disease and amyotrophic lateral sclerosis. Much of this work has focused on mitochondrial-derived reactive oxygen species; however, the contribution of mitochondrial fusion and fission to neuronal health and disease as well as other mitochondrial processes remain to be explored (Lin and Beal, 2006; Westermann, 2010). SCAN1 is emblematic of the interplay between the nuclear and mitochondrial genomes and how dysfunction in both organelles can jointly contribute to disease. This dual nuclear and mitochondrial pathobiology will need to be taken into consideration in experimental design as well as in the classification and clinical management of neurologic disorders.

8. Acknowledgements

We thank William Gibson, Michel Roberge, Fabio Rossi, Alireza Baradaran-Heravi, Marie Morimoto from the University of British Columbia and Camilo Toro from the National Institutes of Health in Bethesda, Maryland for their valuable opinions and critical review of this manuscript.

9. References

Ames, B.N., Shigenaga, M.K., and Hagen, T.M. (1993). Oxidants, antioxidants, and the degenerative diseases of aging. Proc Natl Acad Sci U S A *90*, 7915-7922.

Barekati, Z., Radpour, R., Kohler, C., Zhang, B., Toniolo, P., Lenner, P., Lv, Q., Zheng, H., and Zhong, X.Y. (2010). Methylation profile of TP53 regulatory pathway and mtDNA alterations in breast cancer patients lacking TP53 mutations. Hum Mol Genet *19*, 2936-2946.

Barzilai, A. (2011). The neuro-glial-vascular interrelations in genomic instability symptoms. Mech Ageing Dev *132*, 395-404.

Bender, A., Krishnan, K.J., Morris, C.M., Taylor, G.A., Reeve, A.K., Perry, R.H., Jaros, E., Hersheson, J.S., Betts, J., Klopstock, T., *et al.* (2006). High levels of mitochondrial DNA deletions in substantia nigra neurons in aging and Parkinson disease. Nat Genet *38*, 515-517.

Chen, H., and Chan, D.C. (2009). Mitochondrial dynamics--fusion, fission, movement, and mitophagy--in neurodegenerative diseases. Hum Mol Genet *18*, R169-176.

Chen, H., McCaffery, J.M., and Chan, D.C. (2007). Mitochondrial fusion protects against neurodegeneration in the cerebellum. Cell *130*, 548-562.

Ciccia, A., and Elledge, S.J. (2010). The DNA damage response: making it safe to play with knives. Mol Cell *40*, 179-204.

Connelly, J.C., and Leach, D.R. (2004). Repair of DNA covalently linked to protein. Mol Cell *13*, 307-316.

Cortes Ledesma, F., El Khamisy, S.F., Zuma, M.C., Osborn, K., and Caldecott, K.W. (2009). A human 5'-tyrosyl DNA phosphodiesterase that repairs topoisomerase-mediated DNA damage. Nature *461*, 674-678.

Das, B.B., Antony, S., Gupta, S., Dexheimer, T.S., Redon, C.E., Garfield, S., Shiloh, Y., and Pommier, Y. (2009). Optimal function of the DNA repair enzyme TDP1 requires its phosphorylation by ATM and/or DNA-PK. Embo J *28*, 3667-3680.

Das, B.B., Dexheimer, T.S., Maddali, K., and Pommier, Y. (2010). Role of tyrosyl-DNA phosphodiesterase (TDP1) in mitochondria. Proc Natl Acad Sci U S A *107*, 19790-19795.

de Laat, W.L., Jaspers, N.G., and Hoeijmakers, J.H. (1999). Molecular mechanism of nucleotide excision repair. Genes Dev *13*, 768-785.

Debethune, L., Kohlhagen, G., Grandas, A., and Pommier, Y. (2002). Processing of nucleopeptides mimicking the topoisomerase I-DNA covalent complex by tyrosyl-DNA phosphodiesterase. Nucleic Acids Res *30*, 1198-1204.

Dexheimer, T.S., Antony, S., Marchand, C., and Pommier, Y. (2008). Tyrosyl-DNA phosphodiesterase as a target for anticancer therapy. Anticancer Agents Med Chem *8*, 381-389.

Dexheimer, T.S., Stephen, A.G., Fivash, M.J., Fisher, R.J., and Pommier, Y. (2010). The DNA binding and 3'-end preferential activity of human tyrosyl-DNA phosphodiesterase. Nucleic Acids Res *38*, 2444-2452.

Dunlop, J., Corominas, M., and Serras, F. (2000). The novel gene glaikit, is expressed during neurogenesis in the Drosophila melanogaster embryo. Mechanisms of development *96*, 133-136.

Dunlop, J., Morin, X., Corominas, M., Serras, F., and Tear, G. (2004). glaikit is essential for the formation of epithelial polarity and neuronal development. Curr Biol *14*, 2039-2045.

el-Khamisy, S.F., and Caldecott, K.W. (2007). DNA single-strand break repair and spinocerebellar ataxia with axonal neuropathy-1. Neuroscience *145*, 1260-1266.

El-Khamisy, S.F., Masutani, M., Suzuki, H., and Caldecott, K.W. (2003). A requirement for PARP-1 for the assembly or stability of XRCC1 nuclear foci at sites of oxidative DNA damage. Nucleic Acids Res *31*, 5526-5533.

Embirucu, E.K., Martyn, M.L., Schlesinger, D., and Kok, F. (2009). Autosomal recessive ataxias: 20 types, and counting. Arq Neuropsiquiatr *67*, 1143-1156.

Fishel, M.L., Vasko, M.R., and Kelley, M.R. (2007). DNA repair in neurons: so if they don't divide what's to repair? Mutat Res *614*, 24-36.

Frosina, G., Fortini, P., Rossi, O., Carrozzino, F., Raspaglio, G., Cox, L.S., Lane, D.P., Abbondandolo, A., and Dogliotti, E. (1996). Two pathways for base excision repair in mammalian cells. J Biol Chem *271*, 9573-9578.

Hakonen, A.H., Goffart, S., Marjavaara, S., Paetau, A., Cooper, H., Mattila, K., Lampinen, M., Sajantila, A., Lonnqvist, T., Spelbrink, J.N., *et al.* (2008). Infantile-onset spinocerebellar ataxia and mitochondrial recessive ataxia syndrome are associated with neuronal complex I defect and mtDNA depletion. Hum Mol Genet *17*, 3822-3835.

Harman, D. (1972). The biologic clock: the mitochondria? J Am Geriatr Soc *20*, 145-147.

Harman, D. (1981). The aging process. Proc Natl Acad Sci U S A *78*, 7124-7128.

Hirano, R., Interthal, H., Huang, C., Nakamura, T., Deguchi, K., Choi, K., Bhattacharjee, M.B., Arimura, K., Umehara, F., Izumo, S., *et al.* (2007). Spinocerebellar ataxia with axonal neuropathy: consequence of a Tdp1 recessive neomorphic mutation? EMBO J *26*, 4732-4743.

Hirano, R., Salih, M.A.M., Takashima, H., and Boerkoel, C.F. (1993). Spinocerebellar Ataxia with Axonal Neuropathy, Autosomal Recessive.

Hire, R., Katrak, S., Vaidya, S., Radhakrishnan, K., and Seshadri, M. (2010). Spinocerebellar ataxia type 17 in Indian patients: two rare cases of homozygous expansions. Clin Genet.

Hsiang, Y.H., Lihou, M.G., and Liu, L.F. (1989). Arrest of replication forks by drug-stabilized topoisomerase I-DNA cleavable complexes as a mechanism of cell killing by camptothecin. Cancer Res *49*, 5077-5082.

Hudson, E.K., Hogue, B.A., Souza-Pinto, N.C., Croteau, D.L., Anson, R.M., Bohr, V.A., and Hansford, R.G. (1998). Age-associated change in mitochondrial DNA damage. Free radical research *29*, 573-579.

Interthal, H., Chen, H.J., and Champoux, J.J. (2005a). Human Tdp1 cleaves a broad spectrum of substrates, including phosphoamide linkages. J Biol Chem *280*, 36518-36528.

Interthal, H., Chen, H.J., Kehl-Fie, T.E., Zotzmann, J., Leppard, J.B., and Champoux, J.J. (2005b). SCAN1 mutant Tdp1 accumulates the enzyme--DNA intermediate and causes camptothecin hypersensitivity. Embo J *24*, 2224-2233.

Interthal, H., Pouliot, J.J., and Champoux, J.J. (2001). The tyrosyl-DNA phosphodiesterase Tdp1 is a member of the phospholipase D superfamily. Proc Natl Acad Sci U S A *98*, 12009-12014.

Jeppesen, D.K., Bohr, V.A., and Stevnsner, T. (2011). DNA repair deficiency in neurodegeneration. Progress in neurobiology *94*, 166-200.

Katyal, S., and McKinnon, P.J. (2007). DNA repair deficiency and neurodegeneration. Cell Cycle *6*, 2360-2365.

Kovtun, I.V., Liu, Y., Bjoras, M., Klungland, A., Wilson, S.H., and McMurray, C.T. (2007). OGG1 initiates age-dependent CAG trinucleotide expansion in somatic cells. Nature *447*, 447-452.

Kraemer, K.H., Lee, M.M., and Scotto, J. (1987). Xeroderma pigmentosum. Cutaneous, ocular, and neurologic abnormalities in 830 published cases. Arch Dermatol *123*, 241-250.

Krishnakumar, R., and Kraus, W.L. (2010). The PARP side of the nucleus: molecular actions, physiological outcomes, and clinical targets. Mol Cell *39*, 8-24.

Kruman, II, Wersto, R.P., Cardozo-Pelaez, F., Smilenov, L., Chan, S.L., Chrest, F.J., Emokpae, R., Jr., Gorospe, M., and Mattson, M.P. (2004). Cell cycle activation linked to neuronal cell death initiated by DNA damage. Neuron *41*, 549-561.

Larsen, N.B., Rasmussen, M., and Rasmussen, L.J. (2005). Nuclear and mitochondrial DNA repair: similar pathways? Mitochondrion *5*, 89-108.

Lee, S.Y., Kim, H., Hwang, H.J., Jeong, Y.M., Na, S.H., Woo, J.C., and Kim, S.G. (2010). Identification of tyrosyl-DNA phosphodiesterase as a novel DNA damage repair enzyme in Arabidopsis. Plant Physiol *154*, 1460-1469.

Lehmann, A.R. (2003). DNA repair-deficient diseases, xeroderma pigmentosum, Cockayne syndrome and trichothiodystrophy. Biochimie *85*, 1101-1111.

Lesher, D.T., Pommier, Y., Stewart, L., and Redinbo, M.R. (2002). 8-Oxoguanine rearranges the active site of human topoisomerase I. Proc Natl Acad Sci U S A *99*, 12102-12107.

Lin, M.T., and Beal, M.F. (2006). Mitochondrial dysfunction and oxidative stress in neurodegenerative diseases. Nature *443*, 787-795.

Liu, C., Pouliot, J.J., and Nash, H.A. (2002). Repair of topoisomerase I covalent complexes in the absence of the tyrosyl-DNA phosphodiesterase Tdp1. Proc Natl Acad Sci U S A *99*, 14970-14975.

Lobsiger, C.S., and Cleveland, D.W. (2007). Glial cells as intrinsic components of non-cell-autonomous neurodegenerative disease. Nature neuroscience *10*, 1355-1360.

Macovei, A., Balestrazzi, A., Confalonieri, M., and Carbonera, D. (2010). The tyrosyl-DNA phosphodiesterase gene family in Medicago truncatula Gaertn.: bioinformatic investigation and expression profiles in response to copper- and PEG-mediated stress. Planta *232*, 393-407.

Marchand, C., Lea, W.A., Jadhav, A., Dexheimer, T.S., Austin, C.P., Inglese, J., Pommier, Y., and Simeonov, A. (2009). Identification of phosphotyrosine mimetic inhibitors of human tyrosyl-DNA phosphodiesterase I by a novel AlphaScreen high-throughput assay. Mol Cancer Ther *8*, 240-248.

Nance, M.A., and Berry, S.A. (1992). Cockayne syndrome: review of 140 cases. Am J Med Genet *42*, 68-84.

Owen, B.A., Yang, Z., Lai, M., Gajec, M., Badger, J.D., 2nd, Hayes, J.J., Edelmann, W., Kucherlapati, R., Wilson, T.M., and McMurray, C.T. (2005). (CAG)(n)-hairpin DNA binds to Msh2-Msh3 and changes properties of mismatch recognition. Nat Struct Mol Biol *12*, 663-670.

Pommier, Y., Pourquier, P., Fan, Y., and Strumberg, D. (1998). Mechanism of action of eukaryotic DNA topoisomerase I and drugs targeted to the enzyme. Biochim Biophys Acta *1400*, 83-105.

Pommier, Y., Redon, C., Rao, V.A., Seiler, J.A., Sordet, O., Takemura, H., Antony, S., Meng, L., Liao, Z., Kohlhagen, G., *et al.* (2003). Repair of and checkpoint response to topoisomerase I-mediated DNA damage. Mutat Res *532*, 173-203.

Pourquier, P., and Pommier, Y. (2001). Topoisomerase I-mediated DNA damage. Adv Cancer Res *80*, 189-216.

Proux, E., Studer, R.A., Moretti, S., and Robinson-Rechavi, M. (2009). Selectome: a database of positive selection. Nucleic Acids Res *37*, D404-407.

Sahin, E., and Depinho, R.A. (2010). Linking functional decline of telomeres, mitochondria and stem cells during ageing. Nature *464*, 520-528.

Subba Rao, K. (2007). Mechanisms of disease: DNA repair defects and neurological disease. Nat Clin Pract Neurol *3*, 162-172.

Takashima, H., Boerkoel, C.F., John, J., Saifi, G.M., Salih, M.A., Armstrong, D., Mao, Y., Quiocho, F.A., Roa, B.B., Nakagawa, M., *et al.* (2002). Mutation of TDP1, encoding a topoisomerase I-dependent DNA damage repair enzyme, in spinocerebellar ataxia with axonal neuropathy. Nat Genet *32*, 267-272.

Tsao, Y.P., Russo, A., Nyamuswa, G., Silber, R., and Liu, L.F. (1993). Interaction between replication forks and topoisomerase I-DNA cleavable complexes: studies in a cell-free SV40 DNA replication system. Cancer Res *53*, 5908-5914.

Wang, Y., Dawson, V.L., and Dawson, T.M. (2009). Poly(ADP-ribose) signals to mitochondrial AIF: a key event in parthanatos. Exp Neurol *218*, 193-202.

Wang, Y., Kim, N.S., Haince, J.F., Kang, H.C., David, K.K., Andrabi, S.A., Poirier, G.G., Dawson, V.L., and Dawson, T.M. (2011). Poly(ADP-ribose) (PAR) binding to apoptosis-inducing factor is critical for PAR polymerase-1-dependent cell death (parthanatos). Sci Signal *4*, ra20.

Westermann, B. (2010). Mitochondrial fusion and fission in cell life and death. Nat Rev Mol Cell Biol *11*, 872-884.

Wu, J., and Liu, L.F. (1997). Processing of topoisomerase I cleavable complexes into DNA damage by transcription. Nucleic Acids Res *25*, 4181-4186.

Yakes, F.M., and Van Houten, B. (1997). Mitochondrial DNA damage is more extensive and persists longer than nuclear DNA damage in human cells following oxidative stress. Proc Natl Acad Sci U S A *94*, 514-519.

Zhang, H., Barcelo, J.M., Lee, B., Kohlhagen, G., Zimonjic, D.B., Popescu, N.C., and Pommier, Y. (2001). Human mitochondrial topoisomerase I. Proc Natl Acad Sci U S A *98*, 10608-10613.

Zhang, H.F., Tomida, A., Koshimizu, R., Ogiso, Y., Lei, S., and Tsuruo, T. (2004). Cullin 3 promotes proteasomal degradation of the topoisomerase I-DNA covalent complex. Cancer Res *64*, 1114-1121.

Zhou, T., Akopiants, K., Mohapatra, S., Lin, P.S., Valerie, K., Ramsden, D.A., Lees-Miller, S.P., and Povirk, L.F. (2009). Tyrosyl-DNA phosphodiesterase and the repair of 3'-phosphoglycolate-terminated DNA double-strand breaks. DNA Repair (Amst) *8*, 901-911.

Zong, W.X., and Thompson, C.B. (2006). Necrotic death as a cell fate. Genes Dev *20*, 1-15.

4

Eye Movement Abnormalities in Spinocerebellar Ataxias

Roberto Rodríguez-Labrada and Luis Velázquez-Pérez
Centre for the Research and Rehabilitation of Hereditary Ataxias, Holguin
Cuba

1. Introduction

Spinocerebellar ataxias (SCAs) are a heterogeneous group of autosomal dominant neurodegenerative disorders characterized by a progressive cerebellar syndrome, variably associated to signs of brainstem involvement, pyramidal or extrapyramidal manifestations and cognitive dysfunctions, among other features that confer a remarkable wide range in phenotypes (Harding, 1983; Durr, 2010).

SCAs are associated with at least 31 different genetic loci, but the responsible gene is known in only 19 of them. Causative mutations include coding CAG expansions leading to a long polyglutamine (polyQ) tract in the respective proteins (SCA1, 2, 3, 6, 7 and 17), non-coding trinucleotide or pentanucleotide expansions (SCA8, 10, 12 and 31), as well as conventional mutations (SCA5, 11, 13, 14, 15/16, 20, 27 and 28) (Durr, 2010). The worldwide prevalence of SCAs is estimated near to 5-7 cases per 100 000 inhabitants but it can be higher in some regions due to foundational effects such as SCA2 in Holguín, Cuba (Velazquez-Pérez et al., 2009a) and SCA3 in Azores islands, Portugal (Vale et al., 2010).

Oculomotor disturbances are prominent features of SCA patients as result of cerebellar and brainstem neurodegeneration (Zee et al., 1976; Pula et al., 2010). The study of eye movement abnormalities give us valuable tools to search disease biomarkers because they can be easily accessible to clinical and/or electrophysiological evaluations and their dynamic properties and neurobiological basis are well known (Leigh & Kennard, 2004; Leigh & Zee, 2006; Reilly et al., 2008). The focus of this chapter is to review the state of the art of the eye movement deficits in SCAs, emphasizing in the usefulness of these features as disease biomarkers.

2. Brief overview of eye movements

Eye movements contribute to the clear vision stabilizing images on the retina, especially against movements of the head and body, capturing and keeping particular stimuli on the fovea and aligning the retinal images in the two eyes to guarantee the single vision and stereopsis. These functions can be achieved by 5 basic types of eye movements. For example, the image stabilization on the retina is promoted by the vestibulocular and optokinetic reflexes; the foveation occurs thorough the saccadic and smooth pursuit movements, whereas the binocular alignment is guaranteed by the vergence eye movements (Bruce & Friedman, 2002).

Eye movements differ in many aspects, such as their velocity, reaction time, reflexivity/volitional degree and their neurobiological substrate (Sparks, 2002). Nevertheless all have generic kinematic properties and share a common final path represented by three cranial nerve nuclei and the three pairs of eye muscles that they control (Bruce & Friedman, 2002; Leigh & Zee, 2006). Cranial nerve III (oculomotor) innervates superior, inferior and medial rectus muscles as well as the inferior oblique muscle, whereas troclear (IV) and abducens (VI) nerves innervate the superior oblique and lateral rectus respectively (Leigh & Zee, 2006).

Main features and neurophysiological bases of the 5 basic types of eye movements will be briefly addressed as follow.

2.1 Vestibulocular reflex (VOR)

The vestibulocular reflex (VOR) is elicited by the vestibular system in response to body/head rotations and consists in compensatory eye movements in opposite direction to body/head movement to guarantee the image stabilization on the retina (Aw et al., 1996). VOR depends of two neural circuits: *a)* Basic three neurons circuit and, *b)* Neural integrator circuit.

In the basic three neurons circuit, the head/body rotations are detected and transduced by vestibular ganglion neurons in the semicircular canal. Then, the transduced information is projected to neurons of the vestibular nuclei, located in the pons, and from there to oculomotor neurons (OMN) in one of the three oculomotor nuclei. Nevertheless, the three neurons circuit by itself is unable to adequately stabilize the image on the retina because it only generates phasic innervations of the oculomotor muscles, causing the return of the eye back to the central position due to the pulling of elastic forces. The neural integrator serves to exactly overcome this elastic force producing tonic innervations of oculomotor muscles. It is located in the *prepositus hypoglossi* and medial vestibular nuclei, which receive projections from the vestibular nuclei and have recurrent connections onto themselves. Some vestibular afferents go directly to the floculus/parafloculus cerebellar lobe, which is involved in VOR adaptation (Bruce & Friedman, 2002).

2.2 Optokinetic reflex (OKR)

When head/body rotations are very large and continued the VOR is depressed and thus it is complemented by the optokinetic reflex (OKR), in which the speed and direction of a full-field image motion is computed to develop eye movements with two phases, an slow phase that alternates with resetting quick phase (Tusa & Zee, 1989). Pathway underlying OKR includes the nucleus of the optic tract, which receives visual motion signals from the contralateral eye and striate/extrastriate cortical areas. This information is send to the vestibular nuclei and to the inferior olivary nucleus, and then to the flocular/paraflocular Purkinje cells via their climbing fibers (Bruce & Friedman, 2002).

2.3 Saccadic eye movements

Saccades are ballistic, conjugate eye movements that redirect fovea from one object of interest to another, allowing to explore accurately the visual scenes. For that, the saccadic system processes information about the distance and direction of a target image from the current position of gaze. Saccades are the fastest eye movements, reaching up to 600⁰/s. There are close relationships between saccadic peak velocities, durations and amplitudes, which represent the saccadic main sequence (Bahill et al., 1975, Ramat et al., 2007).

Behaviourally, the saccades may be classified as reflexive guided saccades and intentional or volitional saccades. The first ones are evoked by the suddenly appearing targets, whereas the second ones, called also higher-order saccades, are made purposely, involve high cognitive processing and include voluntary, memory guided and delayed saccades as well as antisaccades (Müri & Nyffeler, 2008; Leigh & Kennard, 2004).

The neural basis of saccadic eye movements system comprises some cortico-cortical and cortico-subcortical networks (Müri & Nyffeler, 2008). Visual information processed in the primary visual cortex is send to higher cortical areas, such as parietal eye field (PEF) and frontal eye field (FEF), which are involved in the preparation and triggering of reflexive and intentional saccades respectively (Pierrot-Deseilligny, et al., 2004). These cortical areas project their output directly or through the basal ganglia, to superior colliculus, a midbrain structure that identifies the target in retinotopic coordinates, generates trigger signal to the brainstem premotor oculomotor circuitry and encodes the magnitude and direction of the desired eye movement. This information is projected to the cerebellum, via a pontine pre-cerebellar nucleus, which guarantees the saccadic accuracy. Premotor burst neurons (PBN) for horizontal saccades lie within the paramedian pontine reticular formation (PPRF) while burst neurons for vertical and torsional saccades lie within the rostral interstitial nucleus of the medial longitudinal fasciculus. Saccade-related cerebellar areas include the oculomotor vermis (lobules VI and VII) and the caudal region of the fastigial nucleus which send saccade commands to the contralateral PBNs leading the activation of motorneurons and oculomotor muscles related with the desired saccadic movement (Leigh & Zee, 2006; Robinson & Fuchs, 2001; Prsa & Their, 2011; Voogd et al., 2011).

2.4 Smooth pursuit movements

Smooth-pursuit eye movements enable us to maintain the image of a moving object relatively stable on or near the fovea by matching eye velocity to target velocity (Leigh & Zee, 2006). Smooth pursuit performance is optimal for target speeds ranging between 15⁰/s and 30⁰/s but pursuit velocity can reach up to 100⁰/s (Lencer & Trillenberg 2008; Bruce & Friedman, 2002). Smooth pursuit system is closely related to other oculomotor systems such as OKR and saccadic system. In fact, the small position errors raised when the tracking velocity is not properly matched to the target are corrected by saccadic movements named "catch up" saccades (Lencer & Trillenberg, 2007).

Neuronal pathways for smooth pursuit movements involve a complex network of cortical and subcortical structures. Extrastriate visual area V5 (divided into middle temporal visual area (MT) and the medial superior temporal visual area (MST)) play a crucial role for motion perception and smooth pursuit control. This area receives visual motion information from the primary visual cortex in a retinotopic and ipsilaterally organized fashion. The MT area encodes image motion in a retinal coordinate system whereas MST area converts the signals into a spatial coordinate system. The signals generated in the V5 area are projected to other cortical areas in the parietal and frontal lobes. Among them, the frontal eye field (FEF) is involved in the generation of oculomotor command for smooth pursuit. Both visual motion signals and oculomotor commands are relayed to oculomotor parts of the cerebellum, through the dorsolateral and medial pontine nuclei. Smooth pursuit-related areas of the cerebellum comprise the paraflocculus, the flocculus, the oculomotor vermis and the uvula, which control the initiation and maintenance of smooth pursuit. Finally, the cerebellar output is projected, via the vestibular nuclei, to the oculomotor nuclei (Lencer & Trillenberg, 2007; Mustari et al., 2009).

2.5 Vergence eye movements

Vergence eye movements are disjunctive movements that provide the binocular alignment in response to changing fixation target distances, requiring that both eyes point in contrary directions (Zee & Levi, 1989). Vergence movements are elicited by retinal disparity (when a fixation target is not on both foveae) and retinal blur (when a target is not in focus) and are closely related to the lens accommodation and pupillary reflexes. Although the neural basis of vergence eye movements are not well understood, it is known that both the retinal disparity and the retinal blur signals are processed by cortical visual areas such as primary visual cortex (V1) and an anterior region of the FEF. Additionally, it is presumed an important role of the oculomotor nucleus (III) for vergence movements, due to its known relation to lens accommodation and pupillary reflexes (Vilis, 1997; Bruce & Friedman, 2002). The cerebellum is involved in the processing of dynamic vergence eye movements (Sander et al., 2009). Cerebellar regions related with these disconjugate eye movements lie on the dorsal paraflocculus, and the floccular lobe, which project to the lateral portion of the posterior interposed nucleus (Voogd et al., 2011).

2.6 Oculomotor disturbances

Oculomotor disturbances can be topographically classified as peripheral or central disturbances. Peripheral abnormalities result from lesions in the oculomotor muscles or nerves, whereas the central disturbances are caused by lesions in the brainstem, cerebellum or other higher-level centers (Karatas, 2009). Oculomotor signs of cerebellar impairment include pathological nystagmus such as downbeat, rebound and periodic alternating nystagmus, as well as abnormal pursuit, VOR/OKR abnormalities and saccadic dysmetria (Robinson & Fuchs, 2001; Strupp et al., 2011). Whereas, brainstem involvement produces slowed vertical, torsional or horizontal saccades, ophthalmoplegia, VOR/OKR impairments and gaze-evoked nystagmus (Rüb et al., 2008, Strupp et al., 2011). Affectations in the basal ganglia can lead to reduced ability to initiate voluntary eye movements and to suppress unwanted saccades, in addition to deficits in memory-guided saccades, eye-head coordination and eye-hand coordination (Hikosaka et al., 2000; Shires et al., 2010). Frontal cortex lesions produce prolongation of saccadic latency, impaired ability to make saccades to remembered target locations and errors on the antisaccade task, as well as delayed initiation of smooth pursuit and increase of catch up saccades (Pierrot-Deseilligny et al., 2004; Thurtell et al., 2007; Karatas, 2009).

3. Oculomotor findings of spinocerebellar ataxias

3.1 Spinocerebellar ataxia type 1 (SCA1)

The main eye movement abnormalities of SCA1 patients include saccadic dysmetria, gaze evoked nystagmus and depressed smooth pursuit (Matilla-Dueñas et al., 2008). Saccadic hypermetria is observed in majority of the cases, appears at an early stage of the disease and progresses quickly (Klostermann et al., 1997; Rivaud-Pechoux et al., 1998; Buttner et al., 1998). The overshoot of saccades may reach values greater than 30% in comparison with normal subjects (Buttner et al., 1998).

Brainstem oculomotor signs such as saccadic slowing or ophthalmoparesis are observed in 74% (Schmitz-Hübsch, et al., 2008). Reduction of saccade velocity can be detected in mildly affected patients and it is accentuated with the disease duration. Advanced patients may show ophthalmoparesis or severe saccadic slowing, so that saccadic hypermetria is less noticeable in comparison to early stages (Klostermann et al., 1997). Abnormal prolongation of saccadic latency occurs in 67% of cases (Buttner et al., 1998), whereas the execution of the antisaccadic task shows increased error rates, suggesting the presence of neurodegenerative changes in the frontal cortex (Rivaud-Pechoux et al., 1998).

Reduced gain of smooth pursuit and OKN is noticed in 92% of SCA1 cases with the lowest smooth pursuit gains in comparison to SCA2 and SCA3 patients and comparable values of OKN gains to SCA2 (Burk et al., 1998). The progressive saccadic slowing causes the diminution of catch up saccades during visual tracking, leading to decrease of the smooth pursuit amplitudes on advanced disease (Buttner et al., 1998, Klostermann et al., 1997). Regarding vestibular functions, SCA1 patients are usually characterized by reduced VOR gains, which distinguish this SCA subtype from SCA2 but neither from SCA3 nor SCA6 (Burk et al., 1998; Buttner et al., 1998).

No oculomotor abnormalities of SCA1 patients correlate with the number of CAG repeats (Burk et al., 1999; Rivaud-Pechoux et al.,1998), suggesting that they are not under significant genetic control but are more dependent on disease duration.

3.2 Spinocerebellar ataxia type 2 (SCA2)

The most common oculomotor sign in patients with SCA2 is a significant reduction in horizontal saccadic eye velocity owing to brainstem involvement. This feature called attention to Wadia and Swami when made the first report of SCA2 in 1971, so that they described the disease as "*a new form of heredofamilial spinocerebellar degeneration with slow eye movements*" (Wadia & Swami, 1971). Several clinical and epidemiological studies have confirmed the high frequency of this saccadic alteration in more than 80% of cases (Velazquez-Pérez et al., 2009a; Orozco et al., 1989; Cancel et al., 1997, Wadia et al., 1998; Schmitz-Hübsch, et al., 2008).

The first electronystagmographical evaluation of SCA2 patients was conducted by Kulkarni & Wadia in 1975 who found a relative decrease of saccadic velocity up to 25% in comparison with controls (Kulkarni & Wadia, 1975). Furthermore, comparative studies of oculomotor phenotypes among patients with cerebellar ataxias demonstrated that saccadic slowing is more prominent in SCA2 patients in comparison with SCA1, SCA3, SCA6 (Burk, et al; 1999; Buttner et al., 1998; Rivaud-Pechoux et al., 1998) and late onset cerebellar ataxia (Rufa & Federighi, 2011) giving an important diagnostic value to this oculomotor feature for SCA2.

A comprehensive electronystagmographical study developed in 82 SCA2 Cuban patients showed little overlap between maximal saccadic velocity (MSV) values of SCA2 patients and controls. This study demonstrated a high sensitivity for SCA2 diagnosis assessed by a receiver operating characteristic (ROC) yielding an area under the curve of 0.99. The most important finding of this work was the significant influence of the number of CAG repeats, but not of disease duration, on saccadic velocity (Figure 1). According to this relationship, patients with larger expansions showed more saccadic slowing, identifying the saccadic velocity as the main variable endophenotype of the SCA2, which is under strong genetic control and therefore it may be considered as a sensitive biomarker for the study of polyglutamine toxicity. Also, MSV was negatively correlated with the total score of a cerebellar ataxia scale suggesting its association with the severity of the cerebellar syndrome (Velázquez et al., 2004). Other study performed in Cuban SCA2 patients revealed a closer relationship between the saccadic velocity and the visuomotor learning capabilities assessed by a prism adaptation task (Fernandez-Ruiz, et al., 2007).

A preliminary follow-up evaluation of saccadic slowing after one year in 30 SCA2 patients revealed no significant changes of MSV (Seifried et al., 2004). Nevertheless, other follow-up study during a larger period time it is being conducted in a large Cuban SCA2 cohort.

The saccadic slowing appears during the presymptomatic stage of the disease only for 60° target amplitude, but asymptomatic subjects carrying full-penetrant CAG expansions (≥36) show reduced MSV values even for 30°. In fact, the MSV reduction is stronger in carriers of large expansions. This preclinical feature progresses insidiously and it correlates with predicted time to clinical manifestation, which classifies this variable as a preclinical biomarker of high values for diagnosis and prognosis of the disease (Velázquez-Pérez et al., 2009b).

The neuroanatomical basis of this disorder has been elucidated by post-mortem studies that demonstrated the marked loss of excitatory PBN in the PPRF (Buttner-Ennever, et al., 1985; Geiner et al., 2008), the structure that coordinates the horizontal saccades (Leigh & Zee, 2006). Early, Gierga et al, 2005 had reported a significant neuronal death in the abducens (cranial nerve VI) and oculomotor nucleus (cranial nerve III), which innervate the oculomotor muscles responsible for eye movements in the horizontal plane (Leigh & Zee, 2006).

Hypometric saccades to extreme gaze positions are usual in SCA2 patients (Velázquez, 2008), nevertheless for short target amplitudes the saccade accuracy is maintained, although some patients can make hypermetric saccades. It has been suggested that as SCA2 patients having slow saccades that are no longer ballistic, visual feedback might be continuously available during the movement execution to guide the eye to its target rendering accurate short saccades (Federighi et al., 2011).

A recent electronystagmographical study in 110 SCA2 patients demonstrated the significant prolongation of saccadic latency in 46% of SCA2 patients. This variable was neither influenced by the CAG repeats, disease duration nor ataxia score, but it was close related with the neuropsychological performance of frontal-executive tasks, which highlights the saccadic latency as sensitive biomarker of cognitive disorders in SCA2 (Rodríguez-Labrada, et al., 2011a). Additionally, SCA2 patients show increased antisaccadic error rate (Rivaud-Pechoux et al., 1998). The delayed saccade onset and antisaccadic deficits could be explained by the severe gyral atrophy and neuronal loss in the frontal lobes and neurodegenerative changes in caudate nucleus and substantia nigra (Orozco et al., 1989; Durr et al., 1995; Estrada et al., 1999; Gierga et al., 2005), as well as deficits in the processing

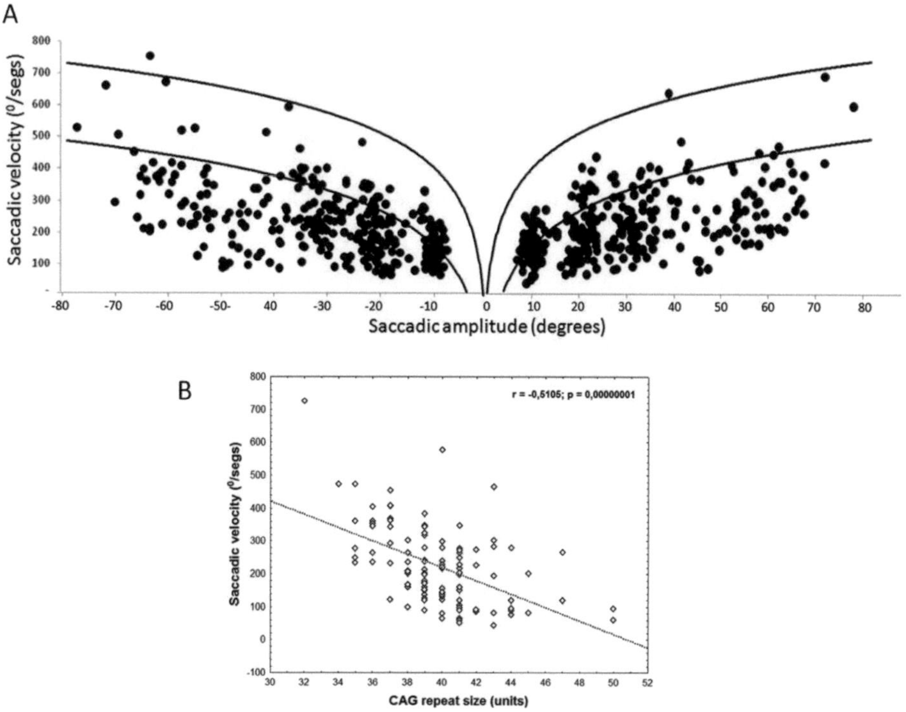

Fig. 1. Saccadic slowing in SCA2. A) Relationship of saccadic velocity and amplitudes in SCA2 patients. Show the significant reduction of saccadic velocity in almost all subjects. Dark lines represent the saccadic velocity ± 2 SD of controls. B) Influence of CAG repeat size on the saccadic velocity.

of visual information (Kremlacek et al., 2011) or in the visual-spatial attention (Le Pira et al., 2002).

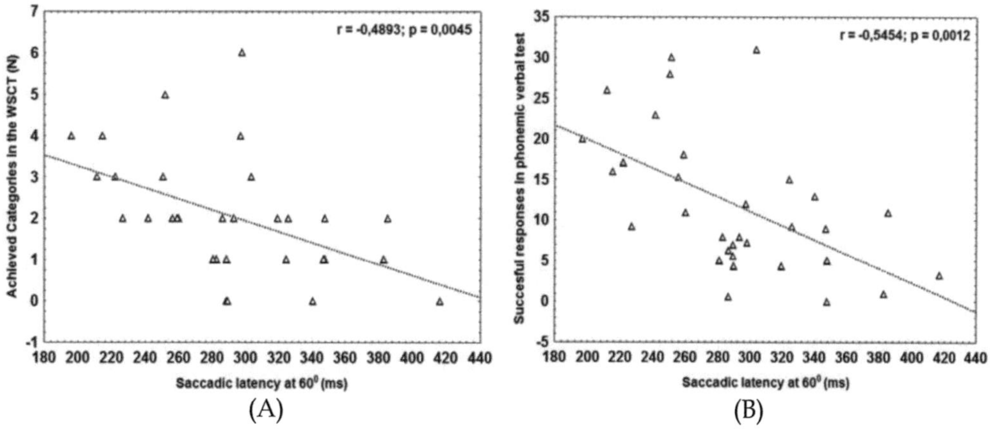

Fig. 2. Saccadic latency correlates with frontal-executive dysfunctions in SCA2 patients. Correlation analyses of saccadic latency with achieved categories in the Wisconsin sort card test (WSCT) and the number of correct responses in the phonemic verbal test.

Other oculomotor alterations include ofthalmoplegia, which usually appears at advanced disease in the 45% of the cases, although the severe saccadic slowing might overlook the frequency of ofthalmoplegia in SCA2. These patients have mild reduction of smooth pursuit gain in correspondence with the atrophy of cerebellar floculus (Ying et al., 2006) and the decrease of catch up saccades. The physiological and pathological nystagmus are very rare in SCA2 due to impaired ability to produce saccadic corrective phases. Some SCA2 patients have VOR responses with reduced gain (Burk et al., 1999; Rivaud-Pechoux et al., 1998; Buttner et al., 1998).

Saccadic eye movements have also been used to evaluate the efficacy of therapeutical alternatives in Cuban SCA2 patients, such as neurorehabilitation (Rodríguez et al., 2008) and oral supplementation with zinc-sulphate (Velázquez-Pérez et al, 2011a). In both cases the saccadic latency decreased significantly after the therapies, but saccadic velocity and dysmetria were unchanged.

For SCA2, the oculomotor function has not only evaluated in wake state, since the density of rapid eye movements (saccadic) during REM sleep was recently assessed. Both symptomatic and presymptomatic subjects show a marked decrease in this parameter, which is negatively correlated with the ataxia score in the patients (Velázquez-Pérez, et al., 2011b; Rodríguez-Labrada et al., 2011b). These findings suggest the usefulness of saccadic density during REM sleep as progression marker of the disease and reflect the extension of the oculomotor brainstem involvement to the sleep.

3.3 Spinocerebellar ataxia type 3 (SCA3)

Pathological nystagmus are prominent oculomotor signs of SCA3 patients. The frequency of gaze evoked and rebound nystagmus is approximately 90% (Jardim et al., 2001) being higher than those in SCA1, SCA2 and SCA6. Square wave jerks are usually reported in SCA3 subjects, unlike SCA1 and SCA2 individuals (Buttner et al, 1998; Burk et al., 1998). This oculomotor sign results from cerebellar disease and consists in small, horizontal, saccade-like movements that lead the eye away from the target trajectory and, after a delay, bring it back onto the target (Leigh & Zee, 2006).

Decreased VOR gain can be detected in majority of SCA3 patients and correlates with the CAG repeats, suggesting the pathologic involvement of the vestibular nuclei in the lateral brainstem. Furthermore, these patients show reduction of smooth pursuit and OKR gains with a presentation frequency above 70% in both cases (Buttner et al, 1998; Burk et al., 1998).

Upon saccades, the main abnormality is saccadic dysmetria. Nevertheless, there are apparently conflicting data regarding the predominant type of dysmetria. Buttner et al., 1998 reported hypermetric saccades in 86% of the cases, while Rivauld-Pechoux et al., 1998, observed a predominance of hypometric (56%) over hypermetric saccades (18%). The disagreement can be explained by differences in the clinical stage of studied patients. In fact, the 81% of the patients recruited by Rivauld-Pechoux and colleagues had a moderate to severe motor disability, which could explain the higher prevalence of saccadic hypometria.

Different to SCA2 and SCA1, decreased saccadic velocity is not a common feature of SCA3 patients (Burk et al., 1999; Rivaud-Pechoux et al., 1998; Buttner et al., 1998). This oculomotor feature appears in advanced disease, perhaps in correspondence with the degenerative changes seen in the raphe interpositus nucleus (Rub et al., 2003), a key structure of the brainstem premotor network that contains the omnipausas neurons, a group of cells that play an important role in determining the size of the velocity command for saccades, beside their well-known role as gating saccades (Miura & Optican, 2006). Also, internuclear and nuclear ophthalmoplegia is observed in 53% and 10% of the cases respectively. The latter is associated with a more severe disease course (Jardim et al., 2001).

Finally, the prolongation of saccadic latency occurs late in few cases (14%) (Buttner et al., 1998) and the performance in the antisaccadic paradigm shows an increase in the number of errors (Rivaud-Pechoux et al., 1998).

3.4 Spinocerebellar ataxia type 6 (SCA6)

Oculomotor function of SCA6 patients is characterized by signs of cerebellar and vestibular impairments such as horizontal and vertical nystagmus, abnormal smooth pursuit, saccadic dysmetria and abnormal VOR (Buttner et al., 1998; Christova et al., 2008; Bour et al., 2008). In comparison with other SCAs, the spontaneous downbeat nystagmus and square-wave jerks have the higher incidence in SCA6 subjects, whereas gaze-evoked nystagmus, rebound nystagmus and periodic alternating nystagmus are common features too (Buttner et al., 1998; Colen et al., 2008; Kim et al., 2010).

Patients with SCA6 have the more severe pursuit, OKN and VOR-fixed deficits among other polyglutamine SCAs but these oculomotor signs are not directly associated to CAG repeats or disease duration (Buttner et al., 1998). Vertical pursuit is impaired more than horizontal whereas downward pursuit more than upward (Bour et al., 2008).

The pattern of saccadic dysmetria in SCA6 is variable since these patients can show both hypometric and hypermetric saccades (Buttner et al., 1998; Bour et al., 2008). Although the decrease of saccadic velocity is not a prominent sign in these patients, it has been reported a mild saccadic slowing in some subjects both for the horizontal and vertical planes (Bour et al., 2008). These findings suggest functional extracerebellar impairment in the saccadic system and therefore are opposed to the paradigm of SCA6 as a "pure cerebellar syndrome." In fact, the screening of non-ataxia signs reveals a 25% of brainstem oculomotor signs (Schmitz-Hübsch, et al., 2008). In these patients the saccadic latency is normal (Buttner et al., 1998).

In 2009, Christova and co-workers studied the eye movement's abnormalities in both symptomatic and asymptomatic SCA6 cohorts and noticed that square-wave jerks, saccadic abnormalities and depressed smooth pursuit can be detected even before the disease onset. Among them, the square-wave jerks were the most prominent with an apparition frequency of 80% (Christova et al., 2008).

3.5 Spinocerebellar ataxia type 7 (SCA7)

The major saccadic alteration in this SCA is the slowing of saccades, together with saccadic dysmetria (Miller et al., 2009; Manrique et al., 2009). The decrease in saccadic velocity in SCA7 is associated with marked pontine atrophy that characterizes these patients from early stages of the disease and progresses to produce significant external ophthalmoplegia in patients with longer disease history (Bang et al., 2004; Martin et al., 1999). These alterations may precede cerebellar and retinal manifestations and are among the earliest signs of the disease (Oh et al., 2001). In addition, some cases have difficulties to initiate the saccadic eye movements and may develop gaze evoked nystagmus (Miller et al., 2009; Manrique et al., 2009).

3.6 Spinocerebellar ataxia type 17 (SCA17)

The patients with SCA17 show hypometric saccades in correspondence with the marked reduction of Purkinje cells in the cerebellum (Hubner et al., 2007). The saccadic hypometria is increased with disease duration but neither with ataxia score nor the number of CAG repeats. In 26% of cases, there are transient saccadic decelerations and accelerations causing hypometric saccades with multiple steps. Clinical assessments have reported normal (Nakamura, 2001) or slowed saccades (Rolfs et al., 2003), although the hypometria or prematurely terminated saccades may conduce to the erroneous classification of slowed saccades. In these patients, the saccadic latency is normal, while antisaccades have a significant increase in the error rate (Hubner et al., 2007).

Smooth pursuit abnormalities in SCA17 patients include decrease of initial eye acceleration, which appears even in the asymptomatic and mildly affected SCA17 mutation carriers, reduced steady state velocity and prolongation of smooth pursuit latency. Smooth pursuit gain decreases with the disease duration and ataxia score, whereas the latency prolongation correlates positively with the ataxia score. Gaze-evoked nystagmus is not a prominent feature in SCA17 patients (Hubner et al., 2007).

3.7 Other spinocerebellar ataxias

With the exception of polyglutamine expansions SCAs, the oculomotor function of remaining SCAs has not been systematically studied while most of data result for clinical assessment. SCA5 is characterized by eye abnormalities owing to cerebellar impairments such as downbeat nystagmus and impaired smooth pursuit movements (Ranum et al., 1994; Ikeda et al., 2002). Similar features occur in SCA8, in addition to saccadic dysmetria (Day et al., 2000; Koob et al., 1999), and SCA10 (Zu et al., 2000; Grewal et al., 2002; Lin & Ashizawa, 2005). SCA11 is associated with horizontal and vertical nystagmus as well as jerky pursuit (Worth et al., 1999), while approximately one third of SCA12 patients can develop saccadic slowing, abnormal smooth pursuits or pathological nystagmus (Worth et al., 1999, Fujigasaki et al., 2001). Besides, in subjects affected with SCA13 is usual to observe horizontal nystagmus (Stevanin et al., 2005; Waters & Pulst, 2008).

Regarding SCA14, the main oculomotor disturbance is the hypermetria of downgaze and horizontal saccades, even from the early stages of the disease. Additionally, upwards gaze evoked nystagmus are common in patients with longer disease duration. Smooth pursuit movements and VOR are also impaired (Yamashita et al, 2000; Brkanac et al, 2002a; Fahey et al., 2005). Eye movement abnormalities of SCA15/16 and SCA18 include nystagmus for all these SCA subtypes associated to saccadic dysmetria in the first one (Miyoshi et al., 2001; Brkanac et al, 2002b; Gardner et al., 2005). In addition, hypermetric saccades into downgaze and lateral gaze are detected in some patients with SCA20 (Knight et al., 2004).

SCA22 patients show nystagmus and impaired smooth pursuit with intermittent corrective saccadic (Chung et al., 2003), while in SCA23 the ocular dysmetria and slowed saccades can be noted (Verbeek et al., 2004; Verbeek, 2009). SCA25, SCA26 and SCA27 are characterized by pathological nystagmus in some patients, associated with slow eye movements in SCA25, abnormal pursuit in SCA26 and saccadic dysmetria in SCA27 (van Swieten, et al., 2003; Stevanin et al. 2004; Yu et al., 2005). SCA28 patients develop gaze-evoked nystagmus at early disease, while subjects with advanced disease have slowed saccades and ophthalmoparesis with frequency estimates of 60% and 80% respectively (Cagnoli et al., 2006). SCA29, which overlap with SCA15, is characterized by bilateral horizontal nystagmus (Dudding et al., 2004). In the case of SCA30, hypermetric saccades and gaze evoked nystagmus can be detected (Storey et al., 2009), as well as abnormal pursuit in SCA31 (Ishikawa et al., 2004). Finally, in a new SCA subtype recently identified by Wang et al., 2010 in two Chinese families, it was observed ocular dysmetria as main oculomotor sign.

4. Conclusions

Eye movement abnormalities are among the most common phenotypic manifestations of patients with SCAs. The most prominent oculomotor feature is the presence of pathological nystagmus in almost all subtypes, which is generally associated to abnormal smooth pursuit, saccadic dysmetria, impaired VOR/OKR, saccadic slowing and ophthalmoplegia. These oculomotor phenotypes are useful, but not determinant, for the differential diagnosis of SCAs. For example, the early and severe saccadic slowing with rare pathological nystagmus distinguishes SCA2 from SCA1, SCA3, SCA6, SCA17 and other SCA subtypes, whereas the marked abnormalities of smooth pursuit, VOR and OKR; in association with pathological nystagmus and rare saccadic slowing may help to define a SCA6 phenotype. Nevertheless, the notable overlapping of oculomotor features between SCA subtypes implies the requirement of other clinical criteria or the genetic testing for sensitively discriminating among these diseases.

The study of eye movement abnormalities allows the identification of several biomarkers useful in the clinical and research practice of SCAs. Some of the oculomotor disturbances precede the ataxia onset, being important preclinical markers to detect the early stages of the neurodegenerative process, to evaluate the genetic susceptibility of the asymptomatic relatives and to identify individuals close to ataxia onset for enrollment in preventive clinical trials and as potential outcome variables in these same trials. As most of the oculomotor abnormalities of SCAs are significantly accentuated with the advance of the disease, these can be used in monitoring clinical progression and therefore to assess the response to symptomatic treatments at short, medium or long term. The number of CAG repeats influences significantly on the saccadic slowing in SCA2 and the reduced VOR gain in SCA3 classifying these oculomotor features as sensitive biomarker of genetic damage, useful to evaluate the effect of modifying factors and therapeutic alternatives on the polyglutamine toxicity.

Despite the above, still is necessary to deep more into the study of oculomotor function in SCAs. For example, vergence movements have not been studied, in spite of the known role of the cerebellum in these eye movements (Robinson & Fuchs, 2001) and the correspondent vergence deficits in patients with circumscribed cerebellar lesions (Sender et al., 2009). Moreover, further neuropathological, imaging and transcranial magnetic stimulation studies are required to focus the oculomotor system in order to provide more insight on eye movement abnormalities and its potential role as therapeutic biomarkers in SCAs.

5. Acknowledgements

We are very indebted to Cuban Ministry of Public Health and to the Iberoamerican Multidisciplinary Network for the Movement Disorders Study: Parkinson disease and Spinocerebellar Ataxias. (RIBERMOV, abbreviation in Spanish).

6. References

Aw ST, Haslwanter T, Halmagyi GM, Curthoys IS, Yavor RA & Todd MJ. (1996). Three-dimensional vector analysis of the human vestibuloocular reflex in response to high-acceleration head rotations. I. Responses in normal subjects. *Journal of Neurophysiology*, Vol.76, pp. 4009-20, ISSN 1522-1598.

Bahill AT, Clark MR & Stark L. (1975) The main sequence, a tool for studying human eye movements. *Mathematical Biosciences*, Vol.24, pp. 191–204, ISSN 0025-5564.

Bang OY, Lee PH, Kim SY, Kim HJ & Huh K. (2004). Pontine atrophy precedes cerebellar degeneration in spinocerebellar ataxia 7: MRI-based volumetric analysis. *Journal of Neurology Neurosurgery and Psychiatry*, Vol.75, No.10, pp. 1452-6, ISSN 1468-330X.

Bour LJ, van Rootselaar AF, Koelman JH & Tijssen MA. (2008). Oculomotor abnormalities in myoclonic tremor: a comparison with spinocerebellar ataxia type 6. *Brain*, Vol.131, pp. 2295-303, ISSN 1460-2156.

Brkanac Z, Bylenok L, Fernandez M, Matsushita M, Lipe H, Wolff J, et al. (2002a). A new dominant spinocerebellar ataxia linked to chromosome 19q13.4-qter. *Archives of Neurology*, Vol.59, No.8, pp. 1291-95, ISSN 1538-3687.

Brkanac Z, Fernandez M, Matsushita M, Lipe H, Wolff J, Bird TD & Raskind WH. (2002b). Autosomal dominant sensory/motor neuropathy with Ataxia (SMNA): Linkage to chromosome 7q22-q32. *American Journal of Medical Genetics*, Vol.114, No.4, pp. 450-57, ISSN 0148-7299.

Bruce CH & Friedman HR. (2002). Eye Movements. *Encyclopedia of the Human Brain*, Vol. 2, pp. 269-97.

Burk K, Fetter M, Abele M, Laccone F, Brice A, Dichgans J, et al. (1999). Autosomal dominant cerebellar ataxia type I: oculomotor abnormalities in families with SCA1, SCA2, and SCA3. *Journal of Neurology*, Vol.246, No.9, pp. 789-97, ISSN 0340-5354.

Buttner JA, Geschwind D, Jen JC, Perlman S, Pulst SM & Baloh RW.(1998). Oculomotor phenotypes in autosomal dominant ataxias. *Archives of Neurology*, Vol.55, No.10, pp. 1353-7, ISSN 1538-3687.

Buttner-Ennever JA, Wadia NH, Sakai H & Schwendeman G. (1985) Neuroanatomy of oculomotor structures in olivopontocerebellar atrophy (OPCA) patient with slow saccades. Journal of Neurology, Vol.232, Suppl 285, ISSN 0340-5354

Cancel G, Durr A, Didierjean O, Imbert G, Burk K, Lezin A, et al. (1997). Molecular and clinical correlations in spinocerebellar ataxia 2: a study of 32 families. *Human Molecular Genetics*, Vol.6, No.5, pp. 709-15, ISSN 1460-2083.

Cagnoli C, Mariotti C, Taroni F, Seri M, Brussino A, Michielotto C, et al. (2006). SCA28, a novel form of autosomal dominant cerebellar ataxia on chromosome 18p11.22-q11.2. *Brain*. Vol.129, pp. 235-42, ISSN 1460-2156.

Carlson KM, Andresen JM & Orr HT. (2009). Emerging pathogenic pathways in the spinocerebellar ataxias. *Current Opinion in Genetics & Development*, Vol.19, No.3, pp. 247-53, ISSN 1879-0380.

Christova P, Anderson JH & Gomez C. (2008). Impaired Eye Movements in Presymptomatic Spinocerebellar Ataxia Type 6. *Archives of Neurology*, Vol.65, No.4, pp. 530-6, ISSN 1538-3687.

Chung MY, Lu YC, Cheng NC & Soong BW. (2003). A novel autosomal dominant spinocerebellar ataxia (SCA22) linked to chromosome 1p21-q23. *Brain*, Vol.126, Pp. 1293-1299, ISSN 0006-8950.

Colen C, Ketko A, George E & Van Stavern G. (2008). Periodic alternating nystagmus and periodic alternating skew deviation in spinocerebellar ataxia type 6. *Journal of Neuro-Ophthalmology*, Vol.28, pp. 287–88, ISSN 1536-5166.

Day JW, Schut LJ, Moseley ML, Durand AC & Ranum LP. (2000). Spinocerebellar ataxia type 8: clinical features in a large family. *Neurology*, Vol.55, No.5, pp.649–57, ISSN 1474-547X.

Dudding TE, Friend K, Schofield PW, Lee S, Wilkinson IA & Richards RI. 2004. Autosomal dominant congenital non-progressive ataxia overlaps with the SCA15 locus. *Neurology*, Vol. 63, pp. 2288-2292, ISSN 0028-3878.

Durr A, Smadja D, Cancel G, Lezin A, Stevanin G, Mikol J, et al. (1995). Autosomal dominant cerebellar ataxia type I in Martinique (French West Indies). Clinical and neuropathological analysis of 53 patients from three unrelated SCA2 families. *Brain*, Vol.118, pp.1573-81, ISSN 1460-2156.

Durr A. (2010). Autosomal dominant cerebellar ataxias: polyglutamine expansions and beyond. *Lancet Neurology*, Vol.9, pp. 885–94, ISSN 1474-4422.

Estrada R, Galarraga J, Orozco G, Nodarse A & Auburger G. (1999). Spinocerebellar ataxia 2 (SCA2): morphometric analyses in 11 autopsies. *Acta Neuropathologica*, Vol.97, No.3, pp. 306-10, ISSN 1432-0533.

Fahey MC, Knight MA, Shaw JH, McK Gardner RJ, du Sart D, Lockhart PJ, et al. (2005). Spinocerebellar ataxia type 14: study of a family with an exon 5 mutation in the PRKCG gene. *Journal of Neurology, Neurosurgery and Psychiatry*, Vol.76, pp. 1720–22, ISSN 1468-330X.

Federighi P, Cevenini G, Dotti MT, Rosini F, Pretegiani E, Federico A, et al. (2011). Differences in saccade dynamics between spinocerebellar ataxia 2 and late-onset cerebellar ataxias. *Brain*, Vol.134, pp. 879–91, ISSN 1460-2156.

Fernández-Ruiz J, Velásquez-Pérez L, Díaz R, Drucker-Colín R, Pérez-González R, et al. (2007). Prism adaptation in spinocerebellar ataxia type 2. *Neuropsychologia*, Vol.45, pp. 2692-98, ISSN 0028-3932.

Fujigasaki H, Verma IC, Camuzat A, Margolis RL, Zander C, Lebre AS, et al. (2001). SCA12 is a rare locus for autosomal dominant cerebellar ataxia: a study of an Indian family. *Annals of Neurology*, Vol.49, pp.117-21, ISSN 0364-5134.

Gardner RJ, Knight MA, Hara K, Tsuji S, Forrest SM & Storey E. (2005). Spinocerebellar ataxia type 15. *The Cerebellum*, Vol.4, No.1, pp. 47–50, ISSN 1473-4230.

Geiner S, Horn AK, Wadia NH, Sakai H & Buttner-Ennever JA. (2008). The neuroanatomical basis of slow saccades in spinocerebellar ataxia type 2 (Wadia-subtype). *Progress in Brain Research*, Vol.171, pp. 575-81. ISSN 1875-7855.

Gierga K, Burk K, Bauer M, Orozco G, Auburger G, Schultz C, et al. (2005). Involvement of the cranial nerves and their nuclei in spinocerebellar ataxia type 2 (SCA2). *Acta Neuropathologica*, Vol.109, pp. 617-31, ISSN 1432-0533.

Grewal RP, Achari M, Matsuura T, et al. (2002). Clinical features and ATTCT repeat expansion in spinocerebellar ataxia type 10. *Archives of Neurology*, Vol.59, pp. 1285–90, ISSN 1538-3687.

Harding AE. (1983). Classification of the hereditary ataxias and paraplegias. *The Lancet*, Vol.1, pp. 1151–55, ISSN 1474-547X.

Hikosaka O, Takikawa Y & Kawagoe R. (2000). Role of the basal ganglia in the control of purposive saccadic eye movements. *Physiological Reviews*, Vol.80, No.3, pp. 953-78, ISSN 0031-9333.

Holmes SE, O'Hearn EE, McInnis MG, Gorelick-Feldman DA, Kleiderlein JJ, Callahan C, et al. (1999). Expansion of a novel CAG trinucleotide repeat in the 5' region of PPP2R2B is associated with SCA12. *Nature Genetics*, Vol.23, pp.391-92, ISSN 1061-4036.

Hubner J, Sprenger A, Klein C, Hagenah J, Rambold H, Zuhlke C, et al. (2007). Eye movement abnormalities in spinocerebellar ataxia type 17 (SCA17). *Neurology*, Vol.69, No.11, pp. 1160-8, ISSN 0028-3878.

Ikeda Y, Dick KA, Weatherspoon MR, Gincel D, Armbrust KR, Dalton JC et al. (2006). Spectrin mutations cause spinocerebellar ataxia type 5. *Nature Genetics*, Vol.38, pp. 184–90, ISSN 1061-4036.

Ishikawa K, Toru S, Tsunemi T, Li M, Kobayashi K, Yokota T, et al. (2005). An autosomal dominant cerebellar ataxia linked to chromosome 16q22.1 is associated with a single-nucleotide substitution in the 5' untranslated region of the gene encoding a protein with spectrin repeat and Rho guanine-nucleotide exchange-factor domains. American Journal of Humab Genetics, Vol.77, No.2, pp. 280-96, ISSN 0002-9297.

Jardim LB, Pereira ML, Silveira I, Ferro A, Sequeiros J & Giugliani R. (2001). Neurologic findings in Machado-Joseph disease: relation with disease duration, subtypes, and (CAG)n. *Archives of Neurology*, Vol.58, No.6, pp. 899-904, ISSN 1538-3687.

Karatas M. (2009). Internuclear and supranuclear disorders of eye movements: clinical features and causes. *European Journal of Neurology*, Vol.16, pp.1265–77, ISSN 1468-1331.

Kim JM, Lee JY, Kim HJ, Kim JS, Kim YK, Park SS, et al. (2010). The wide clinical spectrum and nigrostriatal dopaminergic damage in spinocerebellar ataxia type 6. *Journal of Neurology, Neurosurgery and Psychiatry*, Vol.81, pp. 529–32, ISSN 1468-330X.

Klostermann W, Zuhlke C, Heide W, Kompf D & Wessel K. (1997). Slow saccades and other eye movement disorders in spinocerebellar atrophy type 1. *Journal of Neurology*, Vol.244, No.2, pp.105-11, ISSN 0340-5354.

Knight MA, Gardner RJ, Bahlo M, Matsuura T, Dixon JA, Forrest SM, et al. (2004). Dominantly inherited ataxia and dysphonia with dentate calcification: spinocerebellar ataxia type 20. *Brain*, Vol.127, No. 5, pp. 1172–81, ISSN 1460-2156.

Koob MD, Moseley ML, Schut LJ, Benzow KA, Bird TD, Day JW, et al. (1999). An untranslated CTG expansion causes a novel form of spinocerebellar ataxia (SCA8). *Nature Genetics*, Vol.21, pp. 379–84, ISSN 1061-4036.

Kremlacek J, Valis M, Masopust J, Talab R, Kuba M, Kobova Z, et al. (2011). An Electrophysiological Study of Visual Processing in Spinocerebellar Ataxia Type 2 (SCA2). *The Cerebellum*, Vol.10, pp. 32–42, ISSN 1473-4230.

Kulkarni SA & Wadia NH. (1975) Model of an oculomotor subsystem. *International Journal of Biomedical Computation*, Vol6, pp. 1-21, ISSN 0020-7101.

Le Pira F, Zappala G, Saponara R, Domina E, Restivo DA, Regio E, et al. (2002). Cognitive findings in spinocerebellar ataxia type 2: Relationship to genetic and clinical variables *Journal of the Neurological Sciences*, Vol.201, pp. 53–7, ISSN 0022-510X.

Leigh RJ & Kennard C. (2004). Using saccades as a research tool in the clinical neurosciences. *Brain*, Vol.127, pp. 460–77, ISSN 1460-2156.

Leigh RJ & Zee DS. (2006). *The neurology of eye movements* (4th Ed), Oxford University Press, New York, USA.

Lencer R & Trillenberg P. (2008). Neurophysiology and neuroanatomy of smooth pursuit in humans. *Brain and Cognition*, Vol.68, pp. 219–28, ISSN 1090-2147.

Lin X & Ashizawa T. (2005). Recent progress in spinocerebellar ataxia type-10 (SCA10). *The Cerebellum*, Vol. 4, pp. 37–42, ISSN 1473-4230.

Matilla-Dueñas A, Goold R & Giunti P. (2008) Clinical, genetic, molecular, and pathophysiological insights into spinocerebellar ataxia type 1. *The Cerebellum*, Vol. 7 pp. 106-114, ISSN 1473-4222.

Manrique RK, Noval S, Aguilar-Amat MJ, Arpa J, Rosa I & Contreras I. (2009). Ophthalmic Features of Spinocerebellar Ataxia Type 7. *Journal of Neuro-Opthalmology*, Vol.29, pp. 174-9, ISSN 1536-5166.

Martin J, Van Regemorter N, Del-Favero J, Lofgren A & Van Broeckhoven C. (1999). Spinocerebellar ataxia type 7 (SCA7) - correlations between phenotype and genotype in one large Belgian family. *Journal of the Neurological Sciences*, Vol.168, No.1, pp. 37-46, ISSN 0022-510X.

Miller R, Tewari A, Miller J, Garbern J & Van Stavern GP. (2009). Neuro-ophthalmologic features of spinocerebellar ataxia type 7. *Journal of Neuro-Ophthalmol*, Vol.29, pp. 180–86, ISSN 1536-5166.

Miura K & Optican LM. (2006). Membrane channel properties of premotor excitatory burst neurons may underlie saccade slowing after lesions of omnipause neurons. *Journal of Computational Neuroscience*, Vol.20, pp.25–41, ISSN 1573-6873.

Miyoshi Y, Yamada T, Tanimura M, Taniwaki T, Arakawa K, Ohyagi Y, et al. (2001). A novel autosomal dominant spinocerebellar ataxia (SCA16) linked to chromosome 8q22.1-24.1. *Neurology, Vol.*57, No.1, pp. 96-100, ISSN 1526-632X.

Müri RM & Nyffeler T. (2008) Neurophysiology and neuroanatomy of reflexive and volitional saccades as revealed by lesion studies with neurological patients and transcranial magnetic stimulation (TMS). *Brain and Cognition, Vol.*68, pp. 284–292, ISSN 1090-2147.

Mustari MJ, Ono S & Das VE. (2009) Signal Processing and Distribution in Cortical-Brainstem Pathways for Smooth Pursuit Eye Movements. *Annals of New York Academy of Sciences*, Vol.1164, pp. 147–154, ISSN 0077-8923.

Nakamura K. (2001). SCA17, a novel polyglutamine disease caused by the expansion of polyglutamine tracts in TATA-binding protein. *Rinsho Shinkeigaku*, Vol.41, pp. 1123–25.

Oh AK, Jacobson KM, Jen JC & Baloh RW. (2001). Slowing of voluntary and involuntary saccades: an early sign in spinocerebellar ataxia type 7. *Annals of Neurology*, Vol.49, No.6, pp. 801-4, ISSN 1531-8249.

Orozco DG, Estrada R, Perry T, Araña J & Fernández R. (1989). Dominantly inherited olivopontocerebellar atrophy from eastern Cuba. Clinical, neuropathological and biochemimical findings. *Journal of the Neurological Sciences*, Vol.93, pp. 37-50, ISSN 0022-510X.

Pierrot-Deseilligny C, Mileab D & Müri RM. (2004). Eye movement control by the cerebral cortex. *Current opinion in neurology*, Vol.17, pp. 17-25, ISSN 1350-7540.

Prsa M. & Their P. (2011) The role of the cerebellum in saccadic adaptation as a window into neural mechanisms of motor learning. *European Journal of Neuroscience*, Vol.33, pp. 2114–2128, ISSN 0953-816X.

Pula JH, Gomez CM & Kattah JC. (2010). Ophthalmologic features of the common spinocerebellar ataxias. *Current Opinion in Ophtalmology*, Vol.21, No.6, pp. 447-53, ISSN 1531-7021.

Ramat S, Leigh RJ, Zee DS & Optican LM. (2007). What clinical disorders tell us about the neural control of saccadic eye movements. *Brain*, Vol.130, pp. 10-35, ISSN 1460-2156.

Ranum LP, Schut LJ, Lundgren JK, Orr HT & Livingston DM. (1994). Spinocerebellar ataxia type 5 in a family descended from the grandparents of President Lincoln maps to chromosome 11. *Nature Genetics*, Vol. 8, pp. 280–84, ISSN 1061-4036.

Reilly JL, Lencer R, Bishop JR, Keedy S & Sweeney JA. (2008). Pharmacological treatment effects on eye movement control. *Brain and Cognition*, Vol.68, pp. 415-35, ISSN 1090-2147.

Rivaud-Pechoux S, Durr A, Gaymard B, Cancel G, Ploner CJ, Agid Y, et al. (1998). Eye movement abnormalities correlate with genotype in autosomal dominant cerebellar ataxia type I. *Annals of Neurology*, Vol.43, pp. 297-302, ISSN 1531-8249.

Robinson FR & Fuchs AF. (2001). The role of the cerebellum in voluntary eye movements. *Annual Review of Neuroscience*, Vol.24, pp. 981-1004, ISSN 1545-4126.

Rodríguez Díaz JC, Velázquez-Pérez L, Sanchez Cruz G, Almaguer Gotay D, Rodríguez Labrada R, Aguilera Rodríguez R, et al. (2008). Evaluation of Neurological Restoration in patients with Spinocerebellar Ataxia type 2. *Plasticidad & Restauración Neurológica*, Vol.7, pp. 13-8.

Rodríguez-Labrada R; Velázquez-Pérez L; Seigfried C; Canales-Ochoa N; Auburger G; Medrano-Montero J; et al. (2011a). Saccadic latency is prolonged in Spinocerebellar Ataxia type 2 and correlates with the frontal-executive dysfunctions. *Journal of the Neurological Sciences*, Vol.306, pp. 103-07, ISSN 0022-510X.

Rodríguez-Labrada R, Velázquez-Pérez L, Canales Ochoa N, et al. (2011b). Subtle Rapid Eye Movement sleep abnormalities in presymptomatic Spinocerebellar Ataxia type 2 gene carriers. *Movement Disorders*, Vol.26, pp. 347-50, ISSN 1531-8257.

Rolfs A, Koeppen AH, Bauer I, Bauer P, Buhlmann S, Topka H, et al. (2003). Clinical features and neuropathology of autosomal dominant spinocerebellar ataxia (SCA17). *Annals of Neurology*, Vol.54, pp. 367–75, ISSN 1531-8249.

Rüb U, Brunt ER, Gierga K, Schultz C, Paulson H, de Vos RA, et al. (2003). The nucleus raphe interpositus in spinocerebellar ataxia type 3 (Machado-Joseph disease). *Journal of Chemical Neuroanatomy*, Vol.25, No.2, pp.115-27, ISSN 0891-0618.

Rüb U, Jen JC, Braak H & Deller T. (2008). Functional neuroanatomy of the human premotor oculomotor brainstem nuclei: insights from postmortem and advanced in vivo imaging studies. *Experimental Brain Research*, Vol.187, pp. 167-80, ISSN 0014-4819.

Rufa & Federigh. (2011) Fast versus slow: different saccadic behaviour in cerebellar ataxias. In Basic and Clinical Ocular Motor and Vestibular Research. Rucker J & Zee DS, Eds. Annals of the New York Academy of Sciences, Vol.1233, pp. 148–154. ISSN 0077-8923.

Sander T, Sprenger A, Neumann G, Machner B, Gottschalk S, Rambold H, et al. (2009). Vergence deficits in patients with cerebellar lesions. *Brain*, Vol.132, pp. 103-15, ISSN 1460-2156.

Schmitz-Hübsch T, Coudert M, Bauer P, Giunti P, Globas C, Baliko L, et al. (2008). Spinocerebellar ataxia types 1, 2, 3, and 6: disease severity and nonataxia symptoms. *Neurology*, Vol.71, pp. 982-989, ISSN 1526-632X.

Seifried C, Velazquez-Perez L, Santos-Falcon N, Abele M, Ziemann U, Almaguer LE, et al. (2005). Saccade velocity as a surrogate disease marker in spinocerebellar ataxia type 2. *Annals of New York Academy of Sciences*, Vol.1039, pp. 524-7, ISSN 0077-8923.

Shires J, Joshi S & Basso MA. (2010). Shedding new light on the role of the basal ganglia-superior colliculus pathway in eye movements. *Current Opinion in Neurobiology*, Vol.20, pp. 1–9, ISSN 0959-4388.

Soong BW & Paulson HL. (2007). Spinocerebellar ataxias: an update. *Current Opinion in Neurology*, Vol.20, No.4, pp. 438-46, ISSN 1350-7540.

Sparks DL. (2002). The brainstem control of saccadic eye movements. *Nature Reviews Neuroscience*, Vol.3, No.12, pp. 952-64, ISSN 1471-0048.

Stevanin G, Bouslam N, Thobois S, Azzedine H, Ravaux L, Boland A, et al. (2004). Spinocerebellar ataxia with sensory neuropathy (SCA25) maps to chromosome 2p. *Annals of Neurology*, vol.55, No.1, pp. 97-104, ISSN 0364-5134.

Stevanin G, Durr A, Benammar N & Brice A. (2005). Spinocerebellar ataxia with mental retardation (SCA13). *The Cerebellum*, Vol.4, No.1, pp. 43-46, ISSN 1473-4222.

Storey E, Bahlo M, Fahey M, Sisson O, Lueck CJ & Gardner RJ. (2009). A new dominantly inherited pure cerebellar ataxia, SCA 30. *Journal of Neurology Neurosurgery and Psychiatry*, Vol.80, pp. 408–11, ISSN 1468-330X.

Strupp M, Hüfner K, Sandmann R, Zwergal A, Dieterich M, Jahn K, et al. (2011). Central Oculomotor Disturbances and Nystagmus. A Window Into the Brainstem and Cerebellum. *Deutsches Ärzteblatt International*, Vol.108, No.12, pp. 197–204.

Thurtell MJ, Tomsak RL & Leigh RJ. (2007). Disorders of saccades. *Current neurology and neuroscience reports*,Vol.7, No.5, pp. 407-16, ISSN 1528-4042.

Tusa R. & D. Zee. (1989). Cerebral control of smooth pursuit and optokinetic nystagmus. *Current Opinion in Ophthalmology*. Vol.2, pp. 115–146, ISSN 1531-7021.

Vale J, Bugalho P, Silveira I, Sequeiros J, Guimaraes J & Coutinho P. (2010). Autosomal dominant cerebellar ataxia: frequency analysis and clinical characterization of 45 families from Portugal. *European Journal of Neurology*, Vol.17 pp. 124–28, ISSN 1468-1331.

van Swieten JC, Brusse E, de Graaf BM, Krieger E, van de Graaf R, de Koning I, et al. (2003). A mutation in the fibroblast growth factor 14 gene is associated with autosomal dominant cerebellar ataxia [corrected]. *American Journal of Human Genetics*, Vol.72, No.1, pp. 191-99, ISSN 0002-9297.

Velázquez L (2008). *Ataxia Espinocerebelosa tipo 2. Principales aspectos neurofisiológicos para el diagnóstico y pronóstico de la Enfermedad*, (2nd Ed), Ediciones Holguín, ISBN 959-221-202-3, Holguín, Cuba.

Velazquez Perez L, Cruz GS, Santos Falcon N, Enrique Almaguer Mederos L, Escalona Batallan K, Rodríguez Labrada R, et al. (2009a). Molecular epidemiology of spinocerebellar ataxias in Cuba: insights into SCA2 founder effect in Holguin. *Neuroscience Letters*, Vol.454, No.2, pp. 157-60, ISSN 0304-3940.

Velazquez-Perez L, Seifried C, Abele M, Wirjatijasa F, Rodriguez-Labrada R, Santos-Falcon N, et al. (2009b). Saccade velocity is reduced in presymptomatic spinocerebellar ataxia type 2. *Clinical Neurophysiology*, Vol.120, No.3, pp. 632-35, ISSN 1388-2457.

Velazquez-Perez L, Seifried C, Santos-Falcon N, Abele M, Ziemann U, Almaguer LE, et al. (2004). Saccade velocity is controlled by polyglutamine size in spinocerebellar ataxia 2. *Annals of Neurology*, Vol.56, No.3, pp. 444-47, ISSN 1531-8249.

Velázquez-Pérez L, Rodríguez-Chanfrau J, García-Rodríguez JC, Sánchez-Cruz G, Aguilera-Rodríguez R, et al. (2011a). Oral Zinc Sulphate Supplementation for Six Months in

SCA2 Patients: A Randomized, Double-Blind, Placebo-Controlled Trial. *Neurochemical Research,* In press, ISSN 1573-6903.

Velázquez-Pérez L, Voss U, Rodríguez-Labrada R, Auburger G, Canales Ochoa N, Sánchez Cruz G, Galicia Polo L, et al. (2011b). Sleep Disorders in Spinocerebellar Ataxia Type 2 Patients. *Neurodegenerative Diseases,* Vol.8; pp. 447-454, ISSN 1660-2862.

Verbeek DS, van de Warrenburg BP, Wesseling P, Pearson PL, Kremer HP & Sinke RJ. (2004). Mapping of the SCA23 locus involved in autosomal dominant cerebellar ataxia to chromosome region 20p13-12.3. *Brain,* Vol.127, pp. 2551-57, ISSN 1460-2156.

Verbeek DS. (2009). Spinocerebellar ataxia type 23: a genetic update. *The Cerebellum,* Vol.8, No.2, pp. 104-07, ISSN 1473-4222.

Vilis, T. (1997). Physiology of three-dimensional eye movements: saccades and vergence. In Three-Dimensional Kinematics of Eye, Head, and Limb Movements (M. Fetter, T. Haslwanter, H. Misslisch, and D. Tweed, Eds.), pp. 57–72. Harwood Academic Publishing, Amsterdam.

Voogd J, Schraa-Tam CKL, van der Geest JN & De Zeeuw CI. (2011) Visuomotor Cerebellum in Human and Nonhuman Primates. *The Cerebellum,* In press, ISSN 1473-4222.

Wadia NH & Swami RK. (1971) A new form of heredo-familial spinocerebellar degeneration with slow eye movements (nine families). *Brain,* Vol.94, pp. 359–374, ISSN 1460-2156.

Wadia N, Pang J, Desai J, Mankodi A, Desai M & Chamberlain S. (1998). A clinicogenetic analysis of six Indian spinocerebellar ataxia (SCA2) pedigrees. The significance of slow saccades in diagnosis. *Brain,* Vol.121, pp. 2341-55, ISSN 1460-2156.

Wang JL, Yang X, Xia K, Hu ZM, Weng L, Jin X, et al. (2010). TGM6 identified as a novel causative gene of spinocerebellar ataxias using exome sequencing. *Brain,* Vol.133, pp. 3510–18, ISSN 1460-2156.

Waters MF & Pulst SM. (2008). Sca13. *The Cerebellum, Vol.7,* No.2, pp. 165–169, ISSN 1473-4222.

Worth PF, Giunti P, Gardner-Thorpe C, et al. (1999). Autosomal dominant cerebellar ataxia type III: linkage in a large British family to a 7.6-cM region on chromosome 15q14-21.3. *American Journal of Human Genetics,* Vol.65, No.2, pp. 420–26, ISSN 0002-9297.

Yamashita I, Sasaki H, Yabe I, Fukazawa T, Nogoshi S, Komeichi K, et al. (2000). A novel locus for dominant cerebellar ataxia (SCA14) maps to a 10.2-cM interval flanked by D19S206 and D19S605 on chromosome 19q13.4-qter. *Annals of Neurology,* Vol.48, No.2, pp. 156-163, ISSN 0364-5134.

Ying SH, Choi SI, Perlman SL, Baloh RW, Zee DS &Toga AW. (2006). Pontine and cerebellar atrophy correlate with clinical disability in SCA2. *Neurology,* Vol.66, No.3, pp. 424-426, ISSN 1526-632X.

Yu GY, Howell MJ, Roller MJ, Xie TD & Gomez CM. (2005). Spinocerebellar ataxia type 26 maps to chromosome 19p13.3 adjacent to SCA6. *Annals of Neurology,* Vol.57, No.3, pp. 349-54, ISSN 0364-5134.

Zee DS, Yee RD, Cogan DG, Robinson DA & Engel WK. (1976). Ocular motor abnormalities in hereditary cerebellar ataxia. *Brain,* Vol.99, pp. 207-234, ISSN 1460-2156.

Zee DS & Levi L. (1989) Neurological aspects of vergence eye movements. *Revista de Neurologia (Paris),* Vol.145, No.8-9, pp. 613-2.

Zu L, Figueroa KP, Grewal R & Pulst SM. (1999). Mapping of a new autosomal dominant spinocerebellar ataxia to chromosome 22. *American Journal of Human Genetics,* Vol.64, pp. 594-599, ISSN 0002-9297.

5

Spinocerebellar Ataxia Type 2

Luis Velázquez-Pérez[1], Roberto Rodríguez-Labrada[1],
Hans-Joachim Freund[2] and Georg Auburger[3]
[1]*Centre for the Research and Rehabilitation of Hereditary Ataxias, Holguín,*
[2]*International Neuroscience Institute, Hannover,*
[3]*Section Experimental Neurology, Dept. Neurology,*
Goethe University Medical School, Frankfurt am Main,
[1]*Cuba*
[2,3]*Germany*

1. Introduction

The autosomal dominant cerebellar ataxias (ADCA) are a clinically, pathologically and genetically heterogeneous group of neurodegenerative disorders caused by degeneration of cerebellum and its afferent and efferent connections. The degenerative process may additionally involves the ponto- medullar systems, pyramidal tracts, basal ganglia, cerebral cortex, peripheral nerves (ADCA I) and the retina (ADCA II), or can be limited to the cerebellum (ADCA III) (Harding et al., 1993).

The most common of these dominantly inherited autosomal ataxias, ADCA I, includes many Spinocerebellar Ataxias (SCA) subtypes, some of which are caused by pathological CAG trinucleotide repeat expansion in the coding region on the mutated gene. Such is the case for SCA1, SCA2, SCA3/MJD, SCA6, SCA7, SCA17 and Dentatorubral-pallidoluysian atrophy (DRPLA) (Matilla et al., 2006).

Among the almost 30 SCAs, the variant SCA2 is the second most prevalent subtype worldwide, only surpassed by SCA3 (Schöls et al., 2004; Matilla et al., 2006; Auburger, 2011). The disorder was first recognized in India in 1971 by Wadia and Swami, who was intrigued by the early and marked slowing of saccade movements, associated to the cerebellar syndrome (Wadia & Swami, 1971). Contemporarily, in Cuba some neurologists were describing many families coming from the north-east region of the country with the same distinct clinical picture (Vallés et al., 1978). Subsequent epidemiological surveys in this Cuban region, Holguín province, focusing on the causes of the highest SCA2 prevalence rate worldwide found evidence for a founder effect (Orozco et al., 1989; Auburger et al., 1990; Velázquez-Pérez et al., 2001, 2009a).

2. Epidemiology

The collective worldwide prevalence of SCAs is estimated at about 6 cases per 100,000 people, although much higher figures have been reported in particular populations (Schöls et al., 2004). In the case of SCA2, the global prevalence is unknown because the most of the few existing epidemiological studies have been performed in isolated geographical regions with families not large enough for linkage analysis. Nevertheless, large SCA2 families have been found in India, Martinique, Australia, Tunisia, Germany, Italy, Mexico, Poland and especially in Cuba (Klockgether, 2007; Sulek-Pitkowska, et al., 2010, Velázquez-Pérez et al., 2009a).

SCA2 represents 87% of ADCAs in Cuba, with a national prevalence rate of 6.57 cases per 10^5 inhabitants. If asymptomatic at-risk individuals are included in the prevalence analysis, the prevalence rate increases up to 28.51 cases per 10^5 inhabitants, with remarkable values in various eastern provinces, especially in Holguin (Figure 1A). In fact, there are regions in this province where the prevalence reaches higher values such as Baguanos municipality (141.7 per 10^5 inhabitants) (Figure 1B) (Velázquez-Pérez et al., 2009a).

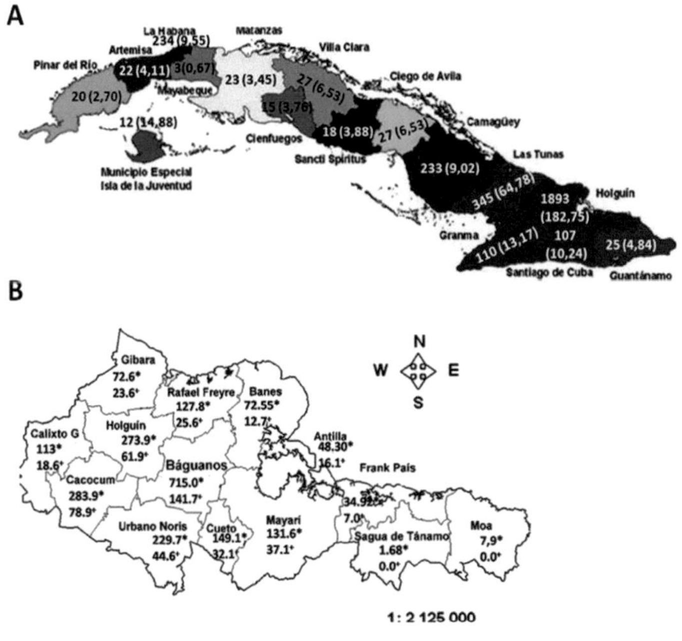

Fig. 1. Epidemiological picture of SCA2 in Cuba. A) Number and prevalence (in parenthesis) of SCA2 mutation carriers in all Cuban provinces. B) Prevalence rates of SCA2 patients (⁺) and SCA2 mutation (*) in Holguin province, Cuba (2006–2007).

3. Clinical features

The clinical picture of SCA2 includes a cerebellar syndrome in all patients, characterized by ataxic gait, cerebellar dysarthria, dysmetria and dysdiadochokinesia (Orozco et al., 1989; Orozco-Diaz et al., 1990). Patients also exhibit abnormal tandem stance (95%), slow saccadic eye movements (91%), limited voluntary ocular movements (88%), loss of vibration sense (73%), areflexia or hyporeflexia (77%) after initial hiperreflexia and abnormal swallowing (76%) (Velazquez-Pérez et al., 2009a).

Autonomic abnormalities (urinary dysfunction, hypohidrosis, constipation, and sexual dysfunction) are present in 78% of the cases and are accentuated in late stages of the disease

(Sánchez-Cruz, et al., 2001; Velázquez-Pérez et al., 2009a, Montes et al., 2010), together with dysphagia, ophthalmoplegia and distal amyotrophy. Sleep disturbances are frequent complaints of SCA2 patients and their relatives. The most prominent sleep disorders are restless legs syndrome (Trojano et al., 1998; Schöls et al., 1998; Abele et al., 2001; Irazno et al., 2007), muscle cramps, insomnia and reduced dream recalls (Velázquez-Pérez et al., 2011a).

Other clinical manifestations of SCA2 are the cognitive dysfunctions, which include frontal-executive impairment, verbal short-term memory deficits as well as reduction of attention and concentration (Storey et al., 1999; Reynaldo-Arminan et al., 2002; Bürk et al., 1999a; 2003). Although neuropsychological pattern of cognitive disturbances of SCA2 patients not necessarily resembling dementia, some studies have reported high frequency of demented patients (Durr et al., 1995, Burk et al., 1999a), but in the SCA2 Cuban population this neuropsychological state is rare (Reynaldo-Arminan et al., 2002; Orozco et al., 1989; 1990). Depression/anxiety/suicide attempts are found in a third of cases (Reynaldo-Arminan et al., 2002). In comparison to other SCAs, the frequency of slowed ocular movements, postural and action tremor and hyporeflexia are distinctive features of SCA2 (Schöls et al., 1997).

Extrapyramidal manifestations are common in SCA2 patients. Myoclonuses are reported in 13.7% whereas dystonia is present in 14.2%. Chorea may appear in approximately 7%. These symptoms are accentuated in patients with larger CAG repeats. Parkinsonian signs appear in some patients with low-range expansions containing CAA interruptions (Gwinn-Hardy et al., 2000; Payami et al., 2003; Lu et al., 2004; Charles et el, 2007). Among these manifestations, resting tremor (14,9%) and rigidity (7,9%) are the most common (Schmitz-Hubsch, et al., 2008). Recently it was reported an unusual case of SCA2 presenting as an ataxia-parkinsonism-motor neuron disease syndrome in a 46-year-old Brazilian man with 40 CAG repeats in the SCA2 gene (Braga-Neto et al., 2011).

The age at onset varies from 3 to 79 years (mean 33). Usually, the first symptom of the disease is the gait ataxia (97%), followed by the cerebellar dysarthria (3%). However some extracerebellar manifestations may occur a decade or more before the onset of gait instability or dysarthria, such as painful muscle cramps in the calf, sleep disturbances, problems with hand writing (Globas et al, 2008), as well as autonomic alterations, consisting in constipation (19.4%) and pollakiuria (17.7%) (Montes-Brown et al, 2011). In the Cuban SCA2 population the anticipation of clinical manifestation age in successive generations is observed in 80% of transmissions, usually upon transmission from an affected father (Velázquez-Pérez et al., 2009a).

Clinical features develop progressively with an increase in cerebellar syndrome, saccade slowing, and other features which confine the patients first to a wheelchair and following to a bed, where they die approximately 15–20 years after the initial symptoms. Nevertheless patients with larger CAG repeats have earlier age at onset, more saccadic slowing, axial tremor, pyramidal-dystonic-choreic signs, mental deficit and in general a faster progression to death (Filla et al 1999, Cancel et al 1997; Schöls et al., 1997; Sasaki et al., 1998; Filla et al., 1999; Velázquez-Pérez et al., 2009a) and the total disease duration from onset to death may vary between 6 and 50 years (Klockgether et al., 1998; Maschke et al., 2005). Also, the female gender is associated with shortened survival (Klockgether et al., 1998). The main cause of death is bronchopneumonia (63%), followed by bronchial aspiration and cardiovascular incidents, among others (Velázquez-Pérez et al, 2011b).

Pediatric-onset SCA2 is associated with large CAG expansions. Infantile phenotype includes rare symptoms such as retinitis pigmentosa, myoclonus-epilepsy, tetraparesis, developmental delay and facial dysmorphism (Babovic-Vuksanovic et al 1998; Rufa et al., 2002; Tan et al., 2004; Di Fabio et al., 2011). Ramocki and coworkers describe a female child who met all developmental milestones until age 3 years, deterioration of expressive language, comprehension, memory, graphomotor skills, and dysarthria. Cranial nerve examination showed bilaterally restricted lateral gaze with oculomotor apraxia (Ramocki, et al., 2008). Abdel-Aleem and Zakiwith reported a male child with progressive extrapyramidal manifestations, developmental delay, slow eye movements and cognitive impairment, trophic changes, vasomotor instability and dysphagia (Aleem and Zakiwith, 2008)

4. Molecular genetics

The underlying mutation of SCA2 consists in the unstable expansion of the trinucleotide repeat $(CAG)_8CAA(CAG)_4CAA(CAG)_8$ within the ATXN2 gene exon 1 located on chromosome 12q24.1. This repeat encodes a polyglutamine (polyQ) tract in the protein ataxin-2 (Gispert et al., 1993; Pulst et al., 1996; Imbert et al., 1996; Sanpei et al., 1996). In normal individuals, the trinucleotide repeat length varies and contains between 13 and 27 units. Intermediate expansions between 28 and 33 units may predispose the individual to an elevated risk for the motor neuron disease ALS or the Parkinson plus syndrome PSP (Elden et al., 2010; Ross et al., 2011). The prevalence of large normal alleles potentially acting as unstable premutation is particularly high in the Cuban province Holguín (Velázquez-Pérez et al., 2009a). Family planning can be aided by presymptomatic molecular genetic diagnostics, but care has to taken to offer psychological treatment together with the genetic counseling.

Pathological alleles in SCA2 have more than 32 CAG repeats, although the repeats range between 32 and 36 units has incomplete penetrance (Pulst et al., 1996; Cancel et al., 1997; Geschwind et al., 1997). The most frequent expanded allele is 37 (72%). The expanded alleles have lost interrupting CAA-triplets, a factor thought to promote the length instability. Expansions occur in 89% and contractions in 11% of the offspring of affected patients. Paternal transmissions show higher variability in repeat lengths compared with the maternal transmissions. (Velázquez-Pérez et al., 2009a). The presence of CAA interruptions in expanded alleles appears to predispose to a phenotype with Parkinson or with motor neuron disease (Charles et al., 2007; Kim et al., 2007; Modoni et al., 2007; Corrado et al., 2011, Yu et al., 2011), although both CAG and CAA code for glutamine, indicating that the neuronal population affected by the pathogenesis is determined by RNA toxicity rather than protein toxicity.

As in other polyQ diseases, in SCA2 the age at onset and symptom severity correlate inversely with the length of the trinucleotide repeat, which accounts for ~80% of variance, whereas the remaining variability suggests the existence of modifier genes, genetic polymorphisms, epigenetic factors and unknown environmental determinants modulating age of onset (Velázquez-Pérez et al., 2009a). Supporting the above mentioned, long normal CAG repeats in the CACNA1A (Pulst et al., 2005) and RAI1 genes (Hayes et al., 2000) as well as the 10398G polymorphism in the mitochondrial complex I gene (Simon et al., 2007) are associated with earlier manifestation age, also in the Cuban SCA2 population.

4.1 The physiological role of ataxin-2 in cell biology

The ataxin-2 protein (ATXN2) is a polypeptide containing 1312 amino acids encoded by 25 exons of the SCA2/ATXN2 gene encompassed within 130 kiloBases of genomic DNA (Sahba et al., 1998), with at least five human isoforms produced by allelic splicing (Nechiporuk et al 1998; Affaitati et al., 2001; Lastres-Becker et al., 2008a) and an expression in many organs, but only selected neurons of the brain (Huynh et al., 1999). It is phosphorylated, but not glycosylated (Turnbull et al., 2004). Currently, the function of ATXN2 is not clear, but several lines of evidence evoke its involvement in RNA metabolism. For example, the protein have sequence motifs related to mRNA processing, most of ATXN2 is associated to polyribosomes, at the rough endoplasmic reticulum (Satterfield and Pallanck, 2006; van de Loo et al., 2009), and this polypeptide interacts with RNA binding proteins such as A2BP1 and PABPC1 (Shibata et al., 2000; Ralser et al., 2005a; Satterfield and Pallanck, 2006).

Interestingly, ATXN2 and its orthologues in other organisms relocalize during periods of cellular stress to mRNP granules where mRNA is stored during translation repression, promote the formation of these stress granules and inhibit cell growth (Swisher and Parker, 2010; Nonhoff et al., 2007). Furthermore, the expression of ATXN2 is induced by specific stressors (Klinkenberg et al., submitted) and ATXN2 levels increase with old age (Huynh et al., 1999). The indirect effects of ATXN2 on RNAs appear to be mediated partially by its interactor DDX6, a RNA helicase (Nonhoff et al., 2007). Also the formation of P-bodies, mRNP granules implicated in RNA degradation, appears to depend on ATXN2, which may localize to these structures and influence the microRNA-mediated deadenylation of silenced RNAs (Nonhoff et al., 2007; Kozlov et al., 2010). There is preliminary evidence that ATXN2 co-sediments and co-localizes with neuronal mRNPs which are responsible for the transport of mRNAs to synaptic sites of local protein synthesis, and indeed ATXN2 is thought to modulate mRNA translation similar to its yeast orthologue Pbp1 (Siddiqui et al., 2007). Thus, ATXN2 might be important for stimulus-dependent local mRNA translation and influence in this way both synaptic strength and long-term potentiation, an electrophysiological finding which was indeed detected in ATXN2-knock-out mice in the amygdala, but not in the hippocampus (Huynh et al., 2009).

Some ATXN2 is also demonstrable at the plasma membrane, and within its protein sequence several proline-rich domains are able to interact with SH3-motif containing proteins. Such an interaction was demonstrated for endophilin A, CIN85 and Src, three components of the endocytosis complex that modulates trophic factor signaling through receptor tyrosine kinases (Ralser et al., 2005b; Nonis et al 2008). In these reports, ATXN2 was found to antagonize the internalization of the receptor for Epidermal Growth Factor. Interestingly, two other neurodegenerative disease proteins are also interactors of this complex, namely Huntingtin and Parkin, which was shown to ubiquitinate ATXN2 directly and to rescue ATXN2-toxicity (Ralser et al., 2005b; Huynh et al., 2007). Furthermore, the deficiency of ATXN2 in knock-out mice was observed to modulate the levels of insulin receptor, resulting in insulin resistance, altered fat metabolism and obesity (Kiehl et al., 2006; Lastres Becker et al., 2008b). Interestingly, the protein family A2D which shares sequence homology with ATXN2 also shows interaction with the cytoplasmic domain of the thrombopoietin and the erythropoietin membrane receptors which lack intrinsic tyrosine kinase activity, but is also internalized to modulate downstream events of cytokine signaling (Meunier et al., 2002). Of course, this physiological influence of ATXN2 on trophic signaling may be important for neural atrophy in SCA2. Finally, recent evidence suggests a localization and role of ATXN2 in the nucleus, acting as interactor of the transcriptional regulator ZBRK1 (Hallen et al., 2011).

4.2 ATXN2 role for different diseases

SCA2 is thought to be caused by a toxic gain-of-function of the ATXN2 protein, but it is not clear to which degree the physiological function of ATXN2 is enhanced and to which degree unspecific toxic effects such as the aggregation of polyQ domain proteins dominate in the pathogenesis. Since polyQ expansions in different disease proteins affect different neuronal populations, and since the overexpression of wild-type ATXN2 and its orthologues in lower species, which lack the polyQ domain completely, is neurotoxic, the specific properties of ATXN2 regarding expression, subcellular localization and interactors seem to be relevant in disease. Intermediate-length expansions of the ATXN2 trinucleotide repeat below the threshold of SCA2 manifestation were shown to have a pathogenic role, increasing the individual risk to manifest the motor neuron degeneration disease ALS (Amyotrophic Lateral Sclerosis) and the basal ganglia degeneration disease within the Parkinson-plus group of disorders PSP (Progressive Supranuclear Palsy) (Elden et al., 2010; Daoud et al., 2011; Ross et al., 2011; Soraru̇ et al., 2011; Lee et al., 2011; van Damme et al., 2011). The RNA metabolism function of ATXN2 may explain this phenomenon, since ALS pathogenesis appears to be mediated mainly by altered mRNA processing (Lagier-Tourenne et al., 2010). ATXN2 gain-of-function also potentiates toxicity of ATXN1 and ATXN3 (the SCA1 and SCA3 disease proteins, respectively) and even toxicity of Tau (the frontotemporal lobar degeneration disease protein) in the fly model (Shulman and Feany, 2003; Al-Ramahi et al., 2007; Lessing and Bonini, 2008; Elden et al., 2010). Conversely, reducing ATXN2 levels is sufficient to mitigate the neurotoxicity triggered by TDP-43, ATXN1 and ATXN3 (Al-Ramahi et al., 2007; Lessing et al., 2008; Elden et al., 2010) in yeast and flies, indicating that these effects are mediated by the physiological function of ATXN2, but not by the polyQ domain which characterizes human ATXN2 and is not conserved until mouse.

Large expansions of ATXN2 were reported to exert a profound effect on intracellular calcium levels through specific binding to the carboxy-terminal region of the type 1 inositol 1,4,5-trisphosphate receptor (IP(3)R1), an intracellular Ca(2+) release channel (Liu et al., 2009), an effect mediated by ATXN2 at its major localization in the cytoplasm.

Several lines of evidence suggest that other alterations of the physiological ATXN2 function influence additional neuron populations and diseases. In neuroblastoma tumors, an upregulation of ATXN2 was found to be a decisive factor to induce apoptosis of the aberrant cells and spontaneous tumor remission (Wiedemeyer et al., 2003). In individuals who reached an age over 100 years, a single nucleotide polymorphism within ATXN2 intron 1 contributes to the genetic signature of exceptional longevity. Moreover, in the general human population the same ATXN2 intron 1 polymorphism determines high blood pressure levels (Levy et al., 2009; Newton-Cheh et al., 2009; Sebastiani et al., 2010).

4.3 Animal models

Animal models have been useful tools to study the polyQ expansion diseases, in particular the brain tissue of early stage pathology. Specifically ATXN2 orthologues are highly conserved until Saccharomyces cerevisiae, permitting high-throughput genetic screens into the function of ATXN2 and revealing the role of ATXN2 as a risk factor for TDP-43 toxicity and motor neuron degeneration (Elden et al., 2010). Again, Drosophila melanogaster studies demonstrated the association of dATX2 with PABP and with polysomes (Satterfield and Pallanck, 2006). The use of RNA interference in Caenorhabditis elegans demonstrated an essential role of the atx-2 gene for early embryonic development (Kiehl et al., 2000).

Taking advantage of the mouse as an organism with genetic versatility and with similarity to man in brain structure, two transgenic models of SCA2 have been generated to date. The first one was produced by Huynh et al., 2000, who reported the use of the murine PcP2 (L7) promoter to direct a strong overexpression of the human ATXN2 gene with an expanded allele of 58 CAG repeats specifically to the cerebellar Purkinje neurons. Using the rotarod test, they found that the animals became ataxic at 26 and 16 weeks for the heterozygous and homozygous transgenic mice, respectively. Also, they described progressive incoordination and morphological alterations of Purkinje cells in this animal model. In 2005, Aguiar and coworkers (Aguiar et al., 2006) generated transgenic mouse lines overexpressing the full-length human ATXN2 gene with 75 CAG units under the control of the human self promoter. A neurological phenotype was reported after 12 weeks for heterozygous and 6 weeks for homozygous mice.

5. Imaging

Magnetic resonance imaging shows early cerebellar and brainstem atrophy (Figure 2) with marked involvement of the cerebellar cortex and the pons/inferior olive region in SCA2, in excellent agreement with the traditional neuropathological nomenclature of olivopontocerebellar atrophy (OPCA). Also, frontotemporal atrophy is observed in advanced disease (Bürk et al., 1996; Giuffrida et al., 1999). Voxel-based morphometry studies have revealed the atrophy of the cerebellar and brainstem white matter as well as the symmetric loss of gray matter in the cerebellar vermis (Brenneis et al., 2003; Brenneis et al., 2005; Della Nave et al., 2008a, b, Goel et al., 2011). Positron emission tomography (PET) studies showed a reduced regional glucose metabolism in the cerebellum, brainstem and parietal cortex, which may occur years before the clinical onset of SCA2 (Inagaki et al., 2005). PET analyses also revealed the loss of striatal dopamine transporter function with nigrostriatal atrophy, similar to the pattern observed in idiopathic Parkinson's disease (Boesch et al., 2004; Wüllner et al 2005; Inagaki et al., 2005). Imaging by proton magnetic resonance spectroscopy demonstrated the loss of choline-containing compounds in SCA2 cerebella, suggesting the decreased production and/or the loss of cell membranes as well as the reduced synthesis of precursors of acetylcholine. The same study demonstrated the increase of lactate levels in the cerebellum suggesting an impairment of glycolysis and mitochondrial function (Boesch et al., 2001).

6. Neuropathology

The macroscopic examination of nervous structures in *post-mortem* samples of SCA2 patients shows a significant atrophy of the cerebellum, brainstem, frontal lobe, as well as pallor of the midbrain *substantia nigra* and a reduction of the cerebral and cerebellar white matter. Microscopically, the cerebellum is characterized by an early and marked neuronal loss in Purkinje cell layer with reduction in the number of dendritic arborizations and torpedo-like deformations of their axons. The number of granular neurons is diminished, usually toward

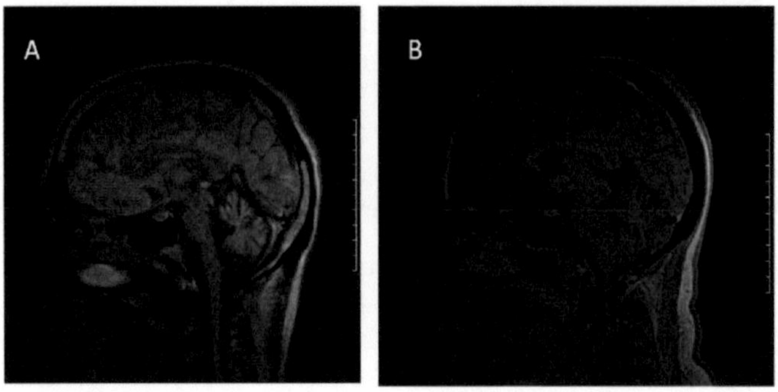

Fig. 2. MRI scans of a SCA2 patient (age 40 years; disease duration 8 years, CAG repeat size 39 units, SARA score 19) (A) and a healthy control (age 40 years, SARA score 0) (B). Note the severe atrophy of cerebellum and brainstem in the SCA2 subject.

late stages of the disease whereas the dentate nucleus is relatively spared. Parallel fibers are sparse and no climbing fibers are observed in the Purkinje cell dendritic trees (Orozco et al., 1989; Ihara et al., 1994; Estrada et al., 1999; Ying et al., 2005). In the brainstem, the most noteworthy microscopic findings are the marked loss of inferior olivary neurons in addition to the degeneration of pontine and other precerebellar brainstem nuclei (Rüb et al., 2005a; Lastres-Becker et al 2008a). The neuropathological evaluation of brainstem and cranial nerves shows that oculomotor, somatomotor, somatosensory, auditory, vestibular and autonomic nuclei are notably affected by neuronal loss and their associated fibers are atrophied and undergo demyelinization (Rüb et al., 2004a, 2004b; Rüb et al., 2006; Gierga et al., 2005; Hoche et al., 2008). Another important neuropathological marker of SCA2 is the notable reduction of neurons of the substantia nigra in the mesencephalon and the extensive degeneration of several thalamic nuclei, such as the reticular, fasciculosus, ventral anterior and posterior, lateral geniculate body and the anterior nuclei (Rüb et al., 2003a, 2003b, 2005b). In the spinal cord, an early and progressive demyelination of the posterior and spinocerebellar columns together with neuronal loss in cuneate and gracile nuclei, dorsal roots and ganglia as well as a reduction of motor neurons, usually in the cervical level and the Clarke's column, are observed (Rüb et al., 2007). Demyelination is severe (Armstrong et al., 2005). The selective neurodegeneration of large neurons affecting multiple regions of the brain with some glial inclusions is quite similar to the pattern of multiple-system atrophy (MSA) (Yagishita and Inoue 1997; Berciano and Ferrer 2005). Polyglutamine inclusion bodies appear to be much less prominent than in Huntington's disease or in SCA3 (Huynh et al., 2000; Uchihara et al., 2001; Koyano et al., 2002; Pang et al., 2002). Also, it is observed a significant loss of giant Betz pyramidal cells in the primary motor cortex. (Hoche et al., 2010). A recent study suggested that either the age at onset or the CAG repeat expansions influence on the distribution pattern of SCA2 neurodegeneration (Ishida et al., 2011).

7. Neurochemistry

The neurochemical findings in SCA2 patients were first recognized by Orozco and co-workers in 1989, (Orozco et al., 1989) who called attention to the significantly decrease of dopamine metabolites such as 3,4-dihydroxyphenylacetic acid (DOPAC) and homovanillic acid (HVA) in cerebrospinal fluid (CSF), likely as result of neuronal depletion in the substancia nigra of autopsied patients. However, the mean concentration of Gamma-amino-butyric acid (GABA), as well as metabolites of noradrenalin and serotonin were similar to normal subjects. Additionally, N-acetyl-aspartate and glutamate are markedly reduced in these patients (Oz et al., 2010).

A pathologically relevant biochemical finding is the significant reduction of zinc, iron and copper levels in the CSF and serum of Cuban SCA2 patients. The reduction of zinc levels could be associated with phenotypic features such as nerve conduction slowing, cognitive dysfunction, and immune-depression at final stages of the disease and could accentuate the dysfunction of cerebellar circuits, based on the important role of this element in the control of synapses in the cerebellum (González et al., 2006). Furthermore, most biomarkers of the antioxidant-prooxidant balance are significantly modified in Cuban SCA2 patients with an increase in malondialdehyde (MDA) as evidence of lipid peroxidation, as well as signs of oxidative damage to protein and DNA and significant reduction of the reduced glutathione (GSH). Also, the activity of glutathione S-transferase (GST), superoxide dismutase (SOD) and catalase (CAT) are depressed in these patients with a disruption of the balance CAT/SOD (Velázquez-Pérez et al, 2003; Almaguer, et al., 2005). A third interesting finding is the decrease of erythropoietin levels in the CSF with a compensatory increase of this molecule in the serum of Cuban SCA2 patients, suggesting the existence of reduced capabilities of neuroprotection in the nervous system (Velazquez-Pérez et al., 2011b). We believe that these biochemical features may contribute to the high phenotypic variability of SCA2 and that they could constitute potential therapeutical targets to design future clinical trials.

8. Neurophysiology

8.1 Nerve conduction and electromyography studies

The most common electrophysiological finding in SCA2 patients is a predominantly sensory axonal neuropathy, expressed by the early and progressive reduction of sensory amplitudes, suggestive of dorsal root ganglionopathy. These alterations are associated with slowing of nerve conduction as sign of demyelination. The progression rate of sensory axonal neuropathy is notably accentuated in patients with large CAG expansion sizes. Motor nerve conduction parameters are usually normal, but in patients with 10-15 years of disease duration it is possible to observe a reduction of motor amplitudes (Kubis et al., 1999; van de Warrenburg et al., 2004; Velázquez-Pérez et al., 2007, 2010). Electromyographical findings reveal motor unit potentials (MUP) with light polyphasic alterations, increased amplitudes and isolated contraction pattern in the first stage of the evolution. In advanced stages of the disease signs of denervation can appear (fibrillations and fasciculations) and the contraction pattern becomes simple oscillations, indicating the loss of motor neurons in the anterior horn of the spinal cord (Velázquez-Pérez et al, 2009b).

8.2 Somatosensory evoked potentials (SSEP)

Tibial nerve SSEPs are characterized by a marked prolongation of the P40 component and central conduction time latencies. In the median nerve SSEP there is a latency prolongation of N20 and N13 components in addition to a reduction of amplitude of Erb potentials. In almost all cases, the SSEPs show abnormal morphology and reduced reproducibility. These alterations get worse quickly in patients with larger CAG repeat number and may be detected even in presymptomatic subjects (Velázquez-Pérez et al., 2007, 2008).

8.3 Brain Stem Auditory Evoked Potentials (BSAEP)

BSAEPs have poor reproducibility and unstable morphology in 95% of the patients, in addition to the increase of latency of the waves III and V and the prolongation of the I–III interpeak interval. These abnormalities are common in patients with disease duration above 10 years but the abnormal reproducibility and morphology can be detected since preclinical stage (Velázquez-Pérez et al., 2007, 2008).

8.4 Visual Evoked Potentials (VEP)

VEP are frequently normal in SCA2 patients, but some patients in advances stages of the disease have prolonged P100 latencies with normal amplitudes. These findings reflect the integrity of the visual pathway in Cuban SCA2 patients, allowing us to distinguish SCA2 from other spinocerebellar ataxias such as SCA1, SCA3 and in particular SCA7 (Velázquez-Pérez et al., 2007, 2008).

8.5 Event-related evoked potentials (ERPs)

ERPs revealed prolongation of visual P300 latencies in 40% of cases with a significant correlation of this variable with the disease duration and clinical affectation (Kremlacek et al., 2011).

8.6 Motor evoked potentials

The study of the corticospinal tract by transcranial magnetic stimulation in SCA2 patients reveals an increase of central motor conduction time and motor threshold. Also, intracortical facilitation may be reduced and the induced cortical silent period prolonged. The progression of these abnormalities is dependent on the disease duration and ataxia severity. They probably reflect the reduced excitability of the motor cortex, disturbed conduction along the pyramidal tract and the loss of facilitatory influences of the cerebellum on the primary motor cortex (Yokota et al., 1998; Restivo et al., 2000, 2004; Schwenkreis et al., 2002)

8.7 Electrooculography

The main oculomotor abnormality in SCA2 is the slowing of horizontal saccadic movements, which is probably the result of early pontine brainstem degeneration. This feature is electrooculographically detectable in 99% of the patients and in several presymptomatic subjects. The maximal saccade velocity is negatively correlated with the polyQ expansion and the ataxia score, but is not significantly influenced by the disease duration. (Rivaud-Pechoux et al., 1998; Bürk et al., 1999b; Velázquez-Pérez et al., 2004, 2008, 2009c). The prolongation of saccadic latency is observed in 46% of the cases, reflecting the cortical/subcortical involvement in SCA2. Although this saccadic feature is not directly influenced by the CAG repeats or the disease duration it is close related with the frontal-executive dysfunctions, identifying it as a promising cognitive biomarker (Rodríguez-Labrada et al., 2011a). Additionally, SCA2 patients showed saccadic dysmetria reflecting the cerebellar involvement (Velázquez-Pérez et al., 2008) although saccades made for short target amplitudes are usually accurate due to the visual feedback might be continuously available during the slow movements (Federighi et al., 2011). Furthermore, gain measurements in smooth pursuit movements and horizontal optokinetic nystagmus are slightly reduced in SCA2 patients, whereas the vestibulo-ocular reflex is normal (Buttner et al., 1998).

8.8 Videopolysomnography and electroencephalography

Sleep disorders are common complaints of SCA2 patients, fundamentally towards the final stages of the disease. Clinically, the most prominent findings are a restless legs syndrome and muscle cramps, which appear in 45 % of the cases. Patients with REM (rapid eye movements) sleep behavior disorder; bruxism and excessive daytime sleepiness are scarse. The polysomnographical evaluation reveals a reduction of REM sleep with decreased REM density in 70% of patients. These REM sleep abnormalities appear before the disease onset and their progression rates depend on ataxia severity and disease duration. (Velazquez-Pérez et al., 2011a; Rodríguez-Labrada et al., 2011b). REM sleep without atonia appears in 31% of SCA2 patients and showed a significant correlation with the ataxia score and CAG expansions (Velazquez-Pérez et al., 2011b). Periodic legs movements (PLMs) are also observed, in the 38% of SCA2 patients (Figure 3). They are directly associated with the clinical severity of the disease and their progression rate is notable (Velazquez-Pérez et al., 2011a). Other less prominent sleep abnormalities are the decrease of sleep efficiency, increase of arousal index and central apnea index. (Boesch et al., 2006; Tuin et al., 2006).

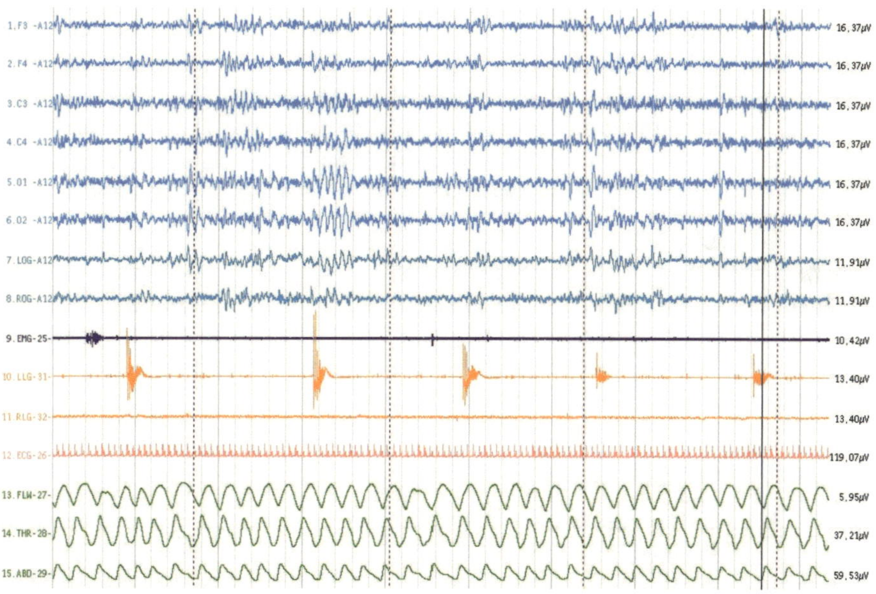

Fig. 3. Two-minute epoch of stage 2 sleep showing periodic leg movements in a SCA2 patient with 44 years old, 12 years of disease duration, 39 CAG repeats in the SCA2 gene and ataxia score in 15 units.

The conventional EEG in SCA2 patients shows a predominantly diffuse theta activity with reduced reactivity to eye opening in 72 % of the cases. In the brain electrical activity mapping a significant increase of absolute power for the theta band with reduction of absolute power for the alpha band is observed (Figure 4).

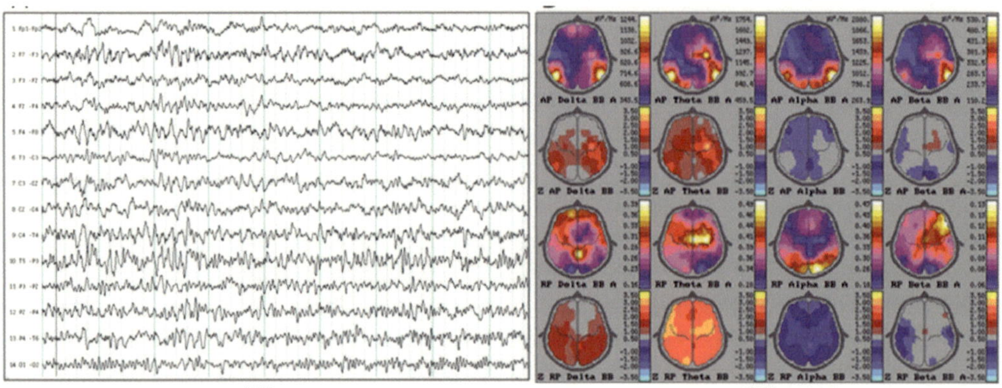

(A) (B)

Fig. 4. Conventional (A) and quantitative (B) EEG from a SCA2 patient with age 40 years, 10 years of disease duration, a repeat expansion to 40 CAG in the SCA2 gene and an ataxia SARA score of 17.

8.9 Other neurophysiological alterations

The study of autonomic control of cardiovascular function by heart rate variability (HRV) in a large group of SCA2 patients reveals the presence of cardiovascular autonomic dysfunction associated to SCA2 (Pradhan et al, 2008; Montes-Brown et al., 2010). Additionally, SCA2 patients show a significant impairment of olfactory threshold, identification and discrimination capabilities. The score of the *University of Pennsylvania smell identification test* (UPSIT) is significantly reduced and it correlates positively with ataxia score but it is not influenced by the age, age at onset, disease duration and CAG repeats (Velázquez et al, 2006).

The prism adaptation task let us identify the impaired adaptation decrement. This alteration is accentuated in patients with larger expansions. Also, the deterioration in the adaptation correlates with the motor performance and saccade velocity, suggesting that structures that degenerate in this disease may contribute to both adaptation and motor performance (Fernandez-Ruiz et al, 2007; Velázquez-Pérez et al, 2009d).

9. Early preclinical signs

The earliest subclinical sign appears even 15 years before the onset of ataxia by the slowing of horizontal saccades at 60^0 of target displacement, with amplitudes and latencies normal. This electrophysiological abnormality is accentuated in subjects with larger CAG repeats and reflects probably the early dysfunction or degeneration of paramedian pontine reticular formation (Velázquez-Pérez et al., 2009c). This alteration is followed by the reduction of REM sleep percentage with decreased rapid eyes movements' density, which may precede the ataxia onset by 10 years although its progression during this stage is insidious (Rodríguez-Labrada et al., 2011b). Other preclinical alterations include decrease of sensory amplitudes (Velázquez-Pérez et al., 2010), increased P40 latency (Velázquez-Pérez et al., 2007), motor performance deficits, shown by the prism adaptation task (Velázquez-Pérez et al., 2009d) and reduced capabilities to identify specific odors in a sensible smell identification test (UPSIT). The comprehensive analysis of these early signs in SCA2 suggests the necessity for revisit the current criteria to define the disease onset delineating the boundaries between presymptomatics and symptomatic states.

10. Therapeutical options

Till now, there is no specific treatment for SCA2. Physiotherapy and neuropsychological rehabilitation have palliative effects on motor and cognitive symptoms. Therefore, Cuban SCA2 patients receive a specialized neurorehabilitation program (Pérez-Avila et al., 2004) since 1998, which has been applied to more than 400 patients and has allowed some recovery of motor, cognitive and antioxidant functions in about 75% of the treated patients (Rodríguez et al., 2008).

Regarding clinical trials, few studies have been conducted. For example, muscle cramps are successfully treated with magnesium and levodopa treatment alleviates the parkinsonian signs in SCA2 patients (Lastres-becker, 2008a), whereas severe myoclonus at advanced stage could be dramatically improved by piracetam (De Rosa et al., 2006). Recently, a randomized, double-blind, placebo-controlled pilot trial using riluzole resulted effective to SCA2 and other subjects with cerebellar ataxias (Ristori et al., 2010). Additionally, a double-blinded and placebo-controlled clinical trial with 50 mg zinc sulphate in 36 Cuban SCA2 patients was effective in increasing the zinc levels in serum and CSF of treated subjects and some benefit of this treatment for the cerebellar syndrome, the peripheral neuropathy and the restoration of antioxidant functions was apparent (Velázquez-Pérez et al., 2011c).

Deep brain stimulation with novel patterned low-frequency stimulation (PLFS) was effective in localizing the tremor generator at a subthalamic-thalamic electrode position, suppressing a coarse postural tremor for several postoperative years in one case (Freund et al., 2007; Barnikol et al., 2008).

11. Conclusions

In conclusion, although we have learnt much since SCA2 was described as a distinct clinical entity (Wadia and Swami, 1971) and since its cause was identified and genetic counseling became available (Imbert et al 1996; Pulst et al., 1996; Sanpei et al 1996), until today we have only taken the first steps towards understanding the pathogenic mechanisms and validating neuroprotective therapies.

12. Acknowledgements

We thank all patients and their family members for the observations and the tissues they contributed to aid to understand this devastating disease. The work was supported by the Cuban Ministry of Health the Deutsche Akademische Austauschdienst, the Deutsche Forschungsgemeinschaft over many years (AU 96/1-1, 1-2, 1-3, 4-1, 9-1 und 9-2, 11-1, 13-1), the Alexander von Humboldt Foundation, and a European Union framework (EuroSCA) (MINSAP). The authors thank Dr. Suzana Gispert for her continuous assistance and Dipl. Biol. Jessica Drost for proofreading the manuscript.

13. References

Abdel-Aleem A, Zaki MS. (2008) Spinocerebellar ataxia type 2 (SCA2) in an Egyptian family presenting with polyphagia and marked CAG expansion in infancy. Journal of Neurology, Vol.255(3), pp. 413–419.

Abele M, Bürk K, Laccone F, Dichgans J & Klockgether T. (2001). Restless legs syndrome in spinocerebellar ataxia types 1, 2, and 3. *Journal of Neurology*, Vol.248, pp. 311-314, ISSN 0340-5354.

Affaitati A, de Cristofaro T, Feliciello A & Varrone S. (2001). Identification of alternative splicing of spinocerebellar ataxia type 2 gene. *Gene*, Vol.267, pp 89–93, ISSN 1879-0038.

Aguiar J, Fernández J, Aguilar A, Mendoza Y, Vázquez M, et al. (2006). Ubiquitous expression of human SCA2 gene under the regulation of the SCA2 self promoter cause specific Purkinje cell degeneration in transgenic mice. *Neuroscience Letter*, Vol.392, pp. 202-206, ISSN 0304-3940.

Almaguer L, Almaguer D, Gonzáles Y, Martínez E & Valcárcel P. (2005). Capacidad antioxidante total de en pacientes cubanos con ataxia Espinocerebelosa tipo 2. *Revista Mexicana de Neurociencias*, Vol.6, pp. 201-206.

Al-Ramahi I, Pérez AM, Lim J, Zhang M, Sorensen R, et al. (2007). dAtaxin-2 mediates expanded Ataxin-1-induced neurodegeneration in a Drosophila model of SCA1. *PLoS Genetic*, Vol.3, No.12, pp. e234, ISSN 1553-7404.

Armstrong J, Bonaventura I, Rojo A, Gonzalez G, Corral J, et al. (2005). Spinocerebellar ataxia type 2 (SCA2) with white matter involvement. *Neuroscience Letter*, Vol.381, pp. 247–51, ISSN 0304-3940.

Auburger G, Díaz GO, Capote RF, Sánchez SG, Pérez MP, et al. (1990). Autosomal dominant ataxia: genetic evidence for locus heterogeneity from a Cuban founder-effect population. *American Journal of Human Genetic*, Vol.46, pp. 1163-77, ISSN 1537-6605.

Auburger, G. (2011). Spinocerebellar Ataxia type 2, In: *Handbook of Clinical Neurology, Third Series*. Aminoff MJ, Boller F, Swaab DF (eds). Subramony SH and Dürr A (volume eds). Amsterdam, Elsevier: Vol 103, chapter 29.

Babovic-Vuksanovic D, Snow K, Patterson MC & Michels VV. (1998). Spinocerebellar ataxia type 2 (SCA 2) in an infant with extreme CAG repeat expansion. *American Journal of Human Genetic* Vol.79, pp. 383–387, ISSN 1537-6605.

Barnikol UB, Popovych OV, Hauptmann C, Sturm V, Freund HJ & Tass PA. (2008). Tremor entrainment by patterned low-frequency stimulation. *Philos. Transact. A Math. Phys. Eng. Sci*, Vol.366, pp. 3545-73.

Berciano J & Ferrer I. (2005) Glial cell cytoplasmic inclusions in SCA2 do not express alpha-synuclein. *Journal of Neurology*, Vol.252, pp. 742–44, ISSN 0340-5354.

Boesch SM, Donnemiller E, Müller J, Seppi K, Weirich-Schwaiger H, et al. (2004). Abnormalities of dopaminergic neurotransmission in SCA2: A combined ^{123} I-ßCIT and ^{123} I-IBZM SPECT study. *Movement Disorders*, Vol.19, pp. 1320–1325, ISSN 1531-8257.

Boesch SM, Frauscher B, Brandauer E, Wenning GK, Hogl B & Poewe W. (2006). Disturbance of rapid eye movement sleep in spinocerebellar ataxia type 2. *Movement Disorders*, Vol.21, pp. 1751-1754, ISSN 1531-8257.

Boesch SM, Schocke M, Bürk K, Hollosi P, Fornai F, et al. (2001). Proton magnetic resonance spectroscopic imaging reveals differences in Spinocerebellar Ataxia Types 2 and 6. *Journal of Magnetic Resonance Imaging,* Vol.13, pp. 553–59, ISSN 1522-2586.

Braga-Neto P, Pedroso JL, Carvalho A, Abrahao A, Alemida L, Escorcio ML, et al. (2011) SCA2 presenting as an ataxia-parkinsonism-motor neuron disease syndrome. *Arquives of Neuropsiquiatry,* Vol.69, pp. 405, ISSN 0004-282X.

Brenneis C, Boesch SM, Egger KE, Seppi K, Scherfler C, et al. (2005). Cortical atrophy in the cerebellar variant of multiple system atrophy: A voxel-based morphometry study. *Movement Disorders,* Vol.21, pp. 159–65, ISSN 1531-8257.

Brenneis C, Bosch SM, Schocke M, Wenning GK & Poewe W. (2003). Atrophy pattern in SCA2 determined by voxelbased morphometry. *Neuroreport* Vol.14, pp. 1799–802, ISSN 0959-4965.

Bürk K, Abele M, Fetter M, Dichgans J, Skalej M, et al. (1996). Autosomal dominant cerebellar ataxia type I clinical features and MRI in families with SCA1, SCA2 and SCA3. *Brain,* Vol.119, pp. 1497–1505, ISSN 1460-2156.

Bürk K, Globas C, Bosch S, Graber S, Abele M, Brice A, et al. (1999a) Cognitive deficits in spinocerebellar ataxia 2. *Brain,* Vol.122, pp. 769-777, ISSN 1460-2156.

Bürk K, Fetter M, Abele M, Laccone F, Brice A, et al. (1999b). Autosomal dominant cerebellar ataxia type I: Oculomotor abnormalities in families with SCA1, SCA2, and SCA3. *Journal of Neurology,* Vol.246, pp. 789–797, ISSN 0340-5354.

Bürk K, Globas C, Bösch S, Klockgether T, Zühlke C, et al. (2003). Cognitive deficits in spinocerebellar ataxia type 1, 2, and 3. *Journal of Neurology,* Vol.250, pp. 207-211, ISSN 0340-5354.

Buttner N, Geschwind D, Jen JC, Perlman S, Pulst SM & Baloh RW. (1998). Oculomotor phenotypes in autosomal dominant ataxias. *Archives of Neurology,* Vol.55, pp. 1353-1357, ISSN 1538-3687.

Cancel G, Dürr A, Didierjean O, Imbert G, Bürk K, et al. (1997). Molecular and clinical correlations in spinocerebellar ataxia 2: A study of 32 families. *Human Molecular Genetics,* Vol.6, pp. 709–715, ISSN 1460-2083.

Charles P, Camuzat A, Benammar N, Sellal F, Destée A, et al. (2007). Are interrupted SCA2 CAG repeat expansions responsible for parkinsonism? *Neurology,* Vol.69, pp. 1970–1975, ISSN 0028-3878.

Corrado L, Mazzini L, Oggioni GD, Luciano B, Godi M, et al. (2011). ATXN-2 CAG repeat expansions are interrupted in ALS patients. *Human Genetics,* (May 3), [Epub ahead of print], ISSN 1432-1203.

Daoud H, Belzil V, Martins S, Sabbagh M, Provencher P, et al. (2011). Association of long ATXN2 CAG repeat sizes with increased risk of Amyotrophic Lateral Sclerosis. *Archives of Neurology,* Vol.68, pp. 739-42, ISSN 1538-3687.

De Rosa A, Striano P, Barbieri F, de Falco A, Rinaldi C, et al. (2006) Suppression of myoclonus in SCA2 by piracetam. *Movement Disorders,* Vol.21 pp. 116-8, ISSN 1531-8257.

Della Nave R, Ginestroni A, Tessa C, Cosottini M, Giannelli M, et al. (2008a). Structural Damage in Spinocerebellar Ataxia Type 2. A Voxel-Based Morphometry Study. *Movement Disorders,* Vol.23, pp. 899-903, ISSN 1531-8257.

Della Nave R, Ginestroni A, Tessa C, Salvatore E, De Grandis D, et al. (2008b). Brain white matter damage in SCA1 and SCA2. An in vivo study using voxel-based morphometry, histogram analysis of mean diffusivity and tract-based spatial statistics. *Neuroimage*, Vol. 43, pp. 10-9, ISSN 1095-9572.

Di Fabio R, Santorelli F, Bertini E, Balestri M, Cursi L, Tessa A, et al. (2011) Infantile Childhood Onset of Spinocerebellar Ataxia Type 2. The cerebellum. In press DOI 10.1007/s12311-011-0315-9. ISSN 1473-4230.

Durr A, Smadja D, Cancel G, Lezin A, Stevanin G, Mikol J, et al. (1995) Autosomal dominant cerebellar ataxia type I in Martinique (French West Indies). Clinical and neuropathological analysis of 53 patients from three unrelated SCA2 families. *Brain*, Vol.118, pp. 1573-1581, ISSN 1460-2156.

Elden AC, Kim HJ, Hart MP, Chen-Plotkin AS, Johnson BS, et al. (2010). Ataxin-2 intermediate-length polyglutamine expansions are associated with increased risk for ALS. *Nature*, Vol.466, pp. 1069-75, ISSN 1476-4687.

Estrada R, Galarraga J, Orozco G, Nodarse A & Auburger G. (1999) Spinocerebellar ataxia 2 (SCA2): morphometric analyses in 11 autopsies characterize it as an olivo-ponto-cerebellar atrophy (OPCA) plus. *Acta Neuropathologica*, Vol.97, pp. 306 -310, ISSN 1432-0533.

Federighi, P., Cevenini, G., Dotti, M. T., Rosini, F., Pretegiani, E., Federico, A. & Rufa, A. (2011). Differences in saccade dynamics between spinocerebellar ataxia 2 and late-onset cerebellar ataxias. *Brain*, Vol.134, pp. 879-91, ISSN 1460-2156.

Fernández-Ruiz J, Velásquez-Pérez L, Díaz R, Drucker-Colín R, Pérez-González R, et al. (2007). Prism adaptation in spinocerebellar ataxia type 2. *Neuropsychologia*, Vol.45, pp. 2692-98, ISSN 0028-3932.

Filla A, De Michele G, Santoro L, Calabrese O, Castaldo I, et al. (1999). Spinocerebellar ataxia type 2 in southern Italy: a clinical and molecular study of 30 families. *Journal of Neurology*, Vol.246, pp. 467–71, ISSN 0340-5354.

Freund H-J, Barnikol UB, Nolte D, Treuer H, Auburger G, et al. (2007). Subthalamic-thalamic DBS in a case with spinocerebellar ataxia type 2 and severe tremor - an unusual clinical benefit. *Movement Disorders*, Vol.22, pp. 732–735, ISSN 1531-8257.

Geschwind DH, Perlman S, Figueroa CP, Treiman LJ & Pulst SM. (1997). The prevalence and wide clinical spectrum of the spinocerebellar ataxia type 2 trinucleotide repeat in patients with autosomal dominant cerebellar ataxia. *American Journal of Human Genetic*, Vol.60, pp. 842–850, ISSN 1537-6605.

Gierga K, Bürk K, Bauer M, Orozco-Díaz G, Auburger G, et al. (2005). Involvement of the cranial nerves and their nuclei in spinocerebellar ataxia type 2 (SCA2). *Acta Neuropathologica (Berl.)*, Vol.109, pp. 617-631, ISSN 1432-0533.

Gispert S, Twells R, Orozco G, Brice A, Weber J, et al. (1993). Chromosomal assignment of the second locus for autosomal dominant cerebellar ataxia (SCA2) to chromosome 12q23-24.1. *Nature Genetics*, Vol.4, pp. 295-299, ISSN 1061-4036.

Giuffrida S, Saponara R, Restivo DA, Trovato Salinaro A, Tomarchio L, et al. (1999). Supratentorial atrophy in spinocerebellar ataxia type 2: MRI study of 20 patients. *Journal of Neurology*, Vol.246, pp. 383–378, ISSN 0340-5354.

Globas C, du Montcel ST, Baliko L, Boesch S, Depondt C, DiDonato S, et al. (2008) Early symptoms in spinocerebellar ataxia type 1, 2, 3, and 6. Movement Disorders, Vol.23, pp. 2232-2238, ISSN 1531-8257.

Goel G, Kumar Pal P, Ravishankar S, Venkatasubramanian G, Jayakumar PN, Krishna N, et al. (2011). Gray matter volume deficits in spinocerebellar ataxia: An optimized voxel based morphometric study. *Parkisonism relat disord.* In press. ISSN 1353-8020.

González C, Sánchez G, González-Quevedo A, et al. (2005). Serum and Cerebrospinal fluid levels of copper, iron and zinc in patients with Ataxia type SCA-2 from the province of Holguín in Cuba. Therapeutic Basic. *Dialogues in Clinical Neuroscience,* Vol.13, pp. 12-16.

Gwinn-Hardy K, Chen JY, Liu HC, Liu TY, Boss M, et al. (2000). Spinocerebellar ataxia type 2 with parkinsonism in ethnic Chinese. *Neurology,* Vol.55, pp. 800-5, ISSN 0028-3878.

Hallen L, Klein H, Stoschek C, Wehrmeyer S, Nonhoff U, et al. (2011). The KRAB-containing zinc-finger transcriptional regulator ZBRK1 activates SCA2 gene transcription through direct interaction with its gene product, ataxin-2. *Human Molecular Genetics,* Vol.20, pp. 104-14, ISSN 1460-2083.

Harding AE. (1993). Clinical features and classification of inherited ataxias. In: *Inherited ataxias,* AE Harding, T Deufel, (eds), 1–14, Raven, New York, USA.

Hayes S, Turecki G, Brisebois K, Lopes-Cendes-I, Gaspar-C, et al. (2000). CAG repeat length in RAI1 is associated with age at onset variability in spinocerebellar ataxia type 2 (SCA2). *Human Molecular Genetics,* Vol.9, pp. 1753-58, ISSN 1460-2083.

Hoche F, Balikó L, den Dunnen W, Steinecker K, Bartos L, Sáfrány E, et al. (2010). Spinocerebellar Ataxia Type 2 (SCA2): Identification of Early Brain Degeneration in One Monozygous Twin in the Initial Disease Stage. *The cerebellum.* In press, ISSN 1473-4230.

Hoche F, Seidel K, Brunt ER, Auburger G, Schöls L, et al. (2008). Involvement of the auditory brainstem system in spinocerebellar ataxia type 2 (SCA2), type 3 (SCA3) and type 7 (SCA7). *Neuropathology and Applied Neurobiology,* Vol.34, pp. 479-91, ISSN 1365-2990.

Huynh DP, Del Bigio MR, Ho DH & Pulst SM. (1999). Expression of ataxin-2 in brains from normal individuals and patients with Alzheimer's disease and spinocerebellar ataxia 2. *Annals of Neurology,* Vol.45, pp. 232-41, ISSN 1531-8249.

Huynh DP, Figueroa K, Hoang N & Pulst SM. (2000). Nuclear localization or inclusion body formation of ataxin-2 are not necessary for SCA2 pathogenesis in mouse or human. *Nature Genetics,* Vol.26, pp. 44–50, ISSN 1061-4036.

Huynh DP, Maalouf M, Silva AJ, Schweizer FE & Pulst SM. (2009). Dissociated fear and spatial learning in mice with deficiency of ataxin-2. *PLoS One.* Vol.4, pp. e6235, ISSN 1932-6203.

Huynh DP, Nguyen DT, Pulst-Korenberg JB, Brice A & Pulst SM. (2007). Parkin is an E3 ubiquitin-ligase for normal and mutant ataxin-2 and prevents ataxin-2-induced cell death. *Experimental Neurology,* Vol.203, pp. 531-41, ISSN 1090-2430.

Ihara T, Sasaki H, Wakisaka A, Takada A, Yoshiki T, et al. (1994). Genetic heterogeneity of dominantly inherited olivopontocerebellar atrophy (OPCA) in the Japanese:

linkage study of two pedigrees and evidence for the disease locus on chromosome 12q (SCA2). *Japanese Journal of Human Genetics*, Vol.39, pp. 305-13.

Imbert G, Saudou F, Yvert G, Devys D, Trottier Y, et al. (1996). Cloning of the gene for spinocerebellar ataxia 2 reveals a locus with high sensitivity to expanded CAG/ glutamine repeats. *Nature Genetics*, Vol.14, pp. 285-291, ISSN 1061-4036.

Inagaki A, Iida A, Matsubara M, Inagaki H. (2005). Positron emission tomography and magnetic resonance imaging in spinocerebellar ataxia type 2: a study of symptomatic and asymptomatic individuals. *European Journal of Neurology*, Vol.12, pp. 725-728, ISSN 1468-1331.

Irazno A, Comella CL, Santamaria J, & Oertel W. (2007). Restless legs syndrome in Parkinson's disease and other neurodegenerative diseases of the central nervous system. *Movement Disorders*, Vol.22, pp. S424-S430, ISSN 1531-8257.

Ishida C, Komai K, Yonezawa K, Sakajiri KI, Nitta E, Kawashima A & Yamada M. (2010). An autopsy case of an aged patient with spinocerebellar ataxia type 2. Neuropathology. In press, ISSN 1440-1789.

Kiehl TR, Nechiporuk A, Figueroa KP, Keating MT, Huynh DP, et al. (2006). Generation and characterization of Sca2 (ataxin-2) knockout mice. *Biochemical and Biophysical Research Communications,* Vol.339, pp. 17–24, ISSN 1090-2104.

Kiehl TR, Shibata H & Pulst SM. (2000). The ortholog of human ataxin-2 is essential for early embryonic patterning in C. elegans. *Journal of Molecular Neurosciences*, Vol.15, pp. 231–241, ISSN 0895-8696.

Kim JM, Hong S, Kim GP, Choi YJ, Kim YK, et al. (2007). Importance of low-range CAG expansion and CAA interruption in SCA2 Parkinsonism. *Archives of Neurology,* Vol.64, pp. 1510-18, ISSN 1538-3687.

Klockgether T, Ludtke R, Kramer B, Abele M, Bürk K, Schöls L, et al. (1998). The natural history of degenerative ataxia: a retrospective study in 466 patients. *Brain,* Vol.121, pp. 589–600, ISSN 1460-2156.

Klockgether T. (2007). Ataxias. In: *Textbook of clinical neurology,* Goetz CG, (Ed.), 741-757, Saunder.

Koyano S, Iwabuchi K, Yagishita S, Kuroiwa Y & Uchihara T. (2002). Paradoxical absence of nuclear inclusion in cerebellar Purkinje cells of hereditary ataxias linked to CAG expansion. *Journal of Neurology Neurosurgery and Psychiatry,* Vol.73, pp. 450–52, ISSN 1468-330X.

Kozlov G, Safaee N, Rosenauer A & Gehring K. (2010) Structural basis of binding of P-body-associated proteins GW182 and ataxin-2 by the Mlle domain of poly(A)-binding protein. *Journal of Biological Chemistry*, Vol.285, pp. 13599-606. ISSN 1083-351X.

Kremlacek J, Valis M, Masopust J, Talab R, Kuba M, Kobova Z, et al. (2011). An Electrophysiological Study of Visual Processing in Spinocerebellar Ataxia Type 2 (SCA2). *The cerebellum,* Vol.10, pp. 32–42, ISSN 1473-4230.

Kubis N, Dürr A, Gugenheim M, Chneiweiss H, Mazzetti P, et al. (1999). Polyneuropathy in autosomal dominant cerebellar ataxias: Phenotype-genotype correlation. *Muscle & Nerve.* Vol.22, pp. 712–7, ISSN 1097-4598.

Lagier-Tourenne C, Polymenidou M & Cleveland DW. (2010). TDP-43 and FUS/TLS: emerging roles in RNA processing and neurodegeneration. *Human Molecular Genetics,* Vol.19, pp. R46-64, ISSN 1460-2083.

Lastres-Becker I, Brodesser S, Lütjohann D, Azizov M, Buchmann J, et al. (2008b) Insulin receptor and lipid metabolism pathology in ataxin-2 knock-out mice. *Human Molecular Genetics,* Vol.17, pp. 1465–1481, ISSN 1460-2083.

Lastres-Becker I, Rüb U & Auburger G. (2008a). Spinocerebellar ataxia (SCA2). *The cerebellum,* Vol.2, No.2, pp. 115-124, ISSN 1473-4230.

Lee T, Li YR, Ingre C, Weber M, Grehl T, et al. (2011). Ataxin-2 intermediate-length polyglutamine expansions in European ALS patients. *Human Molecular Genetics,* Vol. 20, pp. 1697-700, ISSN 1460-2083.

Lessing D & Bonini NM. (2008). Polyglutamine genes interact to modulate the severity and progression of neurodegeneration in Drosophila. *PLoS Biol*ogy, Vol.6 pp. e29, ISSN 1545-7885.

Levy D, Ehret GB, Rice K, Verwoert GC, Launer LJ, et al. (2009). Genome-wide association study of blood pressure and hypertension. *Nature Genetics,* Vol.41, pp. 677-87, ISSN 1061-4036.

Liu J, Tang TS, Tu H, Nelson O, Herndon E, et al. (2009). Deranged calcium signaling and neurodegeneration in spinocerebellar ataxia type 2. *Journal of Neuroscience,* Vol.29, pp. 9148-62, ISSN 1529-2401.

Lu CS, Wu Chou YH, Kuo PC, Chang HC & Weng YH. (2004). The Parkinsonian Phenotype of Spinocerebellar Ataxia Type 2. *Archives of Neurology,* Vol. 61, pp. 35-38, ISSN 1538-3687.

Maschke M, Oehlert G, Xie TD, Perlman S, Subramony SH, et al. (2005). Clinical feature profile of spinocerebellar ataxia type 1-8 predicts genetically defined subtypes. *Movement Disorders,* Vol.20, pp. 1405–12, ISSN 1531-8257.

Matilla A, Goold R & Giunti P. (2006). Molecular pathogenesis of spinocerebellar ataxias. *Brain,* Vol.129, pp. 1357–1370, ISSN 1460-2156.

Medrano J, Velázquez L, Canales N, Rodríguez R & González Y. (2009). Estudio electrofisiológico de pares craneales en enfermos portadores asintomáticos de la SCA2. *Revista de Neurología,* Vol.49, pp. 278-279, ISSN 1576-6578.

Meunier C, Bordereaux D, Porteu F, Gisselbrecht S, Chrétien S & Courtois G. (2002). Cloning and characterization of a family of proteins associated with Mpl. *Journal of Biological Chemistry,* Vol.277, pp. 9139-47, ISSN 1083-351X.

Modoni A, Contarino MF, Bentivoglio AR, Tabolacci E, Santoro M, et al. (2007). Prevalence of spinocerebellar ataxia type 2 mutation among Italian Parkinsonian patients. *Movement Disorders,* Vol.22, pp. 324-27, ISSN 1531-8257.

Montes-Brown J, Estévez BM & Almaguer MLE. (2011). [Dysautonomic features in presymptomatic subjects and patients with spinocerebellar ataxia type 2]. *Revista Mexicana de Neurociencias,* Vol.12 No.2, pp. 76-81.

Montes-Brown J, Gilberto MB, Andrés MG, Mario FB & Luis VP. (2010). Heart rate variability in type 2 spinocerebellar ataxia. *Acta Neurologica Scandinavica,* Vol.122, pp. 329-35, ISSN 1600-0404.

Nechiporuk T, Huynh DP, Figueroa K, Sahba S, Nechiporuk A & Pulst SM. (1998). The mouse SCA2 gene: cDNA sequence, alternative splicing and protein expression. *Human Molecular Genetics,* Vol.7, pp. 1301–9, ISSN 1460-2083.

Newton-Cheh C, Johnson T, Gateva V, Tobin MD, Bochud M, et al. (2009). Genome-wide association study identifies eight loci associated with blood pressure. *Nature Genetics,* Vol.41, pp. 666-76, ISSN 1061-4036.

Nonhoff U, Ralser M, Welzel F, Piccini I & Balzereit D. (2007). Ataxin-2 interacts with the DEAD/H-box RNA helicase DDX6 and interferes with P-bodies and stress granules. *Molecular Biology of the Cell,* Vol.18, pp. 1385-96, ISSN 1059-1524.

Nonis D, Schmidt MH, van de Loo S, Eich F, Dikic I, et al. (2008). Ataxin-2 associates with the endocytosis complex and affects EGF receptor trafficking. *Cell Signal.* Vol.20, pp. 1725-39, ISSN 0898-6568.

Orozco DG, Estrada R, Perry T, Araña J & Fernández R. (1989). Dominantly inherited olivopontocerebellar atrophy from eastern Cuba. Clinical, neuropathological and biochemical findings. *Journal of the Neurological Sciences,* Vol.93, pp. 37-50, ISSN 1300-1817.

Orozco-Díaz G, Nodarse-Fleites A, Cordovés-Sagaz R, Auburger G. (1990). Autosomal dominant cerebellar ataxia: clinical analysis of 263 patients from a homogeneous population in Holguín, Cuba. *Neurology,* Vol.40, pp. 1369-75, ISSN 0028-3878.

Oz G, Iltis I, Hutter D, Thomas W, Bushara KO, Gomez CM. (2010) Distinct Neurochemical Profiles of Spinocerebellar Ataxias 1, 2, 6, and Cerebellar Multiple System Atrophy. Cerebellum DOI 10.1007/s12311-010-0213-6, ISSN 1473-4230.

Pang JT, Giunti P, Chamberlain S, An SF, Vitaliani R, et al. (2002). Neuronal intranuclear inclusions in SCA2: A genetic, morphological and immunohistochemical study of two cases. *Brain,* Vol.125, pp. 656–63, ISSN 1460-2156.

Payami H, Nutt J, Gancher S, Bird T, McNeal MG, et al. (2003). SCA2 may present as levodopa-responsive parkinsonism. *Movement Disorders,* Vol.18, pp. 425-29, ISSN 1531-8257.

Pérez-Ávila I, Fernández-Vieitez JA, Martínez-Góngora E, Ochoa-Mastrapa R & Velázquez-Manresa MG. (2004). Efectos de un programa de ejercicios físicos sobre variables neurológicas cuantitativas en pacientes con ataxia espinocerebelosa tipo 2 en estadio leve. *Revista de Neurología,* Vol.39, pp. 907-10, ISSN 1576-6578.

Pradhan C, Yashavantha BS, Pal PK & Sathyaprabha TN. (2008). Spinocerebellar ataxias type 1, 2 and 3: a study of heart rate variability. *Acta Neurologica Scandinavica,* Vol.117, pp. 337-42, ISSN 1600-0404.

Pulst SM, Nechiporuk A, Nechiporuk T, Gispert S, Chen XN, et al. (1996). Moderate expansion of a normally biallelic trinucleotide repeat in spinocerebellar ataxia type 2. *Nature Genetics,* Vol.14, pp. 269-76, ISSN 1061-4036.

Pulst SM, Santos N, Wang D; Yang H, Huynh D, et al. (2005). Spinocerebellar Ataxia type 2: PolyQ Repeat Variation in the CACNA1A Channel Modifies Age of Onset. *Brain,* Vol.128, pp. 2297-303, ISSN 1460-2156.

Ralser M, Albrecht M, Nonhoff U, Lengauer T, Lehrach H & Krobitsch S. (2005a). An integrative approach to gain insights into the cellular function of human ataxin-2. *Journal of Molecular Biology,* Vol.346, pp. 203-14, ISSN 0022-2836.

Ralser M, Nonhoff U, Albrecht M, Lengauer T, Wanker EE, Lehrach H & Krobitsch S. (2005b). Ataxin-2 and huntingtin interact with endophilin-A complexes to function in plastin-associated pathways. *Human Molecular Genetics,* Vol.14, pp. 2893-909, ISSN 1460-2083.

Ramocki MB, Chapieski L, McDonald RO, Fernandez F, Malphrus AD. (2008) Spinocerebellar ataxia type 2 presenting with cognitive regression in childhood. Journal of Child Neurology, Vol.23, pp. 999–1001.

Restivo DA, Giuffrida S & Rapisarda G (2000). Central motor conduction to lower limb after transcranial magnetic stimulation in spinocerebellar ataxia type 2 (SCA2). *Clinical Neurophysiology,* Vol.111, pp. 630-635, ISSN 1388-2457.

Restivo DA, Lanza S, Giuffrida S, Antonuzzo A, Saponara R, et al. (2004). Cortical silent period prolongation in spinocerebellar ataxia type 2 (SCA2). *Functional Neurology,* Vol.19, pp. 37–41, ISSN 0393-5264

Reynaldo-Arminan RD, Reynaldo-Hernández R, Paneque-Herrera M, Prieto-Avila L & Pérez-Ruiz E. (2002). Mental disorders in patients with spinocerebellar ataxia type 2 in Cuba. *Revista de Neurología,* Vol.35, pp. 818-21, ISSN 1576-6578.

Ristori, G; Romano, S; Visconti, A; Cannoni, S; Spadaro, M; Frontali, M, et al. (2010). Riluzole in cerebellar ataxia: A randomized, double-blind, placebo-controlled pilot trial (CME) (LOE Classification). *Neurology.* Vol.74, No.10, pp. 839-45, ISSN 0028-3878.

Rivaud-Pechoux S, Durr A, Gaymard B, Cancel G, Ploner CJ, et al. (1998). Eye movement abnormalities correlate with genotype in autosomal dominant cerebellar ataxia type I. *Annals of Neurology,* Vol.43, pp. 297–302, ISSN 1531-8249.

Rodríguez JC, Velázquez L, Sánchez G, Almaguer L, Almaguer D, García JC, et al. (2008). Evaluación de la restauración neurológica en pacientes con ataxia SCA2 cubana. *Plasticidad & Restauración Neurológica,* Vol.7, No.1, pp. 13-18.

Rodríguez-Labrada R, Velázquez-Pérez L, Canales Ochoa N, et al. (2011b). Subtle Rapid Eye Movement sleep abnormalities in presymptomatic Spinocerebellar Ataxia type 2 gene carriers. *Movement Disorders,* Vol.26, pp. 347-50, ISSN 1531-8257.

Rodríguez-Labrada R; Velázquez-Pérez L; Seigfried C; Canales N, Auburger G, Medrano J, et al. (2011a). Saccadic latency is prolonged in Spinocerebellar Ataxia type 2 and correlates with the frontal-executive dysfunctions. *Journal of the Neurological Sciences,* Vol.306, pp. 103-07, ISSN 1300-1817.

Ross OA, Rutherford NJ, Baker M, Soto-Ortolaza AI, Carrasquillo MM, et al. (2011). Ataxin-2 repeat-length variation and neurodegeneration. *Human Molecular Genetics,* In press, ISSN 1460-2083.

Rüb U, Brunt ER, de Vos RA, Del Turco D, Del Tredici K, et al. (2004a). Degeneration of the central vestibular system in spinocerebellar ataxia type 3 (SCA3) patients and its possible clinical significance. *Neuropathology and Applied Neurobiology,* Vol.30, pp. 402-14, ISSN 1365-2990.

Rüb U, Brunt ER, Petrasch-Parwez E, Schöls L, Theegarten D, et al. (2006). Degeneration of ingestion-related brainstem nuclei in spinocerebellar ataxia type 2, 3, 6 and 7. *Neuropathology and Applied Neurobiology,* Vol.32, pp. 635-49, ISSN 1365-2990.

Rüb U, Bürk K, Schöls L, Brunt ER, de Vos RA, et al. (2004b). Damage to the reticulotegmental nucleus of the pons in spinocerebellar ataxia type 1, 2, and 3. *Neurology*, Vol.63, pp. 1258-63, ISSN 0028-3878.

Rüb U, Del Turco D, Bürk K, Díaz GO, Auburger G, et al. (2005b). Extended pathoanatomical studies point to a consistent affection of the thalamus in spinocerebellar ataxia type 2. *Neuropathology and Applied Neurobiology*, Vol.31, pp. 127–40, ISSN 1365-2990.

Rüb U, Del Turco D, Del Tredici K, de Vos RA, Brunt ER, et al. (2003b). Thalamic involvement in a spinocerebellar ataxia type 2 (SCA2) and spinocerebellar type 3 (SCA3) patient and its clinical relevance. *Brain*, Vol.126, pp. 1–16, ISSN 1460-2156.

Rüb U, Gierga K, Brunt ER, de Vos RA, Bauer M, et al. (2005a). Spinocerebellar ataxias types 2 and 3: degeneration of the precerebellar nuclei isolates the three phylogenetically defined regions of the cerebellum. *Journal of Neural Transmission*, Vol.112, pp. 1523–45, ISSN 0303-6995.

Rüb U, Schultz C, Del Tredici K, Gierga K, Reifenberger G, de Vos RA, et al. (2003a). Anatomically based guidelines for systematic investigation of the central somatosensory system and their application to a spinocerebellar ataxia type 2 (SCA2) patient. *Neuropathology and Applied Neurobiology*, Vol.29, pp. 418–33, ISSN 1365-2990.

Rüb U, Seidel K, Ozerden I, Gierga K, Brunt ER, et al. (2007). Consistent affection of the central somatosensory system in spinocerebellar ataxia type 2 and type 3 and its significance for clinical symptoms and rehabilitative therapy. *Brain Research Reviews*, Vol.53, pp. 235-49, ISSN 0165-0173.

Rufa A, Dotti MT, Galli L, Orrico A, Sicurelli F & Federico A. (2002). Spinocerebellar ataxia type 2 (SCA2) associated with retinal pigmentary degeneration. *European Neurology*, Vol.47, pp. 128–29, ISSN 1421-9913.

Sahba S, Nechiporuk A, Figueroa KP, Nechiporuk T & Pulst SM. (1998). Genomic structure of the human gene for spinocerebellar ataxia type 2 (SCA2) on chromosome 12q24.1. *Genomics*, Vol.47, pp. 359–64, ISSN 1089-8646.

Sanchez-Cruz G, Velazquez-Perez L, Gomez-Pena L, Martinez-Gongora E, Castellano-Sanchez G & Santos-Falcon N. (2001). Dysautonomic features in patients with Cuban type 2 spinocerebellar ataxia. *Revista de Neurología*, Vol.33, No.5, pp. 428-34, ISSN 1576-6578.

Sanpei K, Takano H, Igarashi S, Sato T, Oyake M, et al. (1996). Identification of the spinocerebellar ataxia type 2 gene using a direct identification of repeat expansion and cloning technique, DIRECT. *Nature Genetics*, Vol.14, pp. 277-84, ISSN 1061-4036.

Sasaki H, Wakisaka A, Sanpei K, Takano H, Igarashi S, et al. (1998). Phenotype variation correlates with CAG repeat length in SCA2 - a study of 28 Japanese patients. *Journal of the Neurological Sciences*, Vol.159, pp. 202-08, ISSN 1300-1817.

Satterfield TF & Pallanck LJ. (2006). Ataxin-2 and its Drosophila homolog, ATX2, physically assemble with polyribosomes. *Human Molecular Genetics*, Vol.15, pp. 2523-32, ISSN 1460-2083.

Schmitz-Hubsch T, Fimmers R, Rakowicz M, Rola R, Zdzienicka E, Fancellu R, et al. (2006) Responsiveness of different rating instruments in spinocerebellar ataxia patients. *Neurology*. Vol.74, pp. 678-g84. ISSN 0028-3878.

Schmitz-Hubsch T, Coudert M, Bauer P, Giunti P, Globas C, Baliko L, et al. (2008) Spinocerebellar ataxia types 1, 2, 3, and 6: disease severity and nonataxia symptoms. *Neurology*, Vol.71, pp.982-989, ISSN 0028-3878.

Schöls L, Haan J, Riess O, Amoiridis G & Przuntek H. (1998). Sleep disturbance in spinocerebellar ataxias: is the SCA3 mutation a cause of restless legs syndrome? *Neurology*. Vol.51, pp. 1603–07, ISSN 0028-3878.

Schöls L, Bauer P, Schmidt T, Schulte T & Riess O. (2004). Autosomal dominant cerebellar ataxias: clinical features, genetics, and pathogenesis. *The Lancet*, Vol. 3, pp. 291-304, ISSN 1474-547X.

Schöls L, Gispert S, Vorgerd M, Menezes Vieira-Saecker AM, Blanke P, et al. (1997). Spinocerebellar ataxia type 2. Genotype and phenotype in German kindreds. *Archives of Neurology*, Vol.54, pp. 1073-80, ISSN 1538-3687.

Schwenkreis P, Tegenthoff M, Witscher K, Börnke C, Przuntek H, et al. (2002). Motor cortex activation by transcranial magnetic stimulation in ataxia patients depends on the genetic defect. *Brain*, Vol.125, pp. 301-05, ISSN 1460-2156.

Sebastiani P, Solovieff N, Puca A, Hartley SW, Melista E, et al. (2010). Genetic Signatures of Exceptional Longevity in Humans. *Science*, (Nov 11), ISSN 0036-8075.

Shibata H, Huynh DP & Pulst SM. (2000). A novel protein with RNA-binding motifs interacts with ataxin-2. *Human Molecular Genetics*, Vol.9, pp. 1303-13, ISSN 1460-2083.

Shulman JM & Feany MB. (2003). Genetic modifiers of tauopathy in Drosophila. *Genetics*, Vol.165, pp. 1233-42, ISSN 0016-6731.

Siddiqui N, Mangus DA, Chang TC, Palermino JM, Shyu AB & Gehring K. (2007) Poly(A) nuclease interacts with the C-terminal domain of polyadenylate-binding protein domain from poly(A)-binding protein. *Journal of Biological Chemistry*, Vol.282, pp. 25067-75, ISSN 1083-351X.

Simon DK, Zheng K, Velázquez L, Figueroa KP, Falcón N, Almaguer LE & Pulst SM. (2007). Mitochondrial complex I gene variant associated with early age of onset in SCA2. *Archives of Neurology*, Vol.64, pp. 1042–44, ISSN 1538-3687.

Sorarù G, Clementi M, Forzan M, Orsetti V, D'Ascenzo C, et al. (2011). ALS risk but not phenotype is affected by ataxin-2 intermediate length polyglutamine expansion. *Neurology*, Vol.76, pp. 2030-31, ISSN 0028-3878.

Storey E, Forrest SM, Shaw JH, Mitchell P & Gardner RJ. (1999) Spinocerebellar ataxia type 2: clinical features of a pedigree displaying prominent frontal-executive dysfunction. *Archives of Neurology*, Vol.56, pp. 43-50, ISSN 1538-3687.

Sulek-Pitkowska A, Zdzienicka E, Raczyñska-Rakowicz M, Krysa W, Rajkiewicz M , Szirkowiec W, et al. (2010). The occurrence of spinocerebellar ataxias in Poland. *Neurologia i Neurochirurgia Polska*, Vol.44, No.3, pp. 238-45.

Swisher KD & Parker R. (2010). Localization to, and effects of Pbp1, Pbp4, Lsm12, Dhh1, and Pab1 on stress granules in Saccharomyces cerevisiae. *PLoS One*. Vol.5, pp. e10006, ISSN 1932-6203.

Tan NC, Zhou Y, Tan AS, Chong SS & Lee WL. (2004). Spinocerebellar ataxia type 2 with focal epilepsy-an unusual association. *Annals of the Academy of Medicine Singapore*, Vol.33, pp. 103–06, ISSN 0304-4602.

Trojano L, Chiacchio L, Grossi D, Pisacreta AI, Calabrese O, Castaldo I, et al. (1998). Determinants of cognitive disorders in Autosomal Dominant Cerebellar Ataxia type 1. *Journal of the Neurological Sciences*, Vol.157, pp. 162-67, ISSN 1300-1817.

Tuin I, Voss U, Kang JS, Kessler K, Rüb U, et al. (2006). Stages of sleep pathology in spinocerebellar ataxia type 2 (SCA2). *Neurology*, Vol.67, pp. 1966-72, ISSN 0028-3878.

Turnbull VJ, Storey E, Tarlac V, Walsh R, Stefani D, et al. (2004). Different ataxin-2 antibodies display different immunoreactive profiles. *Brain Research*, Vol.1027, pp. 103–16, ISSN 0006-8993.

Uchihara T, Fujigasaki H, Koyano S, Nakamura A, Yagishita S & Iwabuchi K. (2001). Non-expanded polyglutamine proteins in intranuclear inclusions of hereditary ataxias - triple-labeling immunofluorescence study. *Acta Neuropathologica*, Vol.102, pp. 149–52, ISSN 1432-0533.

Vallés L, Estrada GL & Bastecherrea SL. (1978). Algunas formas de heredoataxia en una región de Cuba. *Revista de Neurología (Cubana)*, Vol.27, pp. 163-76.

Van Damme P, Veldink JH, van Blitterswijk M, Corveleyn A, van Vught PW, et al. (2011). Expanded ATXN2 CAG repeat size in ALS identifies genetic overlap between ALS and SCA2. *Neurology*, Vol.76, pp. 2066-72, ISSN 0028-3878.

van de Loo S, Eich F, Nonis D, Auburger G & Nowock J. (2009). Ataxin-2 associates with rough endoplasmic reticulum. *Experimental Neurology*. Vol.215, pp. 110-18, ISSN 1090-2430.

van de Warrenburg BP, Notermans NC, Schelhaas HJ, van Alfen N, Sinke RJ, et al. (2004). Peripheral nerve involvement in spinocerebellar ataxias. *Archives of Neurology*, Vol. 61, pp. 257–61, ISSN 1538-3687.

Velázquez PL, Fernández-Ruiz J, Díaz R, González RP, Ochoa NC, et al. (2006) Spinocerebellar ataxia type 2 olfactory impairment shows a pattern similar to other major neurodegenerative diseases. *Journal of Neurology*, Vol.253, No.9, pp. 1165-69, ISSN 0340-5354.

Velázquez-Perez L, Díaz R, Pérez R, Canales N, Rodríguez-Labrada R, et al. (2009d). Motor Decline in Clinically Presymptomatic Spinocerebellar Ataxia Type 2 Gene Carriers. *Plos One*, Vol.4, pp. 5398-5402, ISSN 1932-6203.

Velázquez-Pérez L, Rodríguez-Chanfrau J, García-Rodríguez JC, Sánchez-Cruz G, Aguilera-Rodríguez R, et al. (2011c). Oral Zinc Sulphate Supplementation for Six Months in SCA2 Patients: A Randomized, Double-Blind, Placebo-Controlled Trial. *Neurochemical Research*, In press, ISSN 1573-6903.

Velázquez-Pérez L, Rodríguez-Labrada R, Canales-Ochoa N, Sánchez-Cruz G, Fernández-Ruiz J, et al. (2010) Progression markers of Spinocerebellar Ataxia 2. A twenty years neurophysiological follow up study. *Journal of the Neurological Sciences*, Vol.290, pp. 22-6, ISSN 1300-1817.

Velázquez-Pérez L, Rodríguez-Labrada R, García-Rodríguez JC, Almaguer-Mederos LE, Cruz-Mariño T, Laffita-Mesa JM. (2011b). A Comprehensive Review of

Spinocerebellar Ataxia Type 2 in Cuba. *The Cerebellum*, Vol.10, pp. 184–98, ISSN 1473-4230.

Velázquez-Pérez L, Rodríguez-Labrada R, Medrano-Montero J, Sánchez-Cruz G, Canales-Ochoa N, et al. (2009b). Patrón electromiográfico en enfermos y portadores asintomáticos de la mutación SCA2. *Revista de Neurología*, Vol.49, No.1, pp. 55-6, ISSN 1576-6578.

Velázquez-Pérez L, Sánchez-Cruz G, Canales-Ochoa N, Rodríguez-Labrada R, Rodríguez-Díaz J, et al. (2007). Electrophysiological features in patients and presymptomatic relatives with spinocerebellar ataxia type 2. *Journal of the Neurological Sciences*, Vol.263, No.1-2, pp. 158-64, ISSN 1300-1817.

Velázquez-Pérez L, Sánchez-Cruz G, Santos-Falcón N, Enrique Almaguer-Mederos L, Escalona-Batallán K, et al. (2009a). Molecular epidemiology of spinocerebellar ataxias in Cuba: Insights into SCA2 founder effect in Holguín. *Neuroscience Letters*, Vol.454, pp. 157-60, ISSN 0304-3940.

Velázquez-Pérez L, Santos FN, García R, Paneque HM & Hechavarría PR. (2001). Epidemiología de la Ataxia Cubana. *Revista de Neurología*, Vol.32, pp. 606-11, ISSN 1576-6578.

Velázquez-Perez L, Seifried C, Santos-Falcón N, Abele M, Ziemann U, et al. (2004). Saccade velocity is controlled by polyglutamine size in spinocerebellar ataxia 2. *Annals of Neurology*, Vol.56, No.3, pp. 444-47, ISSN 1531-8249.

Velázquez-Pérez L, Seifried C, Abele M, Wirjatijasa F, Rodríguez-Labrada R, et al. (2009c). Saccade velocity is reduced in presymptomatic spinocerebellar ataxia type 2. *Clinical Neurophysiology*, Vol.120, pp. 632-35, ISSN 1388-2457.

Velázquez-Pérez L, Voss U, Rodríguez-Labrada R, Auburger G, Canales Ochoa N, Sánchez Cruz G, Galicia Polo L, et al. (2011a). Sleep Disorders in Spinocerebellar Ataxia Type 2 Patients. *Neurodegenerative Diseases*. In press, ISSN 1660-2862.

Velázquez-Pérez L. (2008). *Spinocerebellar ataxia type 2. Main neurophysiological aspects into the diagnosis, prognosis and disease evolution* (2nd Ed), Ediciones Holguín, ISBN 959-221-202-3, Holguín, Cuba.

Velázquez L, Sánchez G, García JC, Delgado R, Márquez L, Martínez E, Net al. (2003) Spinocerebellar ataxia type 2 (SCA-2) in Cuba. A study of the clinical electrophysiological and REDOX system variations and its correlation with CAG repeats. *Restorative Neurology and Neurosciences*; 277; 20:(6).

Wadia NH & Swami RK. (1971). A new form of heredo-familial spinocerebellar degeneration with slow eye movements (nine families). *Brain*, Vol.94, pp. 359–74, ISSN 1460-2156.

Wiedemeyer R, Westermann F, Wittke I, Nowock J & Schwab M. (2003). Ataxin-2 promotes apoptosis of human neuroblastoma cells. *Oncogene*, Vol.22, pp. 401-11, ISSN 0950-9232.

Wüllner U, Reimold M, Abele M, Bürk K, Minnerop M, et al. (2005). Dopamine Transporter Positron Emission Tomography in Spinocerebellar Ataxias Type 1, 2, 3, and 6. *Archives of Neurology*, Vol.62, pp. 1280-85, ISSN 1538-3687.

Yagishita S & Inoue M. (1997). Clinicopathology of spinocerebellar degeneration: Its correlation to the unstable CAG repeat of the affected gene. *Pathology International*, Vol.47, pp. 1-15, ISSN 1440-1827.

Ying SH, Choi SI, Lee M, Perlman SL, Baloh RW, et al. (2005). Relative atrophy of the flocculus and ocular motor dysfunction in SCA2 and SCA6. *Annals of the New York Academy of Sciences*, Vol.1039, pp. 430–5, ISSN 0077-8923.

Yokota T, Sasaki H, Iwabuchi K, Shiojiri T, Yoshino A, et al. (1998). Electrophysiological features of central motor conduction in spinocerebellar atrophy type 1, type 2, and Machado-Joseph disease. *Journal of Neurology Neurosurgery and Psychiatry*, Vol.65, pp. 530–34, ISSN 1468-330X.

Yu Z, Zhu Y, Chen-Plotkin AS, Clay-Falcone D, McCluskey L, et al. (2011). PolyQ repeat expansions in ATXN2 associated with ALS are CAA interrupted repeats. *PLoS One*, Vol.6, No.3, pp. e17951, ISSN 1932-6203.

6

Machado-Joseph Disease / Spinocerebellar Ataxia Type 3

Clévio Nóbrega[1] and Luís Pereira de Almeida[1,2]
[1]*CNC - Center for Neurosciences & Cell Biology, University of Coimbra;*
[2]*Faculty of Pharmacy, University of Coimbra, Coimbra, Portugal*

1. Introduction

Spinocerebellar Ataxia type 3 (SCA3) or Machado-Joseph disease (MJD) is one of the most common polyglutamine (polyQ) diseases, which comprise a group of inherited neurodegenerative conditions characterized by the pathological expansion of CAG trinucleotide repeats in the translated regions of unrelated genes. The expansion of a (CAG) tract in the coding region of the causative gene *MJD1,* translates into an expanded polyglutamine tract that confers a toxic gain of function to the ataxin-3 protein. The mutant protein form has 55-84 consecutive glutamines, in contrast to the normal ataxin-3, which carries 10-51 glutamines.

MJD is a fatal disease of the central nervous system (CNS) and a dominant neurodegenerative disorder of adult onset, characterized by a wide range of clinical symptoms, including gait and limb ataxia, peripheral neuropathy, bulging eyes, ophthalmoplegia, postural instability, dystonia, amyotrophy, dysarthria, nystagmus, lingual fasciculation's, facial myokymia and, in some cases, parkinsonism. The expression of mutant ataxin-3 is widespread, although neurodegeneration in MJD has been described in particular brain regions such as the cerebellum, brainstem, substantia nigra, pontine nuclei and striatum. A hallmark of the disease is the presence of neuronal intranuclear inclusions of mutant ataxin-3. The genetic basis of MJD is well described, however, the molecular basis is still poorly understood and controversial. Several pathogenesis mechanisms have been proposed for MJD (as well for other polyQ diseases), which could be explored as potential therapeutic approaches to MJD. Decreasing the expression of mutant ataxin-3 through gene silencing has been shown to be one of the most promising therapeutic approaches to MJD. However, several others are presently under investigation, such as the inhibition of protein cleavage, and the induction of autophagy, as well as strategies based on neuroprotection or regulation of transcriptional dysfunction. The main aim of this chapter is to review the current knowledge about MJD/SCA3, including a short review of clinical and neuropathological aspects of MJD and a particular focus on the pathogenesis and potential therapeutic strategies for the disease.

2. Machado-Joseph disease

Machado-Joseph disease (MJD) or spinocerebellar ataxia type 3 (SCA3) is the most common autosomal subtype of ataxia worldwide (Coutinho and Andrade, 1978; Rosenberg, 1992; Ranum et al., 1995; Schols et al., 2004). It is caused by the unstable expansion of a CAG repeat in the *MJD1* gene, which translates into a polyglutamine tract within the ataxin-3 protein (Takiyama et al., 1993; Kawaguchi et al., 1994). This neurodegenerative disorder of adult onset was named after Antone Joseph and William Machado, of Portuguese Azorean origin, who migrated to USA. MJD was subsequently identified in Brazil, Japan, China, Australia and many other countries. In the islands of the Azores, namely São Miguel and Flores, MJD reaches the highest prevalence (1:140 in the small island of Flores) reported worldwide (Sudarsky and Coutinho, 1995).

3. Clinical and physiological features

MJD is characterized primarily by cerebellar ataxia and pyramidal signs variably associated with a dystonic-rigid extrapyramidal syndrome or peripheral amyotrophy (Lima and Coutinho, 1980; D'Abreu et al., 2010). The clinical hallmark of MJD is progressive ataxia, a dysfunction of motor coordination that can affect gaze, speech, gait, and balance (Taroni and DiDonato, 2004). Other clinical manifestations include external progressive ophthalmoplegia, dystonia, intention fasciculation-like movements of facial and lingual muscles, as well as bulging eyes. Progressive ataxia, hyperreflexia, nystagmus, and dysarthria may occur early in the disease (Lima and Coutinho, 1980; Sudarsky and Coutinho, 1995).

MJD type	Age of onset	Prevalence	Symptoms
I	5-30 years		Limb and gait ataxia, severe dystonia, pyramidal signs, progressive external ophthalmoplegia. Fast progression of symptoms
II	≈ 36 years	The most common	Ataxia, pyramidal deficits and progressive external ophthalmoplegia
III	≈ 50 years	The second most common	Limb and gait ataxia, with marked pyramidal signs. The progressive external ophthalmoplegia can or not manifest. This type has a moderate progression and can evolve to one of the other types
IV	38-47 years	In patients with the fewest CAG-repeats expansion	Slow progressive parkinsonism, responsive to the L-DOPA treatment, fasciculations and peripheral neuropathy
V			Marked spastic paraplegia with or without cerebellar ataxia. This type is usually mis-diagnosed as hereditary spastic paraplegia (HSP)

Table 1. Classification of MJD according to symptoms, prevalence and age of onset.

Recent clinical data has demonstrated increased incidence of non-motor symptoms, which include cognitive and psychiatric disturbances, olfactory dysfunction, and sleep disorders (Rub et al., 2008). Levodopa-responsive parkinsonism symptoms resembling Parkinson's disease were also reported (Gwinn-Hardy et al., 2001). MJD patients present attention and executive dysfunctions, and mildly depressed mood (Klinke et al., 2010). Based on clinical manifestations, MJD was divided into four sub phenotypes (Riess et al., 2008), which in some cases during the progression of the disease can evolve from one type to the other (Fowler, 1984). Recently, an additional MJD type (V) has been proposed based in a homozygous 33-years old patient of Portuguese/Brazilian descent (Lysenko et al., 2010) (Table 1).

4. Neuropathological features

The neuropathological alterations of MJD in the brain consist of widespread neuronal degeneration affecting multiple neuronal systems and not confined to the cerebellum, brain stem, and basal ganglia (Rub et al., 2008). The neuropathology involves cerebellar systems (particularly dentate nucleus and pontine neurons), substantia nigra, and cranial nerve motor nuclei, with relative preservation of cerebellar cortex, particularly Purkinje cells and inferior olive (Sudarsky and Coutinho, 1995; Durr et al., 1996; Yamada et al., 2008). However in some cases, loss of granule and Purkinje cells was found in the cerebellum, mainly in the vermis (Munoz et al., 2002). A marked degeneration of Clarke's column nuclei and vestibular and pontine nuclei is observed (Durr et al., 1996). Marked neuronal loss is also observed in the anterior horn of the spinal cord, and motor nuclei of the brainstem (Rub et al., 2008). Involvement of cerebellar cortex, autonomic ganglia and striatum were also confirmed in MJD (Yamada et al., 2001; Paulson et al., 1997b; Alves et al., 2008b). Recent data based on neuroimaging techniques (magnetic resonance imaging - MRI, and quantitative 3-D volumetry) confirmed a severe atrophy in MJD patients in the whole brainstem (midbrain, pons, and medulla), whole cerebellum, cerebellar hemispheres and cerebellar vermis, putamen and caudate nuclei (Schulz et al., 2010). Significant correlation of both brainstem and cerebellar atrophy with CAG repeat length, age, disease duration and degree of disability has also been recently reported (Camargos et al., 2011). Furthermore, an inverse relationship has been found in MJD patients between posture, gait and limb kinetic subscore (assessed by the Scale for Assessment and Rating Ataxia) and the brainstem and cerebellar hemispheric volumes (Jacobi et al., 2011).

5. The *MJD1* gene

MJD is associated with an unstable expansion of a CAG tract in the coding region of the *MJD1* gene localized on chromosome 14q32.1 (Takiyama et al., 1993; Kawaguchi et al., 1994). *MJD1* encodes ataxin-3, a polyubiquitin-binding protein whose physiological function has been linked to ubiquitin-mediated proteolysis (Burnett et al., 2003; Donaldson et al., 2003; Doss-Pepe et al., 2003; Scheel et al., 2003; Chai et al., 2004; Durcan et al., 2011). The mutation results in an expanded polyglutamine tract at the C-terminus of ataxin-3 (Kawaguchi et al., 1994; Durr et al., 1996). The CAG repeats in the *MJD1* gene range from 10 to 51 in the normal population and from 55 to 87 in MJD patients (Cummings and Zoghbi, 2000; Maciel et al., 2001; Gu et al., 2004; Padiath et al., 2005). This high threshold of pathogenicity is a special characteristic of this disorder, since in most other polyglutamine disorders trinucleotide repeats over 36 to 40 become pathogenic. There is an inverse correlation between the age of onset and the number of CAG repeats, as is the case for other polyglutamine disorders (Maciel et al., 1995; Maruyama et al., 1995; Globas et al., 2008).

6. The ataxin-3 protein

Ataxin-3 is a modular protein with an overall molecular weight of 42 kDa, containing a conserved N-terminal Josephin domain (Masino et al., 2003; Scheel et al., 2003; Albrecht et al., 2004), followed by two ubiquitin-interaction motif (UIM) domains and the polyglutamine repeat region (Figure 1). Alternative splicing of the *MJD1* gene has been shown to result in the production of different isoforms of ataxin-3 varying at the C-terminal portion of the protein (Goto et al., 1997), one of these containing a third UIM domain after the polyglutamine region (Ichikawa et al., 2001). Fifty-six alternative splicing variants of the ataxin-3 mRNA were recently identified, from which 50 had not been previously described, and 26 were only found in MJD patients (Bettencourt et al., 2010). Alternative splicing of ataxin-3 sequences distinct from the trinucleotide repeat may alter the properties of the encoded polyglutamine disease protein and thereby perhaps contribute to selective neurotoxicity (Harris et al., 2010). The protein is expressed in various tissues, suggesting that it plays an important role in eukaryotic cells (see Matos et al., 2011 for an extensive revision of putative ataxin-3 functions).

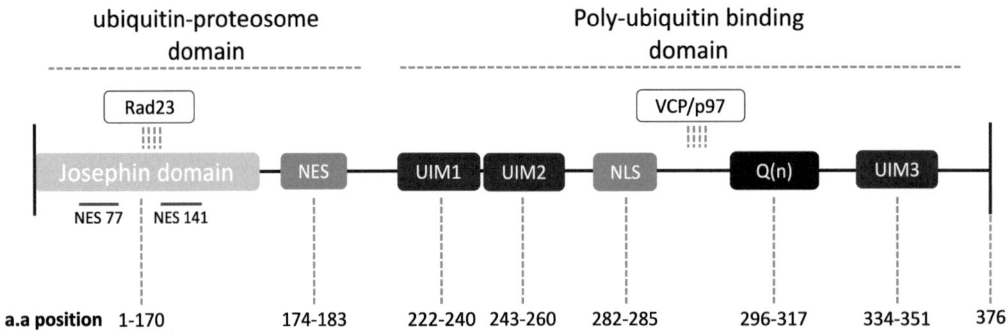

Fig. 1. **Structure of the ataxin-3 protein.** Ataxin-3 is mainly composed of a highly conserved N-terminal domain (Josephin), encoding a predicted ubiquitin-specific protease with the catalytic triad of amino acids (Cys14, His119, and Asn136), a nuclear export signal (NES), followed by a flexible C-terminal tail with 2 or 3 ubiquitin-interacting motifs (UIM), a nuclear localization signal (NLS) and the polyglutamine stretch ($Q_{(n)}$). Rad23 and VCP/p97, the two most frequently described interacting partners of ataxin-3, bind to the Josephin domain and the C-terminal region of the protein, respectively.

Regarding subcellular localization, ataxin-3 has been detected both in the nucleus and in the cytoplasm (Paulson et al., 1997a; Trottier et al., 1998; Ichikawa et al., 2001). A putative nuclear localization signal (NLS) has been identified upstream the polyglutamine repeat region at position 282 (Tait et al., 1998; Albrecht et al., 2004), and shown to have a weak nuclear import activity (Antony et al., 2009). Furthermore, two nuclear export signals (NES) with significant activity were identified in ataxin-3: NES 77 (177-Y99) and NES 141 (E141-E258) (Antony et al., 2009). Ataxin-3 its actively imported to and exported from the cell nucleus, and this nuclear export activity could also be dependent on a motif localized at is N-terminal region (Rodrigues et al., 2007; Macedo-Ribeiro et al., 2009), which is coherent with the hypothesis of the presence of a nuclear export signal (NES 174) following the Josephin domain (Albrecht et al., 2004).

Although the precise cellular role of ataxin-3 and how it is altered upon polyglutamine expansion is presently unknown, ataxin-3 was shown to be a polyubiquitin-binding protein (Donaldson et al., 2003; Doss-Pepe et al., 2003), interacting via the first two UIM domains with K48-linked tetraubiquitin chains (Burnett et al., 2003; Chai et al., 2004). Several lines of evidence suggest that ataxin-3 plays a major role in the ubiquitin proteasomal system, by interacting with ubiquitin and an ubiquitin-like protein called NEDD8 (Ferro et al., 2007). Ataxin-3 was reported to bind and hydrolyze polyubiquitin chains in vitro (Burnett et al., 2003). Recently, it was shown that ataxin-3 deubiquitinates parkin directly (Durcan et al., 2011). The same study argued that compared with wild-type ataxin-3, MJD-linked polyQ-expanded mutant ataxin-3 is more active, possibly owing to its greater efficiency at DUB K27- and K29-linked Ub conjugates on parkin. Ataxin-3 has been also shown to be involved in the regulation of the proteasome by interacting with various substrates (Wang et al., 2006, 2007; Rodrigues et al., 2009). Ataxin-3 deubiquitinating activity is thought to contribute to proteasomal degradation of ubiquitinated proteins by removing the poly-ubiquitin chains from substrates prior to digestion (Boeddrich et al., 2006; Winborn et al., 2008; Todi et al., 2009; Scaglione et al., 2011). Ubiquitination and deubiquitination enzymes help to control neuronal fate determination, axonal path finding and synaptic communication and plasticity (see Todi and Paulson, 2011 for a review). Altogether, these data imply that ataxin-3 modulates ubiquitin-dependent mechanisms, having an active role in the ubiquitin-proteasome pathway.

7. Nuclear inclusions

In MJD, mutant ataxin-3 aggregates into intranuclear inclusions (NIIs) with many affected neurons exhibiting more than one inclusion body, both in and outside areas affected by neurodegeneration (Paulson et al., 1997b; Schimdt et al., 1998; Rub et al., 2006a, b). Aggregates are also found in the cytoplasm of neurons in several affected areas (Hayashi et al., 2003), and in axons within fiber tracts (corpus callosum, the nigrostriatal tract, the olivocerebellar fiber, and others) known to undergo neurodegeneration in MJD (Seidel et al., 2010). The presence of these NIIs is a hallmark of neurodegeneration in the brains of MJD patients (Figure 2A), and to all the CAG repeat diseases except for the spinocerebellar ataxia type 6 (SCA6) (Paulson, 1999; Schols et al., 2004; Soong and Paulson, 2007). NIIs are eosinophilic round structures and vary in size from 0.7 to 3.7 μm. Ultra structurally, NIIs are non-membrane bound, heterogeneous in composition, and contain a mix of granular and filamentous structures. Both normal and expanded ataxin-3, and ubiquitin are components of NIIs of affected neurons in MJD patients (Paulson et al., 1997a), as well as other proteins, including heat shock proteins (HSPs) and transcription factors (Hayashi et al., 2003; Perez et al., 1998; Yamada et al., 2001). Ataxin-2, the protein that upon polyglutamine expansion causes spinocerebellar ataxia type 2 - SCA2, and the TATA box binding protein (TBP) were also found in NIIs of the pontine neurons of MJD patients (Uchihara et al., 2001).

The NIIs in MJD are distributed in many neurons covering a wide range of central and peripheral nervous system regions, including the cerebral cortex (Figure 2B), thalamus and autonomic ganglia (Schilling et al., 1999). The exact role of NIIs in neuronal cell death of MJD patients remains unclear and controversial (Bates, 2003; Michalik and Broeckhoven, 2003; Yamada et al., 2008). However, as NIIs are present in degenerated as well as spared brain regions in advanced MJD patients, NIIs are not thought to be directly pathogenic in affected nerve cells (Rub et al., 2006b). In the other polyglutamine disorders the cytotoxicity of NIIs is also controversial. Several studies raised the possibility that NII formation may be a cellular reaction to reduce the toxic effect of mutant proteins (Klement et al., 1998; Saudou et al., 1998; Cummings et al., 1999). On the other hand, other studies revealed that the presence of transcription factors in NIIs (Yamada et al., 2001; Shimohata et al., 2000a,b), may induce secondarily transcriptional abnormalities in cell nuclei, resulting in slowly progressive neuronal degeneration.

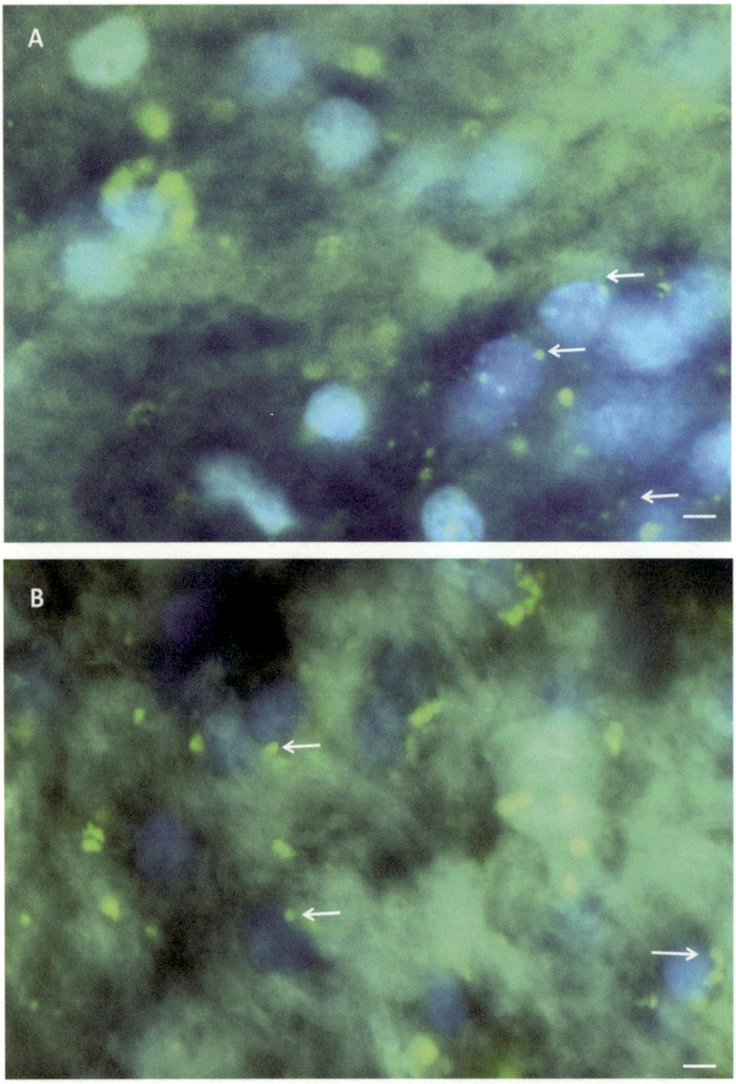

Fig. 2. **Intranuclear inclusions in the striatum of Machado Joseph disease patients.** (A) Fluorescence analysis shows ataxin-3 reaction intranuclear inclusions (green) in the neurons of the striatum of postmortem brain samples of MJD patients (white arrows). (B) Fluorescence microscopy analysis shows ataxin-3 intranuclear inclusions (green) in neurons of the cortex of postmortem brain samples of MJD patients (white arrows). Scale bar: 40μm.

8. Pathogenesis

The genetic basis of MJD is well described, however, the molecular basis is still poorly understood and controversial. It is widely accepted that polyglutamine diseases may share pathogenic mechanisms. In this section several pathogenic mechanisms that could be implicated in MJD are reviewed (Figure 3).

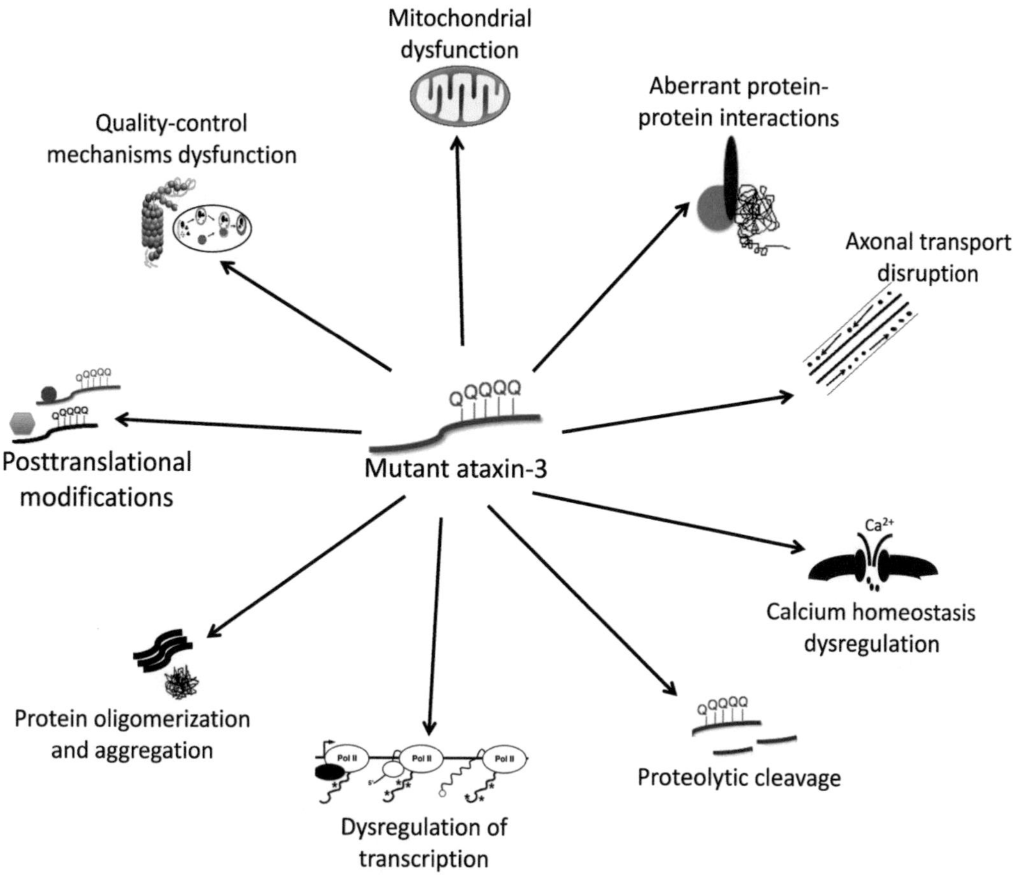

Fig. 3. **Mechanisms of pathogenesis in Machado-Joseph disease**. Several events and mechanisms could contribute to pathogenesis in MJD and other polyglutamine diseases. The presence of mutant ataxin-3 with an expanded tract in the cellular environment, triggers several events that lead to neurodegeneration in selective areas of the brain. For the neuronal cytoxicity and dysfunction several mechanisms related to the toxicity of the expanded polyglutamine stretch are important such as the oligomerization and aggregation, the formation of toxic fragments or posttranslational modifications. Furthermore, the normal function of ataxin-3 in the cell could contribute to the impairment of UPS in MJD, and thus contribute to a dysfunction in cellular quality-control mechanisms. Other mechanisms could also be important to MJD pathogenesis, such as dysregulation of transcription, mitochondrial dysfunction, aberrant protein-protein interactions, calcium homeostasis dysregulation and axonal transport disruption.

8.1 Toxicity of the polyglutamine stretch

A common feature of polyglutamine diseases is the deposition of insoluble intracellular ubiquitinated inclusions containing the misfolded disease protein (Paulson, 1999). These inclusions have long been suspected to be pathologic structures in polyglutamine diseases (Ross, 1997; Martindale et al., 1998; Yamada et al., 2000). Although this correlation is controversial and unclear (Bates, 2003; Michalik and Broeckhoven, 2003; Yamada et al., 2008), the NIIs could physically impair axonal transport or nuclear function (Morfini et al., 2005). Furthermore, the NIIs recruit other proteins, transcription factors and proteasome subunits (Chai et al., 1999a,b), underlying misfolding events that may be critical to pathogenesis (Paulson, 1999; Goti et al., 2004; Jana and Nukina, 2004; Taylor et al., 2002).

Polyglutamine monomers of ataxin-3 acquire β-strand conformations that have been shown to be cytotoxic in cultured cells (Nagai et al., 2007), assembling into oligomers (Bevivino and Loll, 2001; Takahashi et al., 2008), both of ataxin-3 as well as other polyglutamine monomers (Stott et al., 1995; Lathrop et al., 1998; Tanaka et al., 2001; Thakur and Wetzel, 2002), and can also simultaneously dissociate into monomers (Schaffar et al., 2004). Thus, it seems that β-stranded polyglutamine monomers are important for pathogenesis in MJD and other polyglutamine diseases, however its contribution to neurotoxicity is still controversial.

In several neurodegenerative disorders, including Alzheimer's disease, Parkinson's disease, prion diseases, and polyglutamine diseases, including MJD, oligomers of causative proteins have been proposed to be the most toxic structures (Walsh et al., 2002; Kayed et al., 2004) and candidates for a pathogenic intermolecular structure. Polyglutamine oligomers, in particular, have been shown to induce greater toxicity than polyglutamine monomers or inclusion bodies in differentiated neurons (Takahashi et al., 2008). This and other findings support the hypothesis that polyglutamine oligomers may have a crucial role in cytotoxicity (Poirier et al., 2002; Sanchez et al., 2003; Kayed et al., 2003; Ross and Poirier, 2005; Behrends et al., 2006).

The proteolytic cleavage of mutant protein may produce smaller toxic fragments containing an expanded polyglutamine tract, in this way facilitating the entry of cytoplasmic polyglutamine proteins into the nucleus. These toxic cleavage fragments upon release undergo the conformational change required for aggregation formation (Wanker, 2000; Ross et al., 2003). The misfolded expanded fragments may interact with full-length ataxin-3, possibly inducing a misfolding event in the polyQ tract of ataxin-3, which facilitates its stable incorporation into the fibrillar aggregates (Ikeda et al., 1996; Haacke et al., 2006). The proteolytic fragment has been proposed to be a product of caspase enzymes (Wellington et al., 1998; Berke et al., 2004), of autolytic cleavage (Mauri et al., 2006) or of calpains (Haacke et al., 2007). This toxic fragments hypothesis was also proposed for other polyglutamines diseases (Walsh et al., 2005), namely Huntington disease (Goldberg et al., 1996; Schilling et al., 2006) and spinocerebellar ataxia type 7 (SCA7) (Young et al., 2007; Takahashi-Fujigasaki et al., 2011). The mutant ataxin-3 mjd1a putative-cleavage fragment was identified in permanent clones of a transfected cell line (Yamamoto et al., 2001), transgenic mice and MJD patient's brains (Goti et al., 2004). Nevertheless, some controversy remains as other studies failed to identify the proteolytic fragments of ataxin-3 (Cemal et al., 2002; Berke et al., 2004; Chou et al., 2006). Recently, it was reported that the presence of a 259 N-terminal ataxin-3 fragment (without the polyglutamine stretch) was sufficient to induce MJD neurological phenotype in mice (Hubener et al., 2011).

The toxicity of causative gene products in MJD and other polyglutamine diseases has been proposed to be influenced not only by the polyglutamine stretch but also by the post-translational modification of amino acid residues outside the polyglutamine stretch, including phosphorylation (Fei et al., 2007; Tao et al., 2008; Mueller et al., 2009), acetylation (Li et al., 2002; Evert et al., 2006; Chou et al., 2011), ubiquitination (Matsumoto et al., 2004; Jana et al., 2005; de Pril et al., 2007), and sumoylation (Ueda et al., 2002; Shen et al., 2005). These modifications might result in aberrant interactions with other proteins or modification of the properties of causative proteins, including the stability or tendency to form toxic structures.

8.2 Protein interactions

The importance of expanded polyglutamine protein in disease progression is important, however, the toxicity of expanded polyglutamine protein does not fully explain the selective neuronal degeneration in MJD and in other polyglutamine diseases. Mutant ataxin-3 is widely expressed in the brain (Paulson et al., 1997a), even in areas with no significant neuronal degeneration. Thus, the normal function of ataxin-3 or interactions with other proteins in each neuronal subpopulation might explain its selective toxicity (Takahashi et al., 2010). Normal ataxin-3 is found in nuclear inclusions of different polyglutamine diseases, particularly in spinocerebellar ataxia type 1 - SCA1, SCA2, Dentatorubral-pallidoluysian atrophy, (Uchihara et al., 2001) and in neuronal intranuclear hyaline inclusion disease (Takahashi et al., 2001). It is also found in Marinesco bodies under stressful conditions and aging in human and non-human primates brains (Fujigasaki et al., 2000; Fujigasaki et al., 2001; Kettner et al., 2002).

Ataxin-3 recruitment to inclusions raises the possibility that normal ataxin-3 and ubiquitin-mediated pathways may be involved in cellular reactions against stress and misfolded proteins (Fujigasaki et al., 2001). In a *Drosophila* model normal ataxin-3 suppressed the neurotoxicity of mutant ataxin-3 by an ubiquitin-mediated mechanism in association with the proteasome (Warrick et al., 2005). However in a MJD lentiviral rat model the overexpression of normal ataxin-3 did not mitigate the mutant ataxin-3 induced neurodegeneration and even aggravated inclusion generation (Alves et al., 2010).

Several studies have revealed the importance of protein-protein interactions in understanding the normal function of the disease-causing protein (Steffan et al., 2001; Yoshida et al., 2002; Chen et al., 2004; Goehler et al., 2004; Ravikumar et al., 2004; Kaytor et al., 2005; Tsuda et al., 2005). Recently, the normal activity of ataxin-2 was shown to be important to MJD neurodegeneration, suggesting that toxicity of one polyglutamine disease protein could be modulated by the normal activity of another (Lessing and Bonini, 2008). The protein-protein interaction and alteration of the activity of causative proteins was also reported for other neurodegenerative disorders and is therefore an important subject of research (Lim et al., 2006; Zoghbi and Orr, 2009; Elden et al., 2010).

8.3 Dysregulation of transcription

Expanded polyglutamine proteins tend to accumulate in the nucleus, where the high concentration of solutes creates favorable conditions for interaction with transcriptional factors or cofactors (Yamada et al., 2000; Lim et al., 2008). Furthermore, many of the proteins affected by polyglutamine expansion, such as ataxin-1 or ataxin-2 either interact or function as transcription factors (Fernandez-Funez et al., 2000; Lim et al., 2006; Lastres-Becker et al., 2008) suggesting that transcriptional dysregulation may be a central feature of the neurodegenerative mechanism in the polyglutamine disorders (Steffan et al., 2001; Nucifora et al., 2001; Minamiyama et al., 2004; La Spada et al., 2001; Hughes et al., 2001; Yamada et al., 2000; Lim et al., 2008; Godavarthi et al., 2009; Yamanaka et al., 2008, Riley and Orr, 2006). Accordingly, the transcription factor TBP and transcription co-factor CBP were shown to be incorporated into nuclear inclusions of polyglutamine-expanded ataxin-3 (McCampbell et al., 2000). Thus, it is possible that mutant polyglutamine ataxin-3 causes transcriptional dysregulation and resulting neurotoxicity. Downregulation of mRNA levels of genes involved in glutamatergic signaling and signal transduction, but no neurological phenotype, were reported in a MJD transgenic mouse expressing ataxin-3 with 79 CAG repeats in brain regions affected in the disease. This suggests the involvement of transcriptional abnormality in initiating the pathological process of MJD, with expanded ataxin-3 disrupting the normal pattern of gene transcription and contributing to cerebellar dysfunction and ataxia (Chou et al., 2008).

8.4 Ubiquitin-proteasome system dysfunctions

Cells produce a large amount of misfolded proteins, thus protein degradation systems like the UPS or autophagy are crucial to maintain cellular function and viability. A dysfunction in the UPS leads to the accumulation of misfolded proteins, resulting in dysfunction and cell death in neurons. The normal function of ataxin-3 has been linked to protein surveillance pathways (Chai et al., 2004). Ataxin-3 acts as polyubiquitin-binding protein, recruiting poly-ubiquitinated substrates through a carboxy-terminal cluster of ubiquitin interaction motifs (Burnett et al., 2003; Raoul et al., 2005). A loss of mutant ataxin-3 function could affect the UPS and in that way enhance neuronal degeneration and death. Moreover, mutant ataxin-3 nuclear inclusions are ubiquitinated and contain proteasome components, suggesting that the UPS may be disrupted by expanded protein (Paulson et al., 1997b; Chai et al., 1999b).

8.5 Autophagy impairment

There are strong evidences that proteins with a mutant polyglutamine tract are inefficiently degraded by the UPS but could be degraded by macroautophagy, a mechanism with a crucial role in degradation of insoluble aggregate-prone proteins and essential for neuronal survival (Cuervo, 2004a, b; Williams et al., 2006). Recently, our group has shown that important autophagy proteins are sequestered by mutant ataxin-3 inclusions in an MJD lentiviral model and abnormally accumulate in MJD patient's brain (Nascimento-Ferreira et al., 2011). As it happens with the UPS system a disruption in the autophagy system could enhance neurodegeneration and cell death induced by mutant ataxin-3. Accordingly, impairments in the autophagy pathway have been reported in other neurodegenerative diseases (Shibata et al., 2006, Pickford et al., 2008; Crews et al., 2010), as well as a decrease of activity with ageing (Cuervo, 2004b; Vellai, 2009).

8.6 Mitochondrial dysfunction

There is growing evidence that mitochondrial dysfunction may play important roles in neurodegeneration (Knott et al., 2008), and could be implicated in the pathogenesis of MJD

(Yu et al., 2009) and other polyglutamine diseases (Browne et al., 1997; Panov et al., 2002; Cui et al., 2006). In addition, mitochondrial dysfunction has been implicated in ageing, which is a major risk factor of progressive neurodegenerative diseases. Oxidative stress is induced by reactive oxygen species (ROS) or free radicals, and increasing with age, and possibly diminished capacity to deal with oxidative stress may cause modification of cellular macromolecules and lead to cell damage.

8.7 Impairment of axonal transport

The function and survival of neurons demands continuous axonal transport of mRNA and proteins. Several studies suggest that axonal transport disturbance is an attractive hypothesis that could explain the vulnerability of neurons (Gunawardena et al., 2003; Szenbenyi et al., 2003; Caviston et al., 2007). However, currently there is no sufficient evidence to confirm this hypothesis in polyglutamine diseases. Recently, the presence of inclusions in axons was identified in several brain regions of MJD patients affected by neurodegeneration (Seidel et al., 2010). It was hypothesized that the presence of axonal inclusions could be detrimental to axonal transport mechanisms and thereby contribute to degeneration of nerve cells in MJD.

8.8 Dysregulation of intracellular Ca^{2+} homeostasis

Intracellular Ca^{2+} homeostasis is important for the function and survival of neurons, and it has become clear that cellular Ca^{2+} overload, or perturbation of intracellular Ca^{2+} compartmentalization, can cause cytotoxicity and trigger either apoptotic or necrotic cell death (Orrenius et al., 2003). Several studies proposed that deranged Ca^{2+} signaling might play an important role in Huntington's disease (Tang et al., 2003; 2005; Bezprozvanny and Hayden, 2004; Wu et al., 2006). Abnormal Ca^{2+} homeostasis has been reported in mitochondria isolated from lymphoblast's from patients and from brains of the YAC72 HD mouse model (Hodgson et al., 1999; Panov et al., 2002). This Ca^{2+} role could also be important in other polyglutamine diseases, as it is generally assumed that many of these diseases share a common pathogenic mechanism (Cummings and Zoghbi, 2000; Gusella and MacDonald, 2000; Zoghbi and Orr, 2000; Gatchel and Zoghbi, 2005). Accordingly, recent evidence suggests that abnormal neuronal Ca^{2+} signaling might also contribute to pathogenesis in SCAs (Bezprozvanny, 2009; Kasumu and Bezprozvanny, 2010). In MJD, data also suggest that deranged neuronal Ca2+ signaling plays a significant role in pathology onset and progression (Chen et al., 2008). Mutant ataxin-3 has been shown to specifically bind to and activate an intracellular calcium channel, similar to huntingtin. Moreover, long-term feeding of MJD-transgenic mice with a Ca^{2+} stabilizer (dantrolene) alleviated age-dependent motor coordination deficits and prevented neuronal loss in pontine nuclei and substantia nigra regions (Chen et al., 2008).

9. Therapeutic strategies in MJD

Expansion of the polyglutamine tract of ataxin-3 initiates a cascade of events that include the accumulation of insoluble inclusions and culminates in degeneration of specific neurons. The strategies that can be used to treat MJD or other polyglutamine diseases can be grouped into five main approaches: i) reducing the levels of expanded proteins, ii) preventing mutant ataxin-3 cleavage, oligomerization and aggregation, iii) activating the clearance mechanisms, iv) targeting a specific cellular mechanism and v) promoting neuroprotection (Figure 4).

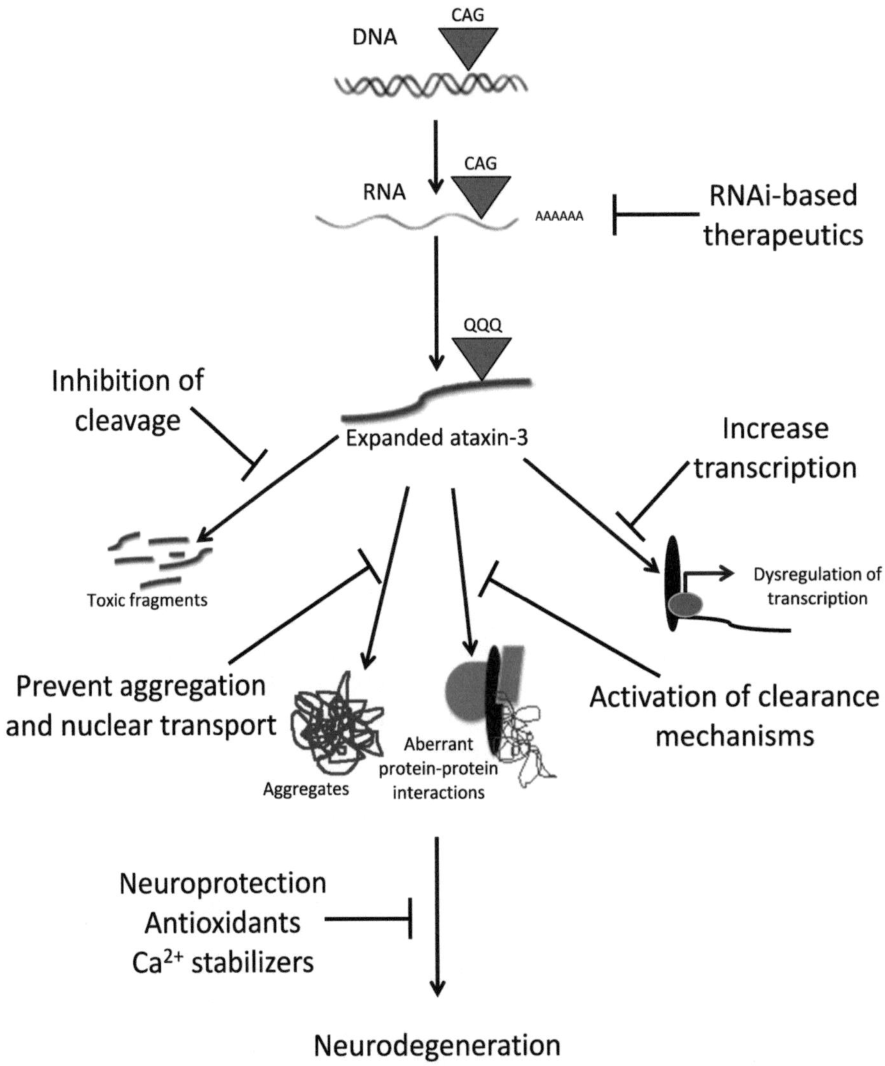

Fig. 4. **Potential therapeutic strategies to Machado-Joseph disease.** Expansion of the polyglutamine tract of ataxin-3 initiates a cascade of events that culminates with the accumulation of insoluble inclusions and degenerations in selected neurons. The strategies that can be used to treat MJD or other polyglutamine diseases can be grouped into five approaches: i) reducing the levels of expanded proteins (using gene silencing by RNAi-based strategies), ii) preventing mutant ataxin-3 cleavage, oligomerization and aggregation (inhibiting proteolysis, using aggregation inhibitors or preventing the nuclear transport), iii) activation of the clearance mechanisms (upregulation of UPS and autophagy), iv) targeting a specific cellular mechanism (increase transcription, stabilize Ca^{2+} homeostasis or inhibit oxidative stress) and v) neuroprotection strategies (using drugs, proteins or factors to protect neurons).

9.1 RNA interference-based therapeutics

Although several approaches could be envisioned to treat MJD and other polyglutamine diseases, the most direct solution to counter these diseases pathogenesis is to reduce the expression of the mutant allele (Kim and Rossi, 2007). RNA interference (RNAi) is a powerful tool for selective knockdown of gene expression. Gene silencing by RNAi has been successfully used to downregulate the expression of mutant genes and rescue phenotype in various neurodegenerative diseases, including Huntington's disease (Harper et al., 2005; Rodriguez-Lebron et al., 2005; DiFiglia et al., 2007, van Bilsen et al., 2008; Lombardi et al., 2009; Pfister et al., 2009), familial forms of amyotrophic lateral sclerosis (ALS) (Raoul et al., 2005; Ralph et al., 2005; Azzouz, 2006), SCA1 (Xia et al., 2004), and MJD (Miller et al., 2003; Alves et al., 2008a, 2010; Hu et al., 2009).

However, a major problem of gene silencing may be the lack of discrimination between normal and mutant forms of the causative protein. In some diseases partial silencing of normal protein could be tolerated; for example in HD transgenic animal models silencing of mutant huntingtin and 75% of endogenous protein led to behavioral enhancement (Boudreau et al., 2009). However, it has been reported that in cellular MJD models absence of wild-type ataxin-3 leads to cytoskeletal disorganization and increased cell death (Rodrigues et al., 2010). This would suggest that for some polyglutamine disorders it might be prudent to preserve the wild-type protein, as prolonged full knockdown of normal protein function could be harmful. This would demand specific targeting of the mutant allele for RNAi.

It was first demonstrated in cell models that RNAi species could be engineered to specifically silence the causative genes while preserving the wild-type, which differed in a single nucleotide (Miller et al., 2003). More recently, our group showed both in vitro and in a rat model of MJD that lentiviral-mediated silencing of the mutant human ataxin-3 was efficient and selective, allowing preservation of wild-type ataxin-3 (Alves et al., 2008a). Specific silencing has also been later reported to SNPs targeting ataxin-7 in SCA7 (Scholefield et al., 2009) and huntingtin in Huntington's disease (Zhang et al., 2009; Hu et al., 2009). This allele-specific silencing of ataxin-3 significantly decreased the severity of the neuropathological abnormalities associated with the disease by targeting a single nucleotide polymorphism (SNPs) that is present in more than 70% of the patients with MJD (Stevanin et al., 1995; Gaspar et al., 1996). These data support the therapeutic potential of RNAi for MJD. However, this therapy would benefit ~70% of MJD patients at best. Whether silencing not discriminating between wild type and mutant alleles would be safe and effective was recently investigated, by either overexpressing or silencing wild-type ataxin-3 in a rat model of MJD. It was shown that (i) overexpression of wild-type ataxin-3 did not protect against MJD pathology, (ii) knockdown of wild-type ataxin-3 did not aggravate MJD pathology and that (iii) non-allele-specific silencing of ataxin-3 strongly reduced neuropathology in a rat model of MJD. These findings indicate that therapeutic strategies involving non-allele-specific silencing to treat MJD patients may also be safe and effective (Alves et al., 2010).

9.2 Preventing the cleavage of ataxin-3

In MJD, it was proposed that production of a cleavage fragment of mutant ataxin-3 contributes to neurotoxicity (Ikeda et al., 1996; Goti et al., 2004; Colomer-Gould, 2005;

Haacke et al., 2006). Thus, blocking the proteases involved in ataxin-3 cleavage and decreasing the concentration of the cleavage fragment bellow a critical level in the brain could be an effective strategy for MJD treatment. This approach has been used for other neurodegenerative diseases, including Alzheimer (Citron, 2004) and Huntington's diseases (Ona et al., 1999; Gafni et al., 2004) and therefore could also be a therapeutic strategy for MJD (Tarlac and Storey, 2003). Nevertheless, the natures of the protease and of the cleavage fragment still need investigation.

9.3 Acceleration of the degradation of misfolded proteins

The acceleration of the proteolysis mechanisms (UPS and autophagy machinery) could promote mutant ataxin-3 degradation and probably prevent or delay the MJD progression. Overexpression of chaperones has been shown to aid in the handling of misfolded or aggregated polyglutamine-expanded ataxin-3 and suppress polyglutamine aggregation with a parallel decrease in toxicity (Chai et al., 1999b). Thus the induction of such molecular chaperones can be envisaged as a strategy for therapy of polyglutamine diseases (Nagai et al., 2010; Robertson et al., 2010). Accordingly, the use of chemical chaperones such as the organic solvent dimethyl sulfoxide - DMSO, cellular osmolytes glycerol, trimethylamine N-oxide - TMAO, and ectoine reduce aggregate formation and cytotoxicity induced by truncated expanded ataxin-3 (Yoshida et al., 2002), alters subcellular localization of inclusions and reduces apoptotic cell death induced by mutant ataxin-3 (Furusho et al., 2005).

It was also shown that overexpression of UPS-related factors or proteins (e.g. E64 or CHIP) increase ubiquitination and degradation rate and decrease aggregation and cell death (Matsumoto et al., 2004; Jana et al., 2005; Miller et al., 2005). Therefore, overexpression of these proteins could be a molecular approach for therapy of MJD. It was shown that CRAG (guanosine triphosphatase) acts as an activator of promylocytic leukaemia protein-associated ubiquitin ligase and leads to the degradation of polyQ through the ubiquitin-proteasome pathway (Qin et al., 2006). Because the expression levels of CRAG decrease in the adult brain (Qin et al., 2006), it was suggested that a reduced level of CRAG could underlie the onset of polyglutamine diseases. In fact, lentiviral-mediated overexpression of CRAG in Purkinje cells of a transgenic mice model extensively cleared polyQ aggregates and re-activated dendritic differentiation, resulting in a striking rescue from ataxia (Torashima et al., 2008). It was also suggested that the activity of normal ataxin-3 could provide a therapeutic approach to MJD, enhancing the cellular pathways in which it participates (Warrick et al., 2005). However, in a lentiviral-based rat model for MJD as well as in double-transgenic mice, the overexpression of normal ataxin-3 did not decrease the pathological abnormalities induced by mutant ataxin-3 (Alves et al., 2010; Hübener et al., 2010).

Another possible therapeutic approach to MJD and to other polyglutamine diseases could be the up-regulation of autophagy, leading to a selective clearance of the mutant protein. Rapamycin, an activator of the autophagy pathway alleviated neurodegeneration in *Drosophila* and in a transgenic mouse model of HD. However, this drug failed to prolong life span in a mouse model (Ravikumar et al., 2004). In MJD, it was recently shown that the administration of a rapamycin esther improves motor coordination in a transgenic model of MJD (Menzies et al., 2010). The rapamycin esther reduced the number of aggregates in the brains of transgenic mice and decreased the levels of cytosolic soluble mutant ataxin-3, while endogenous wild-type protein levels remained unaffected.

Recently, our group showed that lentiviral-mediated overexpression of beclin-1, a crucial protein in early and late steps of autophagy, led to a stimulation of autophagic flux, mutant ataxin-3 clearance and overall neuroprotective effects in neuronal cultures and in a lentiviral-based rat model of MJD (Nascimento-Ferreira et al., 2011). The same study found an abnormal expression of endogenous autophagy markers, accumulation of autophagosomes and decreased levels of beclin in the brain of MJD patients. Overall, these data suggest that up-regulation of UPS or autophagy can be a therapeutic option for MJD and for other polyglutamine diseases.

9.4 Inhibition of nuclear transport

It has been shown that ataxin-3 translocates to the nucleus, and that the polyglutamine expansion is not essential for this transport (Tait et al., 1998). The resulting presence of ataxin-3 in the nucleus has been shown to drastically aggravate the pathology in Machado-Joseph disease (Bichelmeier et al., 2007). Therefore, inhibition of nuclear transport may slow the disease progression, and might be sufficient to ameliorate the disease symptoms, and thus could be explored as therapeutic approach for MJD (Breuer et al., 2010).

9.5 Prevention of protein misfolding, oligomerization and aggregation

Protein misfolding, oligomerization, and formation of insoluble inclusions represent a common physiological response to pathogenic proteins. Thus, different research groups have developed high-throughput screening assays aiming at the discovery of molecules with selective binding affinities for polyglutamine expanded proteins, with the ability to modulate their pathogenic properties and potential therapeutic applications (Desai et al., 2006; Lansbury and Lashuel, 2006). Several compounds have been identified as potential inhibitors of polyglutamine aggregation (Heiser et al., 2000, 2002; Apostol et al., 2003; Sanchéz et al., 2003; Tanaka et al., 2005; Wolfgang et al., 2005; Herbst and Wancker, 2006). The prevention of aggregation and oligomerization by polyglutamine disease can also be promoted by modulation of molecular chaperones (Nagai et al., 2010; Roberston et al., 2010). The Hsp90 inhibitor geldanamycin suppresses aggregation of polyQ-expanded mutant huntingtin through induction of endogenous molecular chaperones (Sittler et al., 2001). In MJD Drosophila models, it was shown that the administration of a less toxic derivative of geldanamycin suppresses polyQ-induced neurodegeneration through the induction of multiple endogenous molecular chaperones (Fujikake et al., 2008).

Another therapeutic approach involves the use of small peptides or molecules with the ability to modulate protein folding, stabilize proteins in their native conformation, and prevent or inhibit aggregation (Tanaka et al., 2005). Several compounds proved to be suitable in preventing polyglutamine proteins aggregation, mainly for Huntington Disease (Table 2). In a screening of 16,000 compounds a small molecule (IC_{50}) that inhibits polyglutamine aggregation in HD neurons and suppresses neurodegeneration *in vivo* was found (Zhang et al., 2005). In a MJD *Drosophila* model a tandem repeat of the polyglutamine binding peptide QBP1, which preferentially binds to polyglutamine stretches, has been shown to decrease aggregate formation and rescue survival (Nagai et al., 2003). More recently a high-content chemical and RNAi screening in a Drosophila primary neuronal culture of HD model identified several compounds that suppress mutant huntingtin aggregate formation (Schulte et al., 2011).

Compound	Disease tested	Study
Geldanamycin	Huntington Disease	Sittler et al., 2001
17-(allylamino)-17-demethoxygeldanamycin (17AAG)	Machado-Joseph Disease	Fujikake et al., 2008
Congo red	Huntington Disease	Frid et al., 2007
C2-8	Huntington Disease	Chopra et al., 2007
Trehalose	Huntington Disease	Tanaka et al., 2005
GW5074	Huntington Disease	Schulte et al., 2011
Juglone	Huntington Disease	Schulte et al., 2011
Radicicol	Huntington Disease	Schulte et al., 2011
Rapamycin	Huntington Disease	Schulte et al., 2011
Rapamycin esther	Machado Joseph disease	Menzies et al., 2010
Camptothecin	Huntington Disease	Schulte et al., 2011
Etoposide	Huntington Disease	Schulte et al., 2011
Ouabain	Huntington Disease	Schulte et al., 2011
Proscillaridin A	Huntington Disease	Schulte et al., 2011
Ethacrynic acid	Huntington Disease	Schulte et al., 2011
IC_{50}	Huntington Disease	Zhang et al., 2005

Table 2. Compounds that have shown to prevent or inhibit polyglutamine proteins aggregation.

9.6 Targeting transcriptional dysfunction

Polyglutamine-expanded ataxin-3 (as other polyglutamine expanded proteins) has been shown to repress transcription. Ataxin-3 acts through distinct mechanisms involving both the polyglutamine-containing C-terminus and the N-terminus of ataxin-3 (Li et al., 2002). Transcriptional dysregulation has been suggested to play a central role in neurodegenerative mechanisms of the polyglutamine disorders (Chou et al., 2008). The overexpression of transcription factors that interact with polyglutamine diseases reduces the cytotoxicity of mutant proteins (Dunah et al., 2002; Taylor et al., 2003). Moreover, it was shown that the use of several reagents that increase transcription reduce the toxicity of expanded polyglutamine (Steffan et al., 2001; Ferrante et al., 2003, 2004; Hockly et al., 2003; Gardian et al., 2005; Shimohata et al., 2005). Recently, it was shown that regulation of transcriptional activity through an inhibition of histone hypoacetylation (Chou et al., 2011) might be a promising therapeutic intervention for MJD. Histone acetylation, which is controlled by histone acetyltransferase and histone deacetylase (HDAC), plays an important role in regulating transcriptional activity (Kurdistani et al., 2004). The H3 and H4 histones were hypoacetylated in the cerebellum of MJD transgenic mice, which displayed transcription downregulation and ataxic symptoms. Daily administration of a HDAC inhibitor (sodium butyrate) reversed histone hypoacetylation and transcriptional downregulation in the cerebellum of the MJD transgenic mice, delaying the onset of ataxic symptoms, ameliorated the neurological phenotype and improved the survival rate of the mice (Chou et al., 2011).

9.7 Targeting the calcium homeostasis

It has been shown that deranged calcium signaling might play an important role in MJD pathology (Chen et al., 2008). The same study found that feeding a MJD transgenic mice with dantrolene, a clinically relevant stabilizer of intracellular Ca^{2+} signaling, improved motor performance and prevented neuronal cell loss in pontine nuclei and *substantia nigra* regions. Therefore, calcium-signaling stabilizers such as dantrolene may be considered as potential therapeutic drugs for the treatment of MJD patients.

9.8 Targeting mitochondrial dysfunctions

Several studies have shown that administration of antioxidants ameliorates motor deficits and prolongs survival in transgenic mouse model of HD (Ferrante et al., 2002). Moreover, drugs that improve transcriptional regulation of genes necessary for energy metabolism also improve HD motor phenotype (Hathorn et al., 2011). In MJD, evidences point to a role of mitochondrial dysfunction in MJD pathogenesis (Yu et al., 2009). Decreased mitochondrial DNA copy numbers were found in mutant cells stably transfected with ataxin-3 with 78 CAG repeats and in MJD patients, compared to normal controls. Furthermore, mitochondrial DNA depletion was higher in MJD patients compared with that in normal individuals. Overall, mutant ataxin-3 may influence the activity of enzymatic components to remove O_{2^*} and H_2O_2 efficiently and promote mitochondrial DNA damage or depletion, which leads to dysfunction of mitochondria (Yu et al., 2009). Therefore, therapies targeting mitochondrial dysfunction in MJD should be further investigated.

9.9 Neuroprotection

The possibility of administration of drugs or molecules with neuroprotective properties in neurodegenerative diseases has also been explored. Many research groups have investigated the use of neurotrophic factors for therapy of polyglutamine disorders over the last decade (Bensadoun et al., 2000; de Almeida et al., 2001; Zala et al., 2004; Xie et al., 2010). In HD the BDNF supply to striatal neurons is compromised. Therefore delivery of this factor has been investigated as a replacement therapy for the missing factor (Zuccato et al., 2001). BDNF replacement was later shown to enhance the motor phenotype (Canals et al., 2004), and BDNF overexpression prevented loss and atrophy of striatal neurons and motor dysfunction (Xie et al., 2010), both in in HD transgenic mice.

Studies in mouse models of Alzheimer's and Parkinson's diseases found that caffeine could alleviate pathological signs and behavior deficits in these neurodegenerative disease paradigms, by antagonizing A2A adenosine receptors (Arendash and Cao, 2010; Prediger, 2010; reviewed in Cunha and Agostinho, 2010). Moreover, administration of caffeine and other stimulants in orexin/ataxin-3 transgenic narcoleptic mice induced an increase in motor activity but the effects on neuropathology remain to be investigated (Okuro et al., 2010) and should be further investigated in MJD models.

Several evidences suggest that neuroprotective compounds could be also explored as a therapeutic strategy in MJD and the drug ability of some of these compounds may contribute to earlier access of patients to much needed disease-modifying therapies.

10. Acknowledgements

CN is supported by the Portuguese Foundation for Science and Technology (SFRH/BPD/62945/2009) and by the Center for Science and Technology of Madeira. Research of LPA group is funded by the Portuguese Foundation for Science and Technology (PTDC/SAUNEU/099307/2008), the National Ataxia Foundation, the Association Française pour les Myopathies, the TREATPOLYQ - FP7-PEOPLE-2010-ITN Marie-Curie Action Initial Training Network and the Richard Chin and Lilly Lock Research Fund.

11. References

Albrecht M, Golatta M, Wullner U, Lengauer T (2004) Structural and functional analysis of ataxin-2 and ataxin-3. Eur J Biochem 271:3155-3170.

Alves S, Nascimento-Ferreira I, Auregan G, Hassig R, Dufour N, Brouillet E, Pedroso de Lima MC, Hantraye P, Pereira de Almeida L, Deglon N (2008a) Allele-specific RNA silencing of mutant ataxin-3 mediates neuroprotection in a rat model of Machado-Joseph disease. PLoS One 3:e3341.

Alves S, Regulier E, Nascimento-Ferreira I, Hassig R, Dufour N, Koeppen A, Carvalho AL, Simoes S, de Lima MC, Brouillet E, Gould VC, Deglon N, de Almeida LP (2008b) Striatal and nigral pathology in a lentiviral rat model of Machado-Joseph disease. Hum Mol Genet 17:2071-2083.

Alves S, Nascimento-Ferreira I, Dufour N, Hassig R, Auregan G, Nobrega C, Brouillet E, Hantraye P, Pedroso de Lima MC, Deglon N, de Almeida LP (2010) Silencing ataxin-3 mitigates degeneration in a rat model of Machado-Joseph disease: no role for wild-type ataxin-3? Hum Mol Genet 19:2380-2394.

Antony PM, Mantele S, Mollenkopf P, Boy J, Kehlenbach RH, Riess O, Schmidt T (2009) Identification and functional dissection of localization signals within ataxin-3. Neurobiol Dis 36:280-292.

Apostol BL, Kazantsev A, Raffioni S, Illes K, Pallos J, Bodai L, Slepko N, Bear JE, Gertler FB, Hersch S, Housman DE, Marsh JL, Thompson LM (2003) A cell-based assay for aggregation inhibitors as therapeutics of polyglutamine-repeat disease and validation in Drosophila. Proc Natl Acad Sci U S A 100:5950-5955.

Arendash GW, Cao C (2010) Caffeine and coffee as therapeutics against Alzheimer's disease. J Alzheimers Dis 20 Suppl 1:S117-126.

Azzouz M (2006) Gene Therapy for ALS: progress and prospects. Biochim Biophys Acta 1762:1122-1127.

Bates G (2003) Huntingtin aggregation and toxicity in Huntington's disease. Lancet 361:1642-1644.

Behrends C, Langer CA, Boteva R, Bottcher UM, Stemp MJ, Schaffar G, Rao BV, Giese A, Kretzschmar H, Siegers K, Hartl FU (2006) Chaperonin TRiC promotes the assembly of polyQ expansion proteins into nontoxic oligomers. Mol Cell 23:887-897.

Bensadoun JC, Deglon N, Tseng JL, Ridet JL, Zurn AD, Aebischer P (2000) Lentiviral vectors as a gene delivery system in the mouse midbrain: cellular and behavioral improvements in a 6-OHDA model of Parkinson's disease using GDNF. Exp Neurol 164:15-24.

Berke SJ, Schmied FA, Brunt ER, Ellerby LM, Paulson HL (2004) Caspase-mediated proteolysis of the polyglutamine disease protein ataxin-3. J Neurochem 89:908-918.

Bettencourt C, Santos C, Montiel R, Costa Mdo C, Cruz-Morales P, Santos LR, Simoes N, Kay T, Vasconcelos J, Maciel P, Lima M (2010) Increased transcript diversity: novel splicing variants of Machado-Joseph disease gene (ATXN3). Neurogenetics 11:193-202.

Bevivino AE, Loll PJ (2001) An expanded glutamine repeat destabilizes native ataxin-3 structure and mediates formation of parallel beta -fibrils. Proc Natl Acad Sci U S A 98:11955-11960.

Bezprozvanny I (2009) Calcium signaling and neurodegenerative diseases. Trends Mol Med 15:89-100.

Bezprozvanny I, Hayden MR (2004) Deranged neuronal calcium signaling and Huntington disease. Biochem Biophys Res Commun 322:1310-1317.

Boeddrich A, Gaumer S, Haacke A, Tzvetkov N, Albrecht M, Evert BO, Muller EC, Lurz R, Breuer P, Schugardt N, Plassmann S, Xu K, Warrick JM, Suopanki J, Wullner U, Frank R, Hartl UF, Bonini NM, Wanker EE (2006) An arginine/lysine-rich motif is crucial for VCP/p97-mediated modulation of ataxin-3 fibrillogenesis. Embo J 25:1547-1558.

Boudreau RL, McBride JL, Martins I, Shen S, Xing Y, Carter BJ, Davidson BL (2009) Nonallele-specific silencing of mutant and wild-type huntingtin demonstrates therapeutic efficacy in Huntington's disease mice. Mol Ther 17:1053-1063.

Breuer P, Haacke A, Evert BO, Wullner U (2010) Nuclear aggregation of polyglutamine-expanded ataxin-3: fragments escape the cytoplasmic quality control. J Biol Chem 285:6532-6537.

Browne SE, Bowling AC, MacGarvey U, Baik MJ, Berger SC, Muqit MM, Bird ED, Beal MF (1997) Oxidative damage and metabolic dysfunction in Huntington's disease: selective vulnerability of the basal ganglia. Ann Neurol 41:646-653.

Burnett B, Li F, Pittman RN (2003) The polyglutamine neurodegenerative protein ataxin-3 binds polyubiquitylated proteins and has ubiquitin protease activity. Hum Mol Genet 12:3195-3205.

Camargos ST, Marques W, Jr., dos Santos AC (2011) Brain stem and cerebellum volumetric analysis of Machado Joseph disease patients. Arq Neuropsiquiatr 69:292-296.

Canals JM, Pineda JR, Torres-Peraza JF, Bosch M, Martin-Ibanez R, Munoz MT, Mengod G, Ernfors P, Alberch J (2004) Brain-derived neurotrophic factor regulates the onset and severity of motor dysfunction associated with enkephalinergic neuronal degeneration in Huntington's disease. J Neurosci 24:7727-7739.

Caviston JP, Ross JL, Antony SM, Tokito M, Holzbaur EL (2007) Huntingtin facilitates dynein/dynactin-mediated vesicle transport. Proc Natl Acad Sci U S A 104:10045-10050.

Cemal CK, Carroll CJ, Lawrence L, Lowrie MB, Ruddle P, Al-Mahdawi S, King RH, Pook MA, Huxley C, Chamberlain S (2002) YAC transgenic mice carrying pathological alleles of the MJD1 locus exhibit a mild and slowly progressive cerebellar deficit. Hum Mol Genet 11:1075-1094.

Chai Y, Berke SS, Cohen RE, Paulson HL (2004) Poly-ubiquitin binding by the polyglutamine disease protein ataxin-3 links its normal function to protein surveillance pathways. J Biol Chem 279:3605-3611.

Chai Y, Koppenhafer SL, Bonini NM, Paulson HL (1999a) Analysis of the role of heat shock protein (Hsp) molecular chaperones in polyglutamine disease. J Neurosci 19:10338-10347.

Chai Y, Koppenhafer SL, Shoesmith SJ, Perez MK, Paulson HL (1999b) Evidence for proteasome involvement in polyglutamine disease: localization to nuclear inclusions in SCA3/MJD and suppression of polyglutamine aggregation in vitro. Hum Mol Genet 8:673-682.

Chen S, Peng GH, Wang X, Smith AC, Grote SK, Sopher BL, La Spada AR (2004) Interference of Crx-dependent transcription by ataxin-7 involves interaction between the glutamine regions and requires the ataxin-7 carboxy-terminal region for nuclear localization. Hum Mol Genet 13:53-67.

Chen X, Tang TS, Tu H, Nelson O, Pook M, Hammer R, Nukina N, Bezprozvanny I (2008) Deranged calcium signaling and neurodegeneration in spinocerebellar ataxia type 3. J Neurosci 28:12713-12724.

Chopra V, Fox JH, Lieberman G, Dorsey K, Matson W, Waldmeier P, Housman DE, Kazantsev A, Young AB, Hersch S (2007) A small-molecule therapeutic lead for Huntington's disease: preclinical pharmacology and efficacy of C2-8 in the R6/2 transgenic mouse. Proc Natl Acad Sci U S A 104:16685-16689.

Chou AH, Chen SY, Yeh TH, Weng YH, Wang HL (2011) HDAC inhibitor sodium butyrate reverses transcriptional downregulation and ameliorates ataxic symptoms in a transgenic mouse model of SCA3. Neurobiol Dis 41:481-488.

Chou AH, Yeh TH, Kuo YL, Kao YC, Jou MJ, Hsu CY, Tsai SR, Kakizuka A, Wang HL (2006) Polyglutamine-expanded ataxin-3 activates mitochondrial apoptotic pathway by upregulating Bax and downregulating Bcl-xL. Neurobiol Dis 21:333-345.

Chou AH, Yeh TH, Ouyang P, Chen YL, Chen SY, Wang HL (2008) Polyglutamine-expanded ataxin-3 causes cerebellar dysfunction of SCA3 transgenic mice by inducing transcriptional dysregulation. Neurobiol Dis 31:89-101.

Citron M (2004) Strategies for disease modification in Alzheimer's disease. Nat Rev Neurosci 5:677-685.

Colomer Gould VF (2005) Mouse models of Machado-Joseph disease and other polyglutamine spinocerebellar ataxias. NeuroRx 2:480-483.

Coutinho P, Andrade C (1978) Autosomal dominant system degeneration in Portuguese families of the Azores Islands. A new genetic disorder involving cerebellar, pyramidal, extrapyramidal and spinal cord motor functions. Neurology 28:703-709.

Crews L, Spencer B, Desplats P, Patrick C, Paulino A, Rockenstein E, Hansen L, Adame A, Galasko D, Masliah E (2010) Selective molecular alterations in the autophagy pathway in patients with Lewy body disease and in models of alpha-synucleinopathy. PLoS One 5:e9313.

Cuervo AM (2004a) Autophagy: in sickness and in health. Trends Cell Biol 14:70-77.

Cuervo AM (2004b) Autophagy: many paths to the same end. Mol Cell Biochem 263:55-72.

Cui L, Jeong H, Borovecki F, Parkhurst CN, Tanese N, Krainc D (2006) Transcriptional repression of PGC-1alpha by mutant huntingtin leads to mitochondrial dysfunction and neurodegeneration. Cell 127:59-69.

Cummings CJ, Reinstein E, Sun Y, Antalffy B, Jiang Y, Ciechanover A, Orr HT, Beaudet AL, Zoghbi HY (1999) Mutation of the E6-AP ubiquitin ligase reduces nuclear inclusion frequency while accelerating polyglutamine-induced pathology in SCA1 mice. Neuron 24:879-892.

Cummings CJ, Zoghbi HY (2000) Trinucleotide repeats: mechanisms and pathophysiology. Annu Rev Genomics Hum Genet 1:281-328.

Cunha RA, Agostinho PM. (2010) Chronic caffeine consumption prevents memory disturbance in different animal models of memory decline. J Alzheimers Dis.;20 Suppl 1:S95-116.

D'Abreu A, Franca MC, Jr., Paulson HL, Lopes-Cendes I (2010) Caring for Machado-Joseph disease: current understanding and how to help patients. Parkinsonism Relat Disord 16:2-7.

de Almeida LP, Zala D, Aebischer P, Deglon N (2001) Neuroprotective effect of a CNTF-expressing lentiviral vector in the quinolinic acid rat model of Huntington's disease. Neurobiol Dis 8:433-446.

de Pril R, Fischer DF, Roos RA, van Leeuwen FW (2007) Ubiquitin-conjugating enzyme E2-25K increases aggregate formation and cell death in polyglutamine diseases. Mol Cell Neurosci 34:10-19.

Desai UA, Pallos J, Ma AA, Stockwell BR, Thompson LM, Marsh JL, Diamond MI (2006) Biologically active molecules that reduce polyglutamine aggregation and toxicity. Hum Mol Genet 15:2114-2124.

DiFiglia M, Sena-Esteves M, Chase K, Sapp E, Pfister E, Sass M, Yoder J, Reeves P, Pandey RK, Rajeev KG, Manoharan M, Sah DW, Zamore PD, Aronin N (2007) Therapeutic silencing of mutant huntingtin with siRNA attenuates striatal and cortical neuropathology and behavioral deficits. Proc Natl Acad Sci U S A 104:17204-17209.

Donaldson KM, Li W, Ching KA, Batalov S, Tsai CC, Joazeiro CA (2003) Ubiquitin-mediated sequestration of normal cellular proteins into polyglutamine aggregates. Proc Natl Acad Sci U S A 100:8892-8897.

Doss-Pepe EW, Stenroos ES, Johnson WG, Madura K (2003) Ataxin-3 interactions with rad23 and valosin-containing protein and its associations with ubiquitin chains and the proteasome are consistent with a role in ubiquitin-mediated proteolysis. Mol Cell Biol 23:6469-6483.

Dunah AW, Jeong H, Griffin A, Kim YM, Standaert DG, Hersch SM, Mouradian MM, Young AB, Tanese N, Krainc D (2002) Sp1 and TAFII130 transcriptional activity disrupted in early Huntington's disease. Science 296:2238-2243.

Durcan TM, Kontogiannea M, Thorarinsdottir T, Fallon L, Williams AJ, Djarmati A, Fantaneanu T, Paulson HL, Fon EA (2011) The Machado-Joseph disease-associated mutant form of ataxin-3 regulates parkin ubiquitination and stability. Hum Mol Genet 20:141-154.

Durr A, Stevanin G, Cancel G, Duyckaerts C, Abbas N, Didierjean O, Chneiweiss H, Benomar A, Lyon-Caen O, Julien J, Serdaru M, Penet C, Agid Y, Brice A (1996)

Spinocerebellar ataxia 3 and Machado-Joseph disease: clinical, molecular, and neuropathological features. Ann Neurol 39:490-499.

Elden AC, Kim HJ, Hart MP, Chen-Plotkin AS, Johnson BS, Fang X, Armakola M, Geser F, Greene R, Lu MM, Padmanabhan A, Clay-Falcone D, McCluskey L, Elman L, Juhr D, Gruber PJ, Rub U, Auburger G, Trojanowski JQ, Lee VM, Van Deerlin VM, Bonini NM, Gitler AD (2010) Ataxin-2 intermediate-length polyglutamine expansions are associated with increased risk for ALS. Nature 466:1069-1075.

Evert BO, Araujo J, Vieira-Saecker AM, de Vos RA, Harendza S, Klockgether T, Wullner U (2006) Ataxin-3 represses transcription via chromatin binding, interaction with histone deacetylase 3, and histone deacetylation. J Neurosci 26:11474-11486.

Fei E, Jia N, Zhang T, Ma X, Wang H, Liu C, Zhang W, Ding L, Nukina N, Wang G (2007) Phosphorylation of ataxin-3 by glycogen synthase kinase 3beta at serine 256 regulates the aggregation of ataxin-3. Biochem Biophys Res Commun 357:487-492.

Fernandez-Funez P, Nino-Rosales ML, de Gouyon B, She WC, Luchak JM, Martinez P, Turiegano E, Benito J, Capovilla M, Skinner PJ, McCall A, Canal I, Orr HT, Zoghbi HY, Botas J (2000) Identification of genes that modify ataxin-1-induced neurodegeneration. Nature 408:101-106.

Ferrante RJ, Andreassen OA, Dedeoglu A, Ferrante KL, Jenkins BG, Hersch SM, Beal MF (2002) Therapeutic effects of coenzyme Q10 and remacemide in transgenic mouse models of Huntington's disease. J Neurosci 22:1592-1599.

Ferrante RJ, Kubilus JK, Lee J, Ryu H, Beesen A, Zucker B, Smith K, Kowall NW, Ratan RR, Luthi-Carter R, Hersch SM (2003) Histone deacetylase inhibition by sodium butyrate chemotherapy ameliorates the neurodegenerative phenotype in Huntington's disease mice. J Neurosci 23:9418-9427.

Ferrante RJ, Ryu H, Kubilus JK, D'Mello S, Sugars KL, Lee J, Lu P, Smith K, Browne S, Beal MF, Kristal BS, Stavrovskaya IG, Hewett S, Rubinsztein DC, Langley B, Ratan RR (2004) Chemotherapy for the brain: the antitumor antibiotic mithramycin prolongs survival in a mouse model of Huntington's disease. J Neurosci 24:10335-10342.

Ferro A, Carvalho AL, Teixeira-Castro A, Almeida C, Tome RJ, Cortes L, Rodrigues AJ, Logarinho E, Sequeiros J, Macedo-Ribeiro S, Maciel P (2007) NEDD8: a new ataxin-3 interactor. Biochim Biophys Acta 1773:1619-1627.

Fowler HL (1984) Machado-Joseph-Azorean disease. A ten-year study. Arch Neurol 41:921-925.

Frid P, Anisimov SV, Popovic N (2007) Congo red and protein aggregation in neurodegenerative diseases. Brain Res Rev 53:135-160.

Fujigasaki H, Uchihara T, Koyano S, Iwabuchi K, Yagishita S, Makifuchi T, Nakamura A, Ishida K, Toru S, Hirai S, Ishikawa K, Tanabe T, Mizusawa H (2000) Ataxin-3 is translocated into the nucleus for the formation of intranuclear inclusions in normal and Machado-Joseph disease brains. Exp Neurol 165:248-256.

Fujigasaki H, Uchihara T, Takahashi J, Matsushita H, Nakamura A, Koyano S, Iwabuchi K, Hirai S, Mizusawa H (2001) Preferential recruitment of ataxin-3 independent of expanded polyglutamine: an immunohistochemical study on Marinesco bodies. J Neurol Neurosurg Psychiatry 71:518-520.

Fujikake N, Nagai Y, Popiel HA, Okamoto Y, Yamaguchi M, Toda T (2008) Heat shock transcription factor 1-activating compounds suppress polyglutamine-induced neurodegeneration through induction of multiple molecular chaperones. J Biol Chem 283:26188-26197.

Furusho K, Yoshizawa T, Shoji S (2005) Ectoine alters subcellular localization of inclusions and reduces apoptotic cell death induced by the truncated Machado-Joseph disease gene product with an expanded polyglutamine stretch. Neurobiol Dis 20:170-178.

Gafni J, Hermel E, Young JE, Wellington CL, Hayden MR, Ellerby LM (2004) Inhibition of calpain cleavage of huntingtin reduces toxicity: accumulation of calpain/caspase fragments in the nucleus. J Biol Chem 279:20211-20220.

Gardian G, Browne SE, Choi DK, Klivenyi P, Gregorio J, Kubilus JK, Ryu H, Langley B, Ratan RR, Ferrante RJ, Beal MF (2005) Neuroprotective effects of phenylbutyrate in the N171-82Q transgenic mouse model of Huntington's disease. J Biol Chem 280:556-563.

Gaspar C, Lopes-Cendes I, DeStefano AL, Maciel P, Silveira I, Coutinho P, MacLeod P, Sequeiros J, Farrer LA, Rouleau GA (1996) Linkage disequilibrium analysis in Machado-Joseph disease patients of different ethnic origins. Hum Genet 98:620-624.

Gatchel JR, Zoghbi HY (2005) Diseases of unstable repeat expansion: mechanisms and common principles. Nat Rev Genet 6:743-755.

Globas C, du Montcel ST, Baliko L, Boesch S, Depondt C, DiDonato S, Durr A, Filla A, Klockgether T, Mariotti C, Melegh B, Rakowicz M, Ribai P, Rola R, Schmitz-Hubsch T, Szymanski S, Timmann D, Van de Warrenburg BP, Bauer P, Schols L (2008) Early symptoms in spinocerebellar ataxia type 1, 2, 3, and 6. Mov Disord 23:2232-2238.

Godavarthi SK, Narender D, Mishra A, Goswami A, Rao SN, Nukina N, Jana NR (2009) Induction of chemokines, MCP-1, and KC in the mutant huntingtin expressing neuronal cells because of proteasomal dysfunction. J Neurochem 108:787-795.

Goehler H, Lalowski M, Stelzl U, Waelter S, Stroedicke M, Worm U, Droege A, Lindenberg KS, Knoblich M, Haenig C, Herbst M, Suopanki J, Scherzinger E, Abraham C, Bauer B, Hasenbank R, Fritzsche A, Ludewig AH, Bussow K, Coleman SH, Gutekunst CA, Landwehrmeyer BG, Lehrach H, Wanker EE (2004) A protein interaction network links GIT1, an enhancer of huntingtin aggregation, to Huntington's disease. Mol Cell 15:853-865.

Goldberg YP, Nicholson DW, Rasper DM, Kalchman MA, Koide HB, Graham RK, Bromm M, Kazemi-Esfarjani P, Thornberry NA, Vaillancourt JP, Hayden MR (1996) Cleavage of huntingtin by apopain, a proapoptotic cysteine protease, is modulated by the polyglutamine tract. Nat Genet 13:442-449.

Goti D, Katzen SM, Mez J, Kurtis N, Kiluk J, Ben-Haiem L, Jenkins NA, Copeland NG, Kakizuka A, Sharp AH, Ross CA, Mouton PR, Colomer V (2004) A mutant ataxin-3 putative-cleavage fragment in brains of Machado-Joseph disease patients and transgenic mice is cytotoxic above a critical concentration. J Neurosci 24:10266-10279.

Goto J, Watanabe M, Ichikawa Y, Yee SB, Ihara N, Endo K, Igarashi S, Takiyama Y, Gaspar C, Maciel P, Tsuji S, Rouleau GA, Kanazawa I (1997) Machado-Joseph disease gene products carrying different carboxyl termini. Neurosci Res 28:373-377.

Gu W, Ma H, Wang K, Jin M, Zhou Y, Liu X, Wang G, Shen Y (2004) The shortest expanded allele of the MJD1 gene in a Chinese MJD kindred with autonomic dysfunction. Eur Neurol 52:107-111.

Gunawardena S, Her LS, Brusch RG, Laymon RA, Niesman IR, Gordesky-Gold B, Sintasath L, Bonini NM, Goldstein LS (2003) Disruption of axonal transport by loss of huntingtin or expression of pathogenic polyQ proteins in Drosophila. Neuron 40:25-40.

Gusella JF, MacDonald ME (2000) Molecular genetics: unmasking polyglutamine triggers in neurodegenerative disease. Nat Rev Neurosci 1:109-115.

Gwinn-Hardy K, Singleton A, O'Suilleabhain P, Boss M, Nicholl D, Adam A, Hussey J, Critchley P, Hardy J, Farrer M (2001) Spinocerebellar ataxia type 3 phenotypically resembling parkinson disease in a black family. Arch Neurol 58:296-299.

Haacke A, Broadley SA, Boteva R, Tzvetkov N, Hartl FU, Breuer P (2006) Proteolytic cleavage of polyglutamine-expanded ataxin-3 is critical for aggregation and sequestration of non-expanded ataxin-3. Hum Mol Genet 15:555-568.

Haacke A, Hartl FU, Breuer P (2007) Calpain inhibition is sufficient to suppress aggregation of polyglutamine-expanded ataxin-3. J Biol Chem 282:18851-18856.

Harper SQ, Staber PD, He X, Eliason SL, Martins IH, Mao Q, Yang L, Kotin RM, Paulson HL, Davidson BL (2005) RNA interference improves motor and neuropathological abnormalities in a Huntington's disease mouse model. Proc Natl Acad Sci U S A 102:5820-5825.

Harris GM, Dodelzon K, Gong L, Gonzalez-Alegre P, Paulson HL (2010) Splice isoforms of the polyglutamine disease protein ataxin-3 exhibit similar enzymatic yet different aggregation properties. PLoS One 5:e13695.

Hathorn T, Snyder-Keller A, Messer A (2011) Nicotinamide improves motor deficits and upregulates PGC-1alpha and BDNF gene expression in a mouse model of Huntington's disease. Neurobiol Dis 41:43-50.

Hayashi M, Kobayashi K, Furuta H (2003) Immunohistochemical study of neuronal intranuclear and cytoplasmic inclusions in Machado-Joseph disease. Psychiatry Clin Neurosci 57:205-213.

Heiser V, Engemann S, Brocker W, Dunkel I, Boeddrich A, Waelter S, Nordhoff E, Lurz R, Schugardt N, Rautenberg S, Herhaus C, Barnickel G, Bottcher H, Lehrach H, Wanker EE (2002) Identification of benzothiazoles as potential polyglutamine aggregation inhibitors of Huntington's disease by using an automated filter retardation assay. Proc Natl Acad Sci U S A 99 Suppl 4:16400-16406.

Heiser V, Scherzinger E, Boeddrich A, Nordhoff E, Lurz R, Schugardt N, Lehrach H, Wanker EE (2000) Inhibition of huntingtin fibrillogenesis by specific antibodies and small molecules: implications for Huntington's disease therapy. Proc Natl Acad Sci U S A 97:6739-6744.

Herbst M, Wanker EE (2006) Therapeutic approaches to polyglutamine diseases: combating protein misfolding and aggregation. Curr Pharm Des 12:2543-2555.

Hockly E, Richon VM, Woodman B, Smith DL, Zhou X, Rosa E, Sathasivam K, Ghazi-Noori S, Mahal A, Lowden PA, Steffan JS, Marsh JL, Thompson LM, Lewis CM, Marks PA, Bates GP (2003) Suberoylanilide hydroxamic acid, a histone deacetylase inhibitor, ameliorates motor deficits in a mouse model of Huntington's disease. Proc Natl Acad Sci U S A 100:2041-2046.

Hodgson JG, Agopyan N, Gutekunst CA, Leavitt BR, LePiane F, Singaraja R, Smith DJ, Bissada N, McCutcheon K, Nasir J, Jamot L, Li XJ, Stevens ME, Rosemond E, Roder JC, Phillips AG, Rubin EM, Hersch SM, Hayden MR (1999) A YAC mouse model for Huntington's disease with full-length mutant huntingtin, cytoplasmic toxicity, and selective striatal neurodegeneration. Neuron 23:181-192.

Hu J, Matsui M, Gagnon KT, Schwartz JC, Gabillet S, Arar K, Wu J, Bezprozvanny I, Corey DR (2009) Allele-specific silencing of mutant huntingtin and ataxin-3 genes by targeting expanded CAG repeats in mRNAs. Nat Biotechnol 27:478-484.

Hubener J, Vauti F, Funke C, Wolburg H, Ye Y, Schmidt T, Wolburg-Buchholz K, Schmitt I, Gardyan A, Driessen S, Arnold HH, Nguyen HP, Riess O (2011) N-terminal ataxin-3 causes neurological symptoms with inclusions, endoplasmic reticulum stress and ribosomal dislocation. Brain 134:1925-1942.

Hughes RE, Lo RS, Davis C, Strand AD, Neal CL, Olson JM, Fields S (2001) Altered transcription in yeast expressing expanded polyglutamine. Proc Natl Acad Sci U S A 98:13201-13206.

Ichikawa Y, Goto J, Hattori M, Toyoda A, Ishii K, Jeong SY, Hashida H, Masuda N, Ogata K, Kasai F, Hirai M, Maciel P, Rouleau GA, Sakaki Y, Kanazawa I (2001) The genomic structure and expression of MJD, the Machado-Joseph disease gene. J Hum Genet 46:413-422.

Ikeda H, Yamaguchi M, Sugai S, Aze Y, Narumiya S, Kakizuka A (1996) Expanded polyglutamine in the Machado-Joseph disease protein induces cell death in vitro and in vivo. Nat Genet 13:196-202.

Jacobi H, Hauser TK, Giunti P, Globas C, Bauer P, Schmitz-Hubsch T, Baliko L, Filla A, Mariotti C, Rakowicz M, Charles P, Ribai P, Szymanski S, Infante J, van de Warrenburg BP, Durr A, Timmann D, Boesch S, Fancellu R, Rola R, Depondt C, Schols L, Zdzienicka E, Kang JS, Ratzka S, Kremer B, Stephenson DA, Melegh B, Pandolfo M, du Montcel ST, Borkert J, Schulz JB, Klockgether T (2011) Spinocerebellar Ataxia Types 1, 2, 3 and 6: the Clinical Spectrum of Ataxia and Morphometric Brainstem and Cerebellar Findings. Cerebellum.

Jana NR, Dikshit P, Goswami A, Kotliarova S, Murata S, Tanaka K, Nukina N (2005) Co-chaperone CHIP associates with expanded polyglutamine protein and promotes their degradation by proteasomes. J Biol Chem 280:11635-11640.

Jana NR, Nukina N (2004) Misfolding promotes the ubiquitination of polyglutamine-expanded ataxin-3, the defective gene product in SCA3/MJD. Neurotox Res 6:523-533.

Kasumu A, Bezprozvanny I (2010) Deranged Calcium Signaling in Purkinje Cells and Pathogenesis in Spinocerebellar Ataxia 2 (SCA2) and Other Ataxias. Cerebellum.

Kawaguchi Y, Okamoto T, Taniwaki M, Aizawa M, Inoue M, Katayama S, Kawakami H, Nakamura S, Nishimura M, Akiguchi I, et al., (1994) CAG expansions in a novel gene for Machado-Joseph disease at chromosome 14q32.1. Nat Genet 8:221-228.

Kayed R, Head E, Thompson JL, McIntire TM, Milton SC, Cotman CW, Glabe CG (2003) Common structure of soluble amyloid oligomers implies common mechanism of pathogenesis. Science 300:486-489.

Kayed R, Sokolov Y, Edmonds B, McIntire TM, Milton SC, Hall JE, Glabe CG (2004) Permeabilization of lipid bilayers is a common conformation-dependent activity of soluble amyloid oligomers in protein misfolding diseases. J Biol Chem 279:46363-46366.

Kaytor MD, Byam CE, Tousey SK, Stevens SD, Zoghbi HY, Orr HT (2005) A cell-based screen for modulators of ataxin-1 phosphorylation. Hum Mol Genet 14:1095-1105.

Kettner M, Willwohl D, Hubbard GB, Rub U, Dick EJ, Jr., Cox AB, Trottier Y, Auburger G, Braak H, Schultz C (2002) Intranuclear aggregation of nonexpanded ataxin-3 in marinesco bodies of the nonhuman primate substantia nigra. Exp Neurol 176:117-121.

Kim DH, Rossi JJ (2007) Strategies for silencing human disease using RNA interference. Nat Rev Genet 8:173-184.

Klement IA, Skinner PJ, Kaytor MD, Yi H, Hersch SM, Clark HB, Zoghbi HY, Orr HT (1998) Ataxin-1 nuclear localization and aggregation: role in polyglutamine-induced disease in SCA1 transgenic mice. Cell 95:41-53.

Klinke I, Minnerop M, Schmitz-Hubsch T, Hendriks M, Klockgether T, Wullner U, Helmstaedter C (2010) Neuropsychological features of patients with spinocerebellar ataxia (SCA) types 1, 2, 3, and 6. Cerebellum 9:433-442.

Knott AB, Perkins G, Schwarzenbacher R, Bossy-Wetzel E (2008) Mitochondrial fragmentation in neurodegeneration. Nat Rev Neurosci 9:505-518.

Kurdistani SK, Tavazoie S, Grunstein M (2004) Mapping global histone acetylation patterns to gene expression. Cell 117:721-733.

La Spada AR, Fu YH, Sopher BL, Libby RT, Wang X, Li LY, Einum DD, Huang J, Possin DE, Smith AC, Martinez RA, Koszdin KL, Treuting PM, Ware CB, Hurley JB, Ptacek LJ, Chen S (2001) Polyglutamine-expanded ataxin-7 antagonizes CRX function and induces cone-rod dystrophy in a mouse model of SCA7. Neuron 31:913-927.

Lansbury PT, Lashuel HA (2006) A century-old debate on protein aggregation and neurodegeneration enters the clinic. Nature 443:774-779.

Lastres-Becker I, Rub U, Auburger G (2008) Spinocerebellar ataxia 2 (SCA2). Cerebellum 7:115-124.

Lathrop RH, Casale M, Tobias DJ, Marsh JL, Thompson LM (1998) Modeling protein homopolymeric repeats: possible polyglutamine structural motifs for Huntington's disease. Proc Int Conf Intell Syst Mol Biol 6:105-114.

Lessing D, Bonini NM (2008) Polyglutamine genes interact to modulate the severity and progression of neurodegeneration in Drosophila. PLoS Biol 6:e29.

Li F, Macfarlan T, Pittman RN, Chakravarti D (2002) Ataxin-3 is a histone-binding protein with two independent transcriptional corepressor activities. J Biol Chem 277:45004-45012.

Lim J, Crespo-Barreto J, Jafar-Nejad P, Bowman AB, Richman R, Hill DE, Orr HT, Zoghbi HY (2008) Opposing effects of polyglutamine expansion on native protein complexes contribute to SCA1. Nature 452:713-718.

Lim J, Hao T, Shaw C, Patel AJ, Szabo G, Rual JF, Fisk CJ, Li N, Smolyar A, Hill DE, Barabasi AL, Vidal M, Zoghbi HY (2006) A protein-protein interaction network for human inherited ataxias and disorders of Purkinje cell degeneration. Cell 125:801-814.

Lima L, Coutinho P (1980) Clinical criteria for diagnosis of Machado-Joseph disease: report of a non-Azorena Portuguese family. Neurology 30:319-322.

Lombardi MS, Jaspers L, Spronkmans C, Gellera C, Taroni F, Di Maria E, Donato SD, Kaemmerer WF (2009) A majority of Huntington's disease patients may be treatable by individualized allele-specific RNA interference. Exp Neurol 217:312-319.

Lysenko L, Grewal RP, Ma W, Peddareddygari LR (2010) Homozygous Machado Joseph Disease: a case report and review of literature. Can J Neurol Sci 37:521-523.

Macedo-Ribeiro S, Cortes L, Maciel P, Carvalho AL (2009) Nucleocytoplasmic shuttling activity of ataxin-3. PLoS One 4:e5834.

Maciel P, Costa MC, Ferro A, Rousseau M, Santos CS, Gaspar C, Barros J, Rouleau GA, Coutinho P, Sequeiros J (2001) Improvement in the molecular diagnosis of Machado-Joseph disease. Arch Neurol 58:1821-1827.

Maciel P, Gaspar C, DeStefano AL, Silveira I, Coutinho P, Radvany J, Dawson DM, Sudarsky L, Guimaraes J, Loureiro JE, et al., (1995) Correlation between CAG repeat length and clinical features in Machado-Joseph disease. Am J Hum Genet 57:54-61.

Martindale D, Hackam A, Wieczorek A, Ellerby L, Wellington C, McCutcheon K, Singaraja R, Kazemi-Esfarjani P, Devon R, Kim SU, Bredesen DE, Tufaro F, Hayden MR (1998) Length of huntingtin and its polyglutamine tract influences localization and frequency of intracellular aggregates. Nat Genet 18:150-154.

Maruyama H, Nakamura S, Matsuyama Z, Sakai T, Doyu M, Sobue G, Seto M, Tsujihata M, Oh-i T, Nishio T, et al., (1995) Molecular features of the CAG repeats and clinical manifestation of Machado-Joseph disease. Hum Mol Genet 4:807-812.

Masino L, Musi V, Menon RP, Fusi P, Kelly G, Frenkiel TA, Trottier Y, Pastore A (2003) Domain architecture of the polyglutamine protein ataxin-3: a globular domain followed by a flexible tail. FEBS Lett 549:21-25.

Matos CA, de Macedo-Ribeiro S, Carvalho AL (2011) Polyglutamine diseases: The special case of ataxin-3 and Machado-Joseph disease. Prog Neurobiol.

Matsumoto M, Yada M, Hatakeyama S, Ishimoto H, Tanimura T, Tsuji S, Kakizuka A, Kitagawa M, Nakayama KI (2004) Molecular clearance of ataxin-3 is regulated by a mammalian E4. Embo J 23:659-669.

Mauri PL, Riva M, Ambu D, De Palma A, Secundo F, Benazzi L, Valtorta M, Tortora P, Fusi P (2006) Ataxin-3 is subject to autolytic cleavage. Febs J 273:4277-4286.

McCampbell A, Taylor JP, Taye AA, Robitschek J, Li M, Walcott J, Merry D, Chai Y, Paulson H, Sobue G, Fischbeck KH (2000) CREB-binding protein sequestration by expanded polyglutamine. Hum Mol Genet 9:2197-2202.

Menzies FM, Huebener J, Renna M, Bonin M, Riess O, Rubinsztein DC (2010) Autophagy induction reduces mutant ataxin-3 levels and toxicity in a mouse model of spinocerebellar ataxia type 3. Brain 133:93-104.

Michalik A, Van Broeckhoven C (2003) Pathogenesis of polyglutamine disorders: aggregation revisited. Hum Mol Genet 12 Spec No 2:R173-186.

Miller VM, Nelson RF, Gouvion CM, Williams A, Rodriguez-Lebron E, Harper SQ, Davidson BL, Rebagliati MR, Paulson HL (2005) CHIP suppresses polyglutamine aggregation and toxicity in vitro and in vivo. J Neurosci 25:9152-9161.

Miller VM, Xia H, Marrs GL, Gouvion CM, Lee G, Davidson BL, Paulson HL (2003) Allele-specific silencing of dominant disease genes. Proc Natl Acad Sci U S A 100:7195-7200.

Minamiyama M, Katsuno M, Adachi H, Waza M, Sang C, Kobayashi Y, Tanaka F, Doyu M, Inukai A, Sobue G (2004) Sodium butyrate ameliorates phenotypic expression in a transgenic mouse model of spinal and bulbar muscular atrophy. Hum Mol Genet 13:1183-1192.

Morfini G, Pigino G, Brady ST (2005) Polyglutamine expansion diseases: failing to deliver. Trends Mol Med 11:64-70.

Mueller T, Breuer P, Schmitt I, Walter J, Evert BO, Wullner U (2009) CK2-dependent phosphorylation determines cellular localization and stability of ataxin-3. Hum Mol Genet 18:3334-3343.

Munoz E, Rey MJ, Mila M, Cardozo A, Ribalta T, Tolosa E, Ferrer I (2002) Intranuclear inclusions, neuronal loss and CAG mosaicism in two patients with Machado-Joseph disease. J Neurol Sci 200:19-25.

Nagai Y, Fujikake N, Ohno K, Higashiyama H, Popiel HA, Rahadian J, Yamaguchi M, Strittmatter WJ, Burke JR, Toda T (2003) Prevention of polyglutamine oligomerization and neurodegeneration by the peptide inhibitor QBP1 in Drosophila. Hum Mol Genet 12:1253-1259.

Nagai Y, Fujikake N, Popiel HA, Wada K (2010) Induction of molecular chaperones as a therapeutic strategy for the polyglutamine diseases. Curr Pharm Biotechnol 11:188-197.

Nagai Y, Inui T, Popiel HA, Fujikake N, Hasegawa K, Urade Y, Goto Y, Naiki H, Toda T (2007) A toxic monomeric conformer of the polyglutamine protein. Nat Struct Mol Biol 14:332-340.

Nascimento-Ferreira I, Santos-Ferreira T, Sousa-Ferreira L, Auregan G, Onofre I, Alves S, Dufour N, Colomer Gould VF, Koeppen A, Deglon N, Pereira de Almeida L (2011) Overexpression of the autophagic beclin-1 protein clears mutant ataxin-3 and alleviates Machado-Joseph disease. Brain 134:1400-1415.

Nucifora FC, Jr., Sasaki M, Peters MF, Huang H, Cooper JK, Yamada M, Takahashi H, Tsuji S, Troncoso J, Dawson VL, Dawson TM, Ross CA (2001) Interference by huntingtin and atrophin-1 with cbp-mediated transcription leading to cellular toxicity. Science 291:2423-2428.

Okuro M, Fujiki N, Kotorii N, Ishimaru Y, Sokoloff P, Nishino S (2010) Effects of paraxanthine and caffeine on sleep, locomotor activity, and body temperature in orexin/ataxin-3 transgenic narcoleptic mice. Sleep 33:930-942.

Ona VO, Li M, Vonsattel JP, Andrews LJ, Khan SQ, Chung WM, Frey AS, Menon AS, Li XJ, Stieg PE, Yuan J, Penney JB, Young AB, Cha JH, Friedlander RM (1999) Inhibition of caspase-1 slows disease progression in a mouse model of Huntington's disease. Nature 399:263-267.

Orrenius S, Zhivotovsky B, Nicotera P (2003) Regulation of cell death: the calcium-apoptosis link. Nat Rev Mol Cell Biol 4:552-565.

Padiath QS, Srivastava AK, Roy S, Jain S, Brahmachari SK (2005) Identification of a novel 45 repeat unstable allele associated with a disease phenotype at the MJD1/SCA3 locus. Am J Med Genet B Neuropsychiatr Genet 133B:124-126.

Panov AV, Gutekunst CA, Leavitt BR, Hayden MR, Burke JR, Strittmatter WJ, Greenamyre JT (2002) Early mitochondrial calcium defects in Huntington's disease are a direct effect of polyglutamines. Nat Neurosci 5:731-736.

Paulson HL (1999) Protein fate in neurodegenerative proteinopathies: polyglutamine diseases join the (mis)fold. Am J Hum Genet 64:339-345.

Paulson HL, Das SS, Crino PB, Perez MK, Patel SC, Gotsdiner D, Fischbeck KH, Pittman RN (1997a) Machado-Joseph disease gene product is a cytoplasmic protein widely expressed in brain. Ann Neurol 41:453-462.

Paulson HL, Perez MK, Trottier Y, Trojanowski JQ, Subramony SH, Das SS, Vig P, Mandel JL, Fischbeck KH, Pittman RN (1997b) Intranuclear inclusions of expanded polyglutamine protein in spinocerebellar ataxia type 3. Neuron 19:333-344.

Perez MK, Paulson HL, Pendse SJ, Saionz SJ, Bonini NM, Pittman RN (1998) Recruitment and the role of nuclear localization in polyglutamine-mediated aggregation. J Cell Biol 143:1457-1470.

Pfister EL, Kennington L, Straubhaar J, Wagh S, Liu W, DiFiglia M, Landwehrmeyer B, Vonsattel JP, Zamore PD, Aronin N (2009) Five siRNAs targeting three SNPs may provide therapy for three-quarters of Huntington's disease patients. Curr Biol 19:774-778.

Pickford F, Masliah E, Britschgi M, Lucin K, Narasimhan R, Jaeger PA, Small S, Spencer B, Rockenstein E, Levine B, Wyss-Coray T (2008) The autophagy-related protein beclin 1 shows reduced expression in early Alzheimer disease and regulates amyloid beta accumulation in mice. J Clin Invest 118:2190-2199.

Poirier MA, Li H, Macosko J, Cai S, Amzel M, Ross CA (2002) Huntingtin spheroids and protofibrils as precursors in polyglutamine fibrilization. J Biol Chem 277:41032-41037.

Prediger RD (2010) Effects of caffeine in Parkinson's disease: from neuroprotection to the management of motor and non-motor symptoms. J Alzheimers Dis 20 Suppl 1:S205-220.

Qin Q, Inatome R, Hotta A, Kojima M, Yamamura H, Hirai H, Yoshizawa T, Tanaka H, Fukami K, Yanagi S (2006) A novel GTPase, CRAG, mediates promyelocytic leukemia protein-associated nuclear body formation and degradation of expanded polyglutamine protein. J Cell Biol 172:497-504.

Ralph GS, Radcliffe PA, Day DM, Carthy JM, Leroux MA, Lee DC, Wong LF, Bilsland LG, Greensmith L, Kingsman SM, Mitrophanous KA, Mazarakis ND, Azzouz M (2005)

Silencing mutant SOD1 using RNAi protects against neurodegeneration and extends survival in an ALS model. Nat Med 11:429-433.

Ranum LP, Lundgren JK, Schut LJ, Ahrens MJ, Perlman S, Aita J, Bird TD, Gomez C, Orr HT (1995) Spinocerebellar ataxia type 1 and Machado-Joseph disease: incidence of CAG expansions among adult-onset ataxia patients from 311 families with dominant, recessive, or sporadic ataxia. Am J Hum Genet 57:603-608.

Raoul C, Abbas-Terki T, Bensadoun JC, Guillot S, Haase G, Szulc J, Henderson CE, Aebischer P (2005) Lentiviral-mediated silencing of SOD1 through RNA interference retards disease onset and progression in a mouse model of ALS. Nat Med 11:423-428.

Ravikumar B, Vacher C, Berger Z, Davies JE, Luo S, Oroz LG, Scaravilli F, Easton DF, Duden R, O'Kane CJ, Rubinsztein DC (2004) Inhibition of mTOR induces autophagy and reduces toxicity of polyglutamine expansions in fly and mouse models of Huntington disease. Nat Genet 36:585-595.

Riess O, Rub U, Pastore A, Bauer P, Schols L (2008) SCA3: neurological features, pathogenesis and animal models. Cerebellum 7:125-137.

Riley BE, Orr HT (2006) Polyglutamine neurodegenerative diseases and regulation of transcription: assembling the puzzle. Genes Dev 20:2183-2192.

Robertson AL, Headey SJ, Saunders HM, Ecroyd H, Scanlon MJ, Carver JA, Bottomley SP (2010) Small heat-shock proteins interact with a flanking domain to suppress polyglutamine aggregation. Proc Natl Acad Sci U S A 107:10424-10429.

Rodrigues AJ, do Carmo Costa M, Silva TL, Ferreira D, Bajanca F, Logarinho E, Maciel P (2010) Absence of ataxin-3 leads to cytoskeletal disorganization and increased cell death. Biochim Biophys Acta 1803:1154-1163.

Rodrigues AJ, Neves-Carvalho A, Ferro A, Rokka A, Corthals G, Logarinho E, Maciel P (2009) ATX-3, CDC-48 and UBXN-5: a new trimolecular complex in Caenorhabditis elegans. Biochem Biophys Res Commun 386:575-581.

Rodriguez-Lebron E, Denovan-Wright EM, Nash K, Lewin AS, Mandel RJ (2005) Intrastriatal rAAV-mediated delivery of anti-huntingtin shRNAs induces partial reversal of disease progression in R6/1 Huntington's disease transgenic mice. Mol Ther 12:618-633.

Rosenberg RN (1992) Machado-Joseph disease: an autosomal dominant motor system degeneration. Mov Disord 7:193-203.

Ross CA (1997) Intranuclear neuronal inclusions: a common pathogenic mechanism for glutamine-repeat neurodegenerative diseases? Neuron 19:1147-1150.

Ross CA, Poirier MA (2005) Opinion: What is the role of protein aggregation in neurodegeneration? Nat Rev Mol Cell Biol 6:891-898.

Ross CA, Poirier MA, Wanker EE, Amzel M (2003) Polyglutamine fibrillogenesis: the pathway unfolds. Proc Natl Acad Sci U S A 100:1-3.

Rub U, Brunt ER, Deller T (2008) New insights into the pathoanatomy of spinocerebellar ataxia type 3 (Machado-Joseph disease). Curr Opin Neurol 21:111-116.

Rub U, Brunt ER, Petrasch-Parwez E, Schols L, Theegarten D, Auburger G, Seidel K, Schultz C, Gierga K, Paulson H, van Broeckhoven C, Deller T, de Vos RA (2006a)

Degeneration of ingestion-related brainstem nuclei in spinocerebellar ataxia type 2, 3, 6 and 7. Neuropathol Appl Neurobiol 32:635-649.

Rub U, de Vos RA, Brunt ER, Sebesteny T, Schols L, Auburger G, Bohl J, Ghebremedhin E, Gierga K, Seidel K, den Dunnen W, Heinsen H, Paulson H, Deller T (2006b) Spinocerebellar ataxia type 3 (SCA3): thalamic neurodegeneration occurs independently from thalamic ataxin-3 immunopositive neuronal intranuclear inclusions. Brain Pathol 16:218-227.

Sanchez I, Mahlke C, Yuan J (2003) Pivotal role of oligomerization in expanded polyglutamine neurodegenerative disorders. Nature 421:373-379.

Saudou F, Finkbeiner S, Devys D, Greenberg ME (1998) Huntingtin acts in the nucleus to induce apoptosis but death does not correlate with the formation of intranuclear inclusions. Cell 95:55-66.

Scaglione KM, Zavodszky E, Todi SV, Patury S, Xu P, Rodriguez-Lebron E, Fischer S, Konen J, Djarmati A, Peng J, Gestwicki JE, Paulson HL (2011) Ube2w and Ataxin-3 Coordinately Regulate the Ubiquitin Ligase CHIP. Mol Cell 43:599-612.

Schaffar G, Breuer P, Boteva R, Behrends C, Tzvetkov N, Strippel N, Sakahira H, Siegers K, Hayer-Hartl M, Hartl FU (2004) Cellular toxicity of polyglutamine expansion proteins: mechanism of transcription factor deactivation. Mol Cell 15:95-105.

Scheel H, Tomiuk S, Hofmann K (2003) Elucidation of ataxin-3 and ataxin-7 function by integrative bioinformatics. Hum Mol Genet 12:2845-2852.

Schilling B, Gafni J, Torcassi C, Cong X, Row RH, LaFevre-Bernt MA, Cusack MP, Ratovitski T, Hirschhorn R, Ross CA, Gibson BW, Ellerby LM (2006) Huntingtin phosphorylation sites mapped by mass spectrometry. Modulation of cleavage and toxicity. J Biol Chem 281:23686-23697.

Schilling G, Becher MW, Sharp AH, Jinnah HA, Duan K, Kotzuk JA, Slunt HH, Ratovitski T, Cooper JK, Jenkins NA, Copeland NG, Price DL, Ross CA, Borchelt DR (1999) Intranuclear inclusions and neuritic aggregates in transgenic mice expressing a mutant N-terminal fragment of huntingtin. Hum Mol Genet 8:397-407.

Schmidt T, Landwehrmeyer GB, Schmitt I, Trottier Y, Auburger G, Laccone F, Klockgether T, Volpel M, Epplen JT, Schols L, Riess O (1998) An isoform of ataxin-3 accumulates in the nucleus of neuronal cells in affected brain regions of SCA3 patients. Brain Pathol 8:669-679.

Scholefield J, Greenberg LJ, Weinberg MS, Arbuthnot PB, Abdelgany A, Wood MJ (2009) Design of RNAi hairpins for mutation-specific silencing of ataxin-7 and correction of a SCA7 phenotype. PLoS One 4:e7232.

Schols L, Bauer P, Schmidt T, Schulte T, Riess O (2004) Autosomal dominant cerebellar ataxias: clinical features, genetics, and pathogenesis. Lancet Neurol 3:291-304.

Schulte J, Sepp KJ, Wu C, Hong P, Littleton JT (2011) High-Content Chemical and RNAi Screens for Suppressors of Neurotoxicity in a Huntington's Disease Model. PLoS One 6:e23841.

Schulz JB, Borkert J, Wolf S, Schmitz-Hubsch T, Rakowicz M, Mariotti C, Schols L, Timmann D, van de Warrenburg B, Durr A, Pandolfo M, Kang JS, Mandly AG, Nagele T, Grisoli M, Boguslawska R, Bauer P, Klockgether T, Hauser TK (2010) Visualization, quantification and correlation of brain atrophy with clinical symptoms in spinocerebellar ataxia types 1, 3 and 6. Neuroimage 49:158-168.

Seidel K, den Dunnen WF, Schultz C, Paulson H, Frank S, de Vos RA, Brunt ER, Deller T, Kampinga HH, Rub U (2010) Axonal inclusions in spinocerebellar ataxia type 3. Acta Neuropathol 120:449-460.

Shen L, Tang JG, Tang BS, Jiang H, Zhao GH, Xia K, Zhang YH, Cai F, Tan LM, Pan Q (2005) Research on screening and identification of proteins interacting with ataxin-3. Zhonghua Yi Xue Yi Chuan Xue Za Zhi 22:242-247.

Shibata M, Lu T, Furuya T, Degterev A, Mizushima N, Yoshimori T, MacDonald M, Yankner B, Yuan J (2006) Regulation of intracellular accumulation of mutant Huntingtin by Beclin 1. J Biol Chem 281:14474-14485.

Shimohata M, Shimohata T, Igarashi S, Naruse S, Tsuji S (2005) Interference of CREB-dependent transcriptional activation by expanded polyglutamine stretches--augmentation of transcriptional activation as a potential therapeutic strategy for polyglutamine diseases. J Neurochem 93:654-663.

Shimohata T, Nakajima T, Yamada M, Uchida C, Onodera O, Naruse S, Kimura T, Koide R, Nozaki K, Sano Y, Ishiguro H, Sakoe K, Ooshima T, Sato A, Ikeuchi T, Oyake M, Sato T, Aoyagi Y, Hozumi I, Nagatsu T, Takiyama Y, Nishizawa M, Goto J, Kanazawa I, Davidson I, Tanese N, Takahashi H, Tsuji S (2000a) Expanded polyglutamine stretches interact with TAFII130, interfering with CREB-dependent transcription. Nat Genet 26:29-36.

Shimohata T, Onodera O, Tsuji S (2000b) Interaction of expanded polyglutamine stretches with nuclear transcription factors leads to aberrant transcriptional regulation in polyglutamine diseases. Neuropathology 20:326-333.

Sittler A, Lurz R, Lueder G, Priller J, Lehrach H, Hayer-Hartl MK, Hartl FU, Wanker EE (2001) Geldanamycin activates a heat shock response and inhibits huntingtin aggregation in a cell culture model of Huntington's disease. Hum Mol Genet 10:1307-1315.

Soong BW, Paulson HL (2007) Spinocerebellar ataxias: an update. Curr Opin Neurol 20:438-446.

Steffan JS, Bodai L, Pallos J, Poelman M, McCampbell A, Apostol BL, Kazantsev A, Schmidt E, Zhu YZ, Greenwald M, Kurokawa R, Housman DE, Jackson GR, Marsh JL, Thompson LM (2001) Histone deacetylase inhibitors arrest polyglutamine-dependent neurodegeneration in Drosophila. Nature 413:739-743.

Stevanin G, Cancel G, Durr A, Chneiweiss H, Dubourg O, Weissenbach J, Cann HM, Agid Y, Brice A (1995) The gene for spinal cerebellar ataxia 3 (SCA3) is located in a region of approximately 3 cM on chromosome 14q24.3-q32.2. Am J Hum Genet 56:193-201.

Stott K, Blackburn JM, Butler PJ, Perutz M (1995) Incorporation of glutamine repeats makes protein oligomerize: implications for neurodegenerative diseases. Proc Natl Acad Sci U S A 92:6509-6513.

Sudarsky L, Coutinho P (1995) Machado-Joseph disease. Clin Neurosci 3:17-22.

Szebenyi G, Morfini GA, Babcock A, Gould M, Selkoe K, Stenoien DL, Young M, Faber PW, MacDonald ME, McPhaul MJ, Brady ST (2003) Neuropathogenic forms of huntingtin and androgen receptor inhibit fast axonal transport. Neuron 40:41-52.

Tait D, Riccio M, Sittler A, Scherzinger E, Santi S, Ognibene A, Maraldi NM, Lehrach H, Wanker EE (1998) Ataxin-3 is transported into the nucleus and associates with the nuclear matrix. Hum Mol Genet 7:991-997.

Takahashi J, Tanaka J, Arai K, Funata N, Hattori T, Fukuda T, Fujigasaki H, Uchihara T (2001) Recruitment of nonexpanded polyglutamine proteins to intranuclear aggregates in neuronal intranuclear hyaline inclusion disease. J Neuropathol Exp Neurol 60:369-376.

Takahashi T, Katada S, Onodera O (2010) Polyglutamine diseases: where does toxicity come from? what is toxicity? where are we going? J Mol Cell Biol 2:180-191.

Takahashi T, Kikuchi S, Katada S, Nagai Y, Nishizawa M, Onodera O (2008) Soluble polyglutamine oligomers formed prior to inclusion body formation are cytotoxic. Hum Mol Genet 17:345-356.

Takahashi-Fujigasaki J, Breidert T, Fujigasaki H, Duyckaerts C, Camonis JH, Brice A, Lebre AS (2011) Amyloid precursor-like protein 2 cleavage contributes to neuronal intranuclear inclusions and cytotoxicity in spinocerebellar ataxia-7 (SCA7). Neurobiol Dis 41:33-42.

Takiyama Y, Nishizawa M, Tanaka H, Kawashima S, Sakamoto H, Karube Y, Shimazaki H, Soutome M, Endo K, Ohta S, et al., (1993) The gene for Machado-Joseph disease maps to human chromosome 14q. Nat Genet 4:300-304.

Tanaka M, Machida Y, Nukina N (2005) A novel therapeutic strategy for polyglutamine diseases by stabilizing aggregation-prone proteins with small molecules. J Mol Med 83:343-352.

Tanaka M, Morishima I, Akagi T, Hashikawa T, Nukina N (2001) Intra- and intermolecular beta-pleated sheet formation in glutamine-repeat inserted myoglobin as a model for polyglutamine diseases. J Biol Chem 276:45470-45475.

Tang TS, Slow E, Lupu V, Stavrovskaya IG, Sugimori M, Llinas R, Kristal BS, Hayden MR, Bezprozvanny I (2005) Disturbed Ca2+ signaling and apoptosis of medium spiny neurons in Huntington's disease. Proc Natl Acad Sci U S A 102:2602-2607.

Tang TS, Tu H, Chan EY, Maximov A, Wang Z, Wellington CL, Hayden MR, Bezprozvanny I (2003) Huntingtin and huntingtin-associated protein 1 influence neuronal calcium signaling mediated by inositol-(1,4,5) triphosphate receptor type 1. Neuron 39:227-239.

Tao RS, Fei EK, Ying Z, Wang HF, Wang GH (2008) Casein kinase 2 interacts with and phosphorylates ataxin-3. Neurosci Bull 24:271-277.

Tarlac V, Storey E (2003) Role of proteolysis in polyglutamine disorders. J Neurosci Res 74:406-416.

Taroni F, DiDonato S (2004) Pathways to motor incoordination: the inherited ataxias. Nat Rev Neurosci 5:641-655.

Taylor JP, Hardy J, Fischbeck KH (2002) Toxic proteins in neurodegenerative disease. Science 296:1991-1995.

Taylor JP, Tanaka F, Robitschek J, Sandoval CM, Taye A, Markovic-Plese S, Fischbeck KH (2003) Aggresomes protect cells by enhancing the degradation of toxic polyglutamine-containing protein. Hum Mol Genet 12:749-757.

Thakur AK, Wetzel R (2002) Mutational analysis of the structural organization of polyglutamine aggregates. Proc Natl Acad Sci U S A 99:17014-17019.

Todi SV, Winborn BJ, Scaglione KM, Blount JR, Travis SM, Paulson HL (2009) Ubiquitination directly enhances activity of the deubiquitinating enzyme ataxin-3. Embo J 28:372-382.

Todi SV, Paulson HL (2011) Balancing act: deubiquitinating enzymes in the nervous system. Trends Neurosci.

Torashima T, Koyama C, Iizuka A, Mitsumura K, Takayama K, Yanagi S, Oue M, Yamaguchi H, Hirai H (2008) Lentivector-mediated rescue from cerebellar ataxia in a mouse model of spinocerebellar ataxia. EMBO Rep 9:393-399.

Trottier Y, Cancel G, An-Gourfinkel I, Lutz Y, Weber C, Brice A, Hirsch E, Mandel JL (1998) Heterogeneous intracellular localization and expression of ataxin-3. Neurobiol Dis 5:335-347.

Tsuda H, Jafar-Nejad H, Patel AJ, Sun Y, Chen HK, Rose MF, Venken KJ, Botas J, Orr HT, Bellen HJ, Zoghbi HY (2005) The AXH domain of Ataxin-1 mediates neurodegeneration through its interaction with Gfi-1/Senseless proteins. Cell 122:633-644.

Uchihara T, Fujigasaki H, Koyano S, Nakamura A, Yagishita S, Iwabuchi K (2001) Non-expanded polyglutamine proteins in intranuclear inclusions of hereditary ataxias--triple-labeling immunofluorescence study. Acta Neuropathol 102:149-152.

Ueda H, Goto J, Hashida H, Lin X, Oyanagi K, Kawano H, Zoghbi HY, Kanazawa I, Okazawa H (2002) Enhanced SUMOylation in polyglutamine diseases. Biochem Biophys Res Commun 293:307-313.

van Bilsen PH, Jaspers L, Lombardi MS, Odekerken JC, Burright EN, Kaemmerer WF (2008) Identification and allele-specific silencing of the mutant huntingtin allele in Huntington's disease patient-derived fibroblasts. Hum Gene Ther 19:710-719.

Vellai T (2009) Autophagy genes and ageing. Cell Death Differ 16:94-102.

Walsh DM, Klyubin I, Fadeeva JV, Cullen WK, Anwyl R, Wolfe MS, Rowan MJ, Selkoe DJ (2002) Naturally secreted oligomers of amyloid beta protein potently inhibit hippocampal long-term potentiation in vivo. Nature 416:535-539.

Walsh R, Storey E, Stefani D, Kelly L, Turnbull V (2005) The roles of proteolysis and nuclear localisation in the toxicity of the polyglutamine diseases. A review. Neurotox Res 7:43-57.

Wang H, Jia N, Fei E, Wang Z, Liu C, Zhang T, Fan J, Wu M, Chen L, Nukina N, Zhou J, Wang G (2007) p45, an ATPase subunit of the 19S proteasome, targets the polyglutamine disease protein ataxin-3 to the proteasome. J Neurochem 101:1651-1661.

Wang Q, Li L, Ye Y (2006) Regulation of retrotranslocation by p97-associated deubiquitinating enzyme ataxin-3. J Cell Biol 174:963-971.

Wanker EE (2000) Protein aggregation and pathogenesis of Huntington's disease: mechanisms and correlations. Biol Chem 381:937-942.

Warrick JM, Morabito LM, Bilen J, Gordesky-Gold B, Faust LZ, Paulson HL, Bonini NM (2005) Ataxin-3 suppresses polyglutamine neurodegeneration in Drosophila by a ubiquitin-associated mechanism. Mol Cell 18:37-48.

Wellington CL, Ellerby LM, Hackam AS, Margolis RL, Trifiro MA, Singaraja R, McCutcheon K, Salvesen GS, Propp SS, Bromm M, Rowland KJ, Zhang T, Rasper D, Roy S, Thornberry N, Pinsky L, Kakizuka A, Ross CA, Nicholson DW, Bredesen DE, Hayden MR (1998) Caspase cleavage of gene products associated with triplet expansion disorders generates truncated fragments containing the polyglutamine tract. J Biol Chem 273:9158-9167.

Williams A, Jahreiss L, Sarkar S, Saiki S, Menzies FM, Ravikumar B, Rubinsztein DC (2006) Aggregate-prone proteins are cleared from the cytosol by autophagy: therapeutic implications. Curr Top Dev Biol 76:89-101.

Winborn BJ, Travis SM, Todi SV, Scaglione KM, Xu P, Williams AJ, Cohen RE, Peng J, Paulson HL (2008) The deubiquitinating enzyme ataxin-3, a polyglutamine disease protein, edits Lys63 linkages in mixed linkage ubiquitin chains. J Biol Chem 283:26436-26443.

Wolfgang WJ, Miller TW, Webster JM, Huston JS, Thompson LM, Marsh JL, Messer A (2005) Suppression of Huntington's disease pathology in Drosophila by human single-chain Fv antibodies. Proc Natl Acad Sci U S A 102:11563-11568.

Wu J, Tang T, Bezprozvanny I (2006) Evaluation of clinically relevant glutamate pathway inhibitors in in vitro model of Huntington's disease. Neurosci Lett 407:219-223.

Xia H, Mao Q, Eliason SL, Harper SQ, Martins IH, Orr HT, Paulson HL, Yang L, Kotin RM, Davidson BL (2004) RNAi suppresses polyglutamine-induced neurodegeneration in a model of spinocerebellar ataxia. Nat Med 10:816-820.

Xie Y, Hayden MR, Xu B (2010) BDNF overexpression in the forebrain rescues Huntington's disease phenotypes in YAC128 mice. J Neurosci 30:14708-14718.

Yamada M, Hayashi S, Tsuji S, Takahashi H (2001) Involvement of the cerebral cortex and autonomic ganglia in Machado-Joseph disease. Acta Neuropathol 101:140-144.

Yamada M, Sato T, Tsuji S, Takahashi H (2008) CAG repeat disorder models and human neuropathology: similarities and differences. Acta Neuropathol 115:71-86.

Yamada M, Tsuji S, Takahashi H (2000) Pathology of CAG repeat diseases. Neuropathology 20:319-325.

Yamamoto Y, Hasegawa H, Tanaka K, Kakizuka A (2001) Isolation of neuronal cells with high processing activity for the Machado-Joseph disease protein. Cell Death Differ 8:871-873.

Yamanaka T, Miyazaki H, Oyama F, Kurosawa M, Washizu C, Doi H, Nukina N (2008) Mutant Huntingtin reduces HSP70 expression through the sequestration of NF-Y transcription factor. Embo J 27:827-839.

Yoshida H, Yoshizawa T, Shibasaki F, Shoji S, Kanazawa I (2002) Chemical chaperones reduce aggregate formation and cell death caused by the truncated Machado-Joseph disease gene product with an expanded polyglutamine stretch. Neurobiol Dis 10:88-99.

Young JE, Gouw L, Propp S, Sopher BL, Taylor J, Lin A, Hermel E, Logvinova A, Chen SF, Chen S, Bredesen DE, Truant R, Ptacek LJ, La Spada AR, Ellerby LM (2007)

Proteolytic cleavage of ataxin-7 by caspase-7 modulates cellular toxicity and transcriptional dysregulation. J Biol Chem 282:30150-30160.

Yu YC, Kuo CL, Cheng WL, Liu CS, Hsieh M (2009) Decreased antioxidant enzyme activity and increased mitochondrial DNA damage in cellular models of Machado-Joseph disease. J Neurosci Res 87:1884-1891.

Zala D, Bensadoun JC, Pereira de Almeida L, Leavitt BR, Gutekunst CA, Aebischer P, Hayden MR, Deglon N (2004) Long-term lentiviral-mediated expression of ciliary neurotrophic factor in the striatum of Huntington's disease transgenic mice. Exp Neurol 185:26-35.

Zhang X, Smith DL, Meriin AB, Engemann S, Russel DE, Roark M, Washington SL, Maxwell MM, Marsh JL, Thompson LM, Wanker EE, Young AB, Housman DE, Bates GP, Sherman MY, Kazantsev AG (2005) A potent small molecule inhibits polyglutamine aggregation in Huntington's disease neurons and suppresses neurodegeneration in vivo. Proc Natl Acad Sci U S A 102:892-897.

Zhang Y, Engelman J, Friedlander RM (2009) Allele-specific silencing of mutant Huntington's disease gene. J Neurochem 108:82-90.

Zoghbi HY, Orr HT (2000) Glutamine repeats and neurodegeneration. Annu Rev Neurosci 23:217-247.

Zoghbi HY, Orr HT (2009) Pathogenic mechanisms of a polyglutamine-mediated neurodegenerative disease, spinocerebellar ataxia type 1. J Biol Chem 284:7425-7429.

Zuccato C, Ciammola A, Rigamonti D, Leavitt BR, Goffredo D, Conti L, MacDonald ME, Friedlander RM, Silani V, Hayden MR, Timmusk T, Sipione S, Cattaneo E (2001) Loss of huntingtin-mediated BDNF gene transcription in Huntington's disease. Science 293:493-498.

7

Spinocerebellar Ataxia Type 12 (SCA 12): Clinical Features and Pathogenetic Mechanisms

Ronald A. Merrill, Andrew M. Slupe and Stefan Strack
University of Iowa Carver College of Medicine
USA

1. Introduction

Spinocerebellar Ataxia 12 (SCA12) is a rare disease that was first identified in a family in the United States. Patients suffered from classical spinocerebellar ataxia symptoms with an age of disease onset ranging from 8-55 years. A trinucleotide (CAG) repeat expansion was confirmed in all the affected individuals. The CAG expansion mapped to the 5′ untranslated region (UTR) of the PPP2R2B gene. This gene encodes a regulatory subunit, Bβ, of the heterotrimeric protein phosphatase 2A (PP2A). The function of this particular PP2A complex is not well understood, and the underlying molecular mechanism of SCA12 remains unclear. Additional pedigrees have been identified throughout the world but SCA12 remains a rare disease. In this chapter we will discuss the clinical manifestation of the disease and the known functions of the PP2A regulator Bβ.

2. Molecular genetics and Incidence

SCA12 is defined as an autosomal dominant cerebellar ataxia (ADCA) of otherwise unknown cause concurrent with a CAG repeat expansion within chromosome 5q31-33 upstream of the PPP2R2B gene (Holmes et. al., 1999). The PPP2R2B gene product, termed Bβ, is a neuron specific regulatory subunit of the heterotrimeric PP2A (Strack et. al., 1998). PP2A has been shown to play an essential role in many cellular functions (Janssens & Goris, 2001). The CAG repeat expansion associated with SCA12 was first identified through an unbiased repeat expansion detection study and found to occur within the noncoding region of the PPP2R2B gene (Holmes et. al., 1999). The nonpathalogical range of allele expansion is quite large (7-45 repeats) and is highly dependent on ethnic background (Fujigasaki et. al., 2001; Holmes et. al., 1999). The lower extreme of the range of pathological allele expansion has been established as 51 repeats. As is common to all ADCA disorders, inheritance of SCA12 follows an autosomal dominant pattern wherein a CAG repeat expansion of pathological length in just one allele is sufficient to induce the SCA12 disease state. Unlike other neurodegenerative diseases associated with a CAG repeat expansion, such as Huntingon disease, the number of CAG repeats associated with SCA12 does not correlate with the age of disease onset (Srivastava et. al., 2001). In addition, nondirectional vertical instability in the length of the expanded allele has been observed, however its clinical significance is unknown (Srivastava et. al., 2001). One individual has been identified with pathological repeat expansions in both alleles; however, due to the young age of this patient, it is unclear what effect homozygosity will have on the disease phenotype (Bahl et. al., 2005).

The world-wide incidence of SCA12 is quite low. Nonetheless, SCA12 has been identified across the globe in independent populations. The results of ADCA population screens that have examined the CAG repeat of the PPP2R2B gene are summarized below (Table 1), regardless of whether a SCA12 pathological CAG repeat expansion was identified. The well characterized SCA12 patient populations will hereafter be referred to as the American, Indian, Italian and Chinese cohorts when referencing the work by Holmes, et. al. (1999) and O'Hearn, et. al. (2001); Fujigaski, et. al. (2001), Srivastava, et. al. (2001) and Bahl, et. al. (2005); Brusco et al. (2002) and Brussino, et. al. (2010); and Jiang, et. al. (2005-1), Jiang, et. al. (2005-2) and Wang, J., et. al. (2011).

Study	County	Affected families (individuals)	Pathalogical $(CAG)_n$ repeat expansion (range)	Healthy Population $(CAG)_n$ repeat expansion (range)	Age range in years of disease onset (mean)
(Holmes, 1999) & (O'Hearn, 2001)	United States	1 (10)	66 - 78	7 - 28	8-55 (34)
(Fujigasaki, 2001)	Indian	1 (9)	55 - 61	9 - 45	39-41 (40)
(Srivastava, 2001)	Indian	5 (6)	55 - 69	7 - 31	26 - 50 (37.2)
(Bahl, 2005)	Indian	20 (81)	51 - 69	8 - 23	26 - 56 (40.2)
(Brussino, 2010)	Italian	2 (3)	57 - 58	NA	45-60 (52)
(Jiang, 2005 - 1)	Chinese	1 (NA)	NA	NA	NA
(Wang, J., 2011)	Chinese	1 (9)	51-52	NA	34
(Brusco, 2002)	Italian	0	NA	8 - 21	NA
(Jiang, 2005 - 2)	Chinese	0	NA	NA	NA
(Silveira, 2002)	Portugal and Brazil	0	NA	8 - 28	NA
(Tsai, 2004)	Taiwan	0	NA	7 - 25	NA
(van de Warrenburg, 2002)	Netherlands	0	NA	NA	NA
(Worth, 2001)	United Kingdom	0	NA	7 - 30	NA
(Cholfin, 2001)	United States	0	NA	9 - 22	NA

Table 1. Summary of SCA12 descriptions available in the primary literature.

3. Clinical features

At present, SCA12 confirmed by genetic testing remains a very rare illness. However, as genetic testing, including whole genome sequencing, becomes common practice, the true incidence of SCA12 may prove to be much higher among previously categorized ADCA patients of unknown cause. Indeed, among a cohort of ADCA patients in India the incidence of SCA12 has proven to be much higher than in other geographical locales (Bahl et. al., 2005; Srivastava et. al., 2001). Given this observation, those who encounter ADCA patients should be aware of SCA12 and develop an index of suspicion informed by careful history taking, detailed neurological examination and deliberate laboratory testing.

As SCA12 has only been recognized as a distinct pathology for the last decade and, at present, only a very few patients have been described in the primary literature, an appreciation for the natural history of the disease is still evolving. By careful consideration of those cases that have been well characterized in the American, Indian, Italian and Chinese cohorts, a clinical picture of the SCA12 patient will be developed here. The descriptions provided here are intended to inform the clinician who encounters ADCA patients of unknown cause and to guide clinical decision-making.

3.1 Patient reported history of illness

Early in the course of the disease the prototypical SCA12 patient will present with postural and action tremor of the upper limbs. Age of onset of this tremor is highly variable with a range between 8 and 55 years, but seems to cluster primarily between the third and fifth decade of life (Brussino et. al., 2010; Fujigasaki et. al., 2001; Holmes et. al., 1999; O'Hearn et. al., 2001; Srivastava et. al., 2001). The first manifestations of the action tremor of the upper limbs have been described by patients as difficulty with activities requiring fine motor coordination, such as writing, as well as difficulties with activities requiring gross motor coordination such as attempting to hold and purposefully manipulate objects like a cup (Fujigasaki et. al., 2001; O'Hearn et. al., 2001). Observers describe the tremor as slowly progressive in nature with an increase in amplitude and involvement of the head and neck have been observed over the course of a decade (O'Hearn et. al., 2001). The action tremor of the upper limbs as the harbinger of the disease is unique to SCA12 and differentiates SCA12 from other ADCA disorders (Schols et. al., 2004; Teive, 2009). This tremor is not, however, universal among SCA12 patients, and its absence does not rule out SCA12 (Srivastava et. al., 2001; Wang, J et. al., 2011). Presentation of the upper limb action tremor is very similar to that of essential tremor and has previously been misdiagnosed as such early in the SCA12 course (O'Hearn et. al., 2001). Differentiating the SCA12 associated upper limb action tremor from isolated essential tremor requires an appreciation of the complete constellation of SCA12 associated symptoms as well as a family history consistent with ADCA.

3.2 Neurological examination

The time elapsed since disease onset has been reported to directly correlate with the number of neurological abnormalities (O'Hearn et. al., 2001). The examination of an SCA12 patient should therefore be informed by the patient reported history. To fully characterize the constellation of symptoms associated with SAC12 early in the course of the disease, care should be taken to elicit mild neurological abnormalities that may otherwise be subclinical in nature. Characterizing the gross neurological deficits present late in the course of the disease can serve to chart disease progression.

3.2.1 Motor skills deficits

As indicated above, the action tremor associated with SCA12 is one of the earliest hallmarks of the disease. Action tremor features include postural and kinetic properties, as well as a low frequency (3 Hz)(O'Hearn et. al., 2001), and are similar to a tremor subset associated with cerebellar lesion termed "cerebellar postural tremor"(Hallett, 1991). As such, the postural features of the tremor can be elicited in the clinical setting by asking the patient to maintain their arms in an outstretched position and observing for limb tremor. The kinetic features of the tremor can be assessed by having the patient engage in a goal-directed movement of the upper limbs, such as finger-to-nose testing. Tremor should disappear completely while the upper limbs are at rest and not maintaining position against the force of gravity.

Loss of motor coordination due to cerebellar dysfunction associated with SCA12 manifests when the patient engages in a number of activities. During finger-to-nose testing, rather than smooth, rapid, accurate movements, the SCA12 patient will display slow, hesitant, inaccurate movements consistent with upper limb dysmetria. Further, the SCA12 patient has been reported to be unable to engage in rapid alternating movements (dysdiadochokinesia) such as alternating between turning the palms or the back of the hand face up (O'Hearn et. al., 2001). Motor deficits also disrupt speech and can result in dysarthria (O'Hearn et. al., 2001; Srivastava et. al., 2001).

Parkinsonain features have also been described in SCA12 patients from the American Cohort. These manifest as paucity of spontaneous movements, mild bradykinesia, upper limb rigidity and postural anteroflexion (O'Hearn et. al., 2001).

A great deal of heterogeneity has been observed in the symptoms of SCA12 patients from different ethnic backgrounds. Unique to the Indian cohort, facial myokymia has also been described in a small number of SCA12 patients (Srivastava et. al., 2001). Although the proband of the Chinese cohort developed generalized ataxia during the third decade of life, action tremor has not been observed (Wang, J et. al., 2011).

3.2.2 Gait abnormalities

The ataxic gait of the SCA12 patient has been described as being very similar to that observed in other diseases with cerebellar dysfunction. The SCA12 patient maintains stability by adopting a broad based stance. Parkinsonian features have also manifest in the gait among individuals of the American Cohort (O'Hearn et. al., 2001). Initiation of movement is delayed. Steps have been described as hesitant, small and slow. When turning, the SCA12 patient has been described as engaging in an "en bloc" approach. A mild ataxic phenotype can be exaggerated by having the patient maintain a tandem gait, wherein the patient walks in a straight line with the heel of the front foot touching the toes of the back foot at each step.

3.2.3 Cranial nerve assessment

With the exception of oculomotor nerve (CNIII) abnormalities, the cranial nerves are largely intact and function without deficit in the SCA12 patient. Horizontal nystagmus has been described and may represent an early manifestation of the disease (Fujigasaki et. al., 2001; Holmes et. al., 2003; O'Hearn et. al., 2001; Srivastava et. al., 2001). In addition slow saccades and broken pursuit have been described in SCA12 patients from the Indian cohort (Fujigasaki et. al., 2001; Srivastava et. al., 2001).

3.2.4 Assessment of reflexes

Diffuse hyperreflexia has been described for SCA12 patients from the American, Indian and Italian cohorts (Brussino et. al., 2010; Fujigasaki et. al., 2001; O'Hearn et. al., 2001; Srivastava et. al., 2001). A return of primitive reflexes in the otherwise mature SCA12 patient has also been described. These reflexes include an extensor plantar response (positive Babinski sign), grasp reflex, rooting reflex and glabellar blink reflex (Myerson sign).

3.2.5 Mental Status

Psychiatric disorders have been reported to occur concurrently with SCA12. Anxiety and depression have been reported in members of the American cohort, but not the Indian or Italian cohorts (Brussino et. al., 2010; O'Hearn et. al., 2001; Srivastava et. al., 2001). Whether these disorders result as a direct consequence of the SCA12 disease process or represent an individual response to the presence of the disease is unclear. Paranoid delusions have also been reported in one SCA12 patient (O'Hearn et. al., 2001). A decline in cognition has been described in SCA12 patients two to three decades after initial onset of the disease (Fujigasaki et. al., 2001; O'Hearn et. al., 2001).

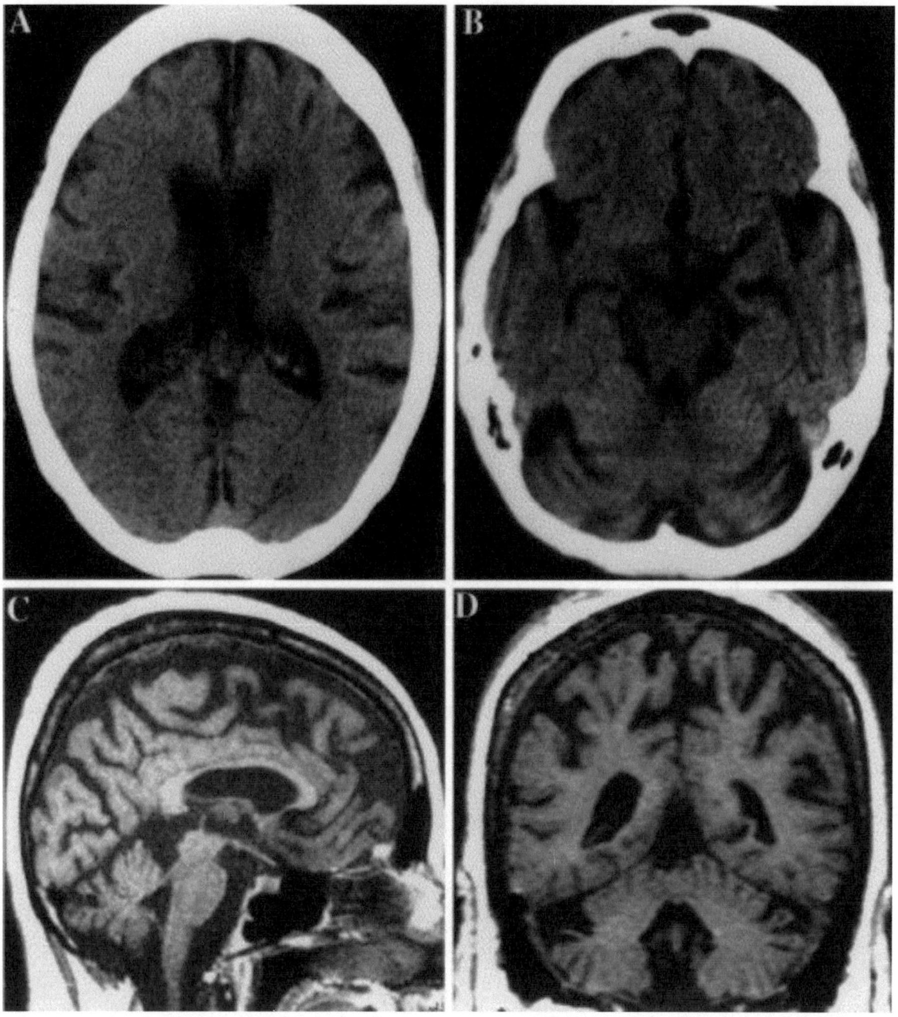

Fig. 1. Neuroradiologic images from two patients with spinocerebellar ataxia type 12. (A,B) Coronal computed tomography of the proband at age 62 years reveals cerebellar and diffuse cerebral cortical atrophy. (C) (sagittal), (D) (coronal): T-1 weighted magnetic resonance images of a 59-year-old affected woman also shows cerebellar and cortical atrophy. Reproduced from Holmes et. al. (2001), with permission from Elsevier Science.

3.3 Neuroimaging studies

Computerized tomography (CT) and magnetic resonance imaging (MRI) studies of symptomatic SCA12 patients reveal that mild to moderate cerebellar and cortical atrophy is a near universal finding of the disease (Brussino et. al., 2010; Fujigasaki et. al., 2001; O'Hearn et. al., 2001; Srivastava et. al., 2001; Wang, J et. al., 2011). An example of these findings from imaging studies performed on members of the American cohort of SCA12 patients is shown (Figure 1). The cerebellar vermis appears to be more vulnerable to atropy than the cerebellar hemispheres (O'Hearn et. al., 2001). Atrophy of subcortical structures has not been described. Additional characterization by single-proton emission computed tomography (SPECT) revealed metabolic deficiencies in atrophic cortical areas; however, the value of this test is uncertain in the symptomatic patient (Fujigasaki et. al., 2001). Proton magnetic resonance spectroscopy has been used to demonstrate neurometabolic and microstructural changes in the SCA12 patient (Brussino et. al., 2010), and this technique represents a noninvasive method that may longitudinally describe the asymptomatic SCA12 patient.

3.4 Genetic testing

Genetic testing for the presence of CAG repeat expansion is available. The reader is directed to the GeneTests Laboratory Directory available online (http://www.ncbi.nlm.nih.gov/sites/GeneTests/lab) for a list of available testing centers. The small sample size of affected individuals currently identified has left the question of penetrance of the disease open. Therefore, a great deal of care should be exercised when interpreting the results of a genetic test from an asymptomatic patient.

3.5 Medical management

Currently, management of SCA12 is limited to providing symptomatic relief for the action tremor. Treatment of the SCA12 action tremor is very similar to that provided for essential tremor. A reduction in tremor amplitude has been achieved with beta-blockers and barbiturates (O'Hearn et. al., 2001). When appropriate, pharmacological relief for symptoms associated with the disease such as depression and anxiety should be offered to the SCA12 patient.

4. PPP2R2B gene regulation and protein function

4.1 PP2A and B regulatory subunit

Protein phosphorylation is the most common posttranslational modification of proteins, and it plays a role in nearly every cellular function. The addition of phosphate is mediated through a large group (>500) of enzymes called kinases and requires ATP as a substrate. The reverse reaction is mediated by a smaller number of protein phosphatases in which, in most cases, specificity is provided through the formation of multimeric protein complexes. One of the most abundant protein phosphatase is PP2A, which is an essential, ubiquitously expressed phosphatase that targets phospho-serine and phospho-threonine. PP2A exists as a heterotrimer composed of one member of four diverse families of regulatory subunits (B), a scaffolding subunit (A) and a catalytic subunit (C) (Figure 2). Humans express 4 families of regulatory subunits termed B, B′, B′′, and B′′′, which determine both cellular localization and substrate specificity (Slupe et. al., 2011). The B family, also known B55, consists of 4 distinct genes (α, β, γ, δ) that encode proteins containing a highly conserved core WD40 domain, which has propeller like structure, with over 90% amino acid identity among the family members (Figure 2B). The Bβ regulatory subunit is encoded by the PPP2R2B gene, which has several splice-variants that are expressed exclusively in neuronal tissue.

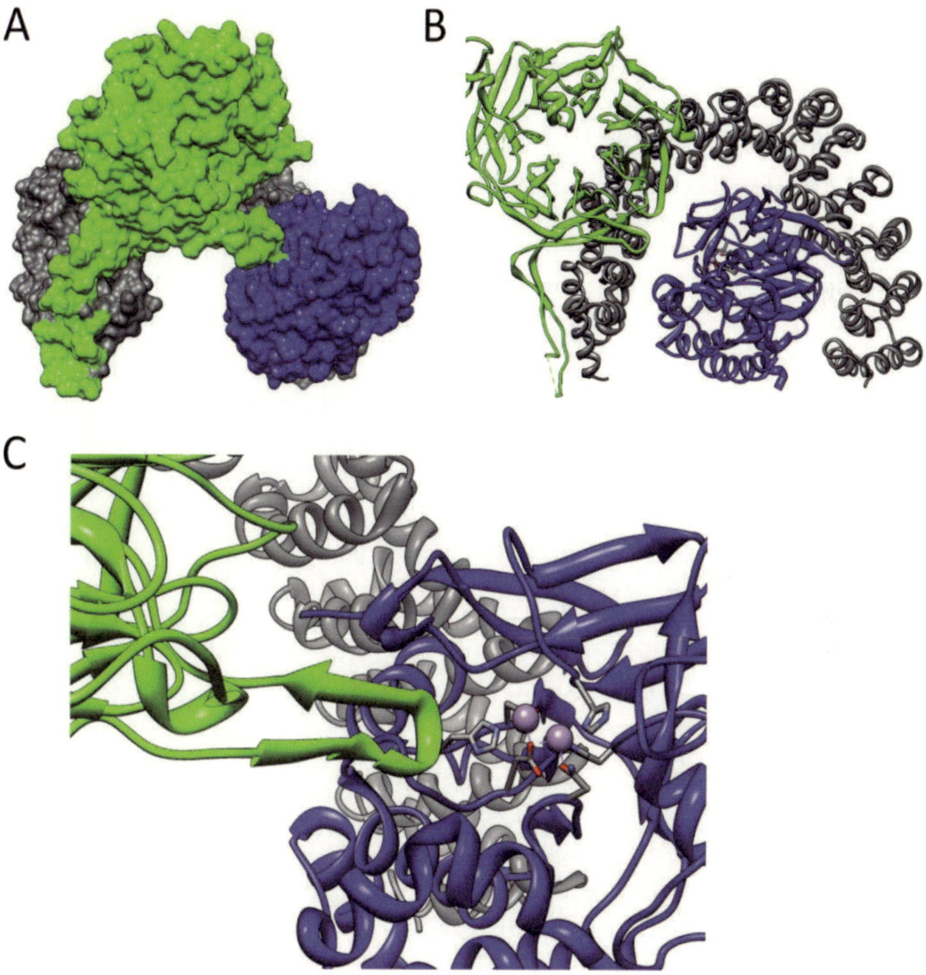

Fig. 2. Models of PP2A/Bα prepared from PDB 3DW8. The subunits of the heterotrimeric complex are color coded with the catalytic subunit (C) in blue, the scaffold subunit (A) in gray, and the regulatory subunit (B) in green. A, "top-down" view of the heterotrimer suface. B, "end-on" view of the heterotrimer ribbon diagram. C, Close of view of the PP2A active site highlighting infiltration of a regulatory subunit loop into the catalytic cleft.

4.2 Gene structure and expression

The exon arrangement of the PPP2R2B gene is highly conserved among mammals and spread over more than 500,000 base pairs (Dagda et. al., 2003; Schmidt et. al., 2002). Exon 1.1 and 1.2 are alternatively expressed first exons containing the ATG start site for the splice variants Bβ1 and Bβ2, respectively. These first exons, which contain the unique amino-termini, are spliced to common exons 2-9 that encode the WD40 domain found in all the B family of regulatory subunits (Figure 3) (Dagda et. al., 2003). At the mRNA level, Bβ1 and Bβ2 are expressed prominently in brain tissue, and Bβ1 can also be found in the testis (Dagda et. al., 2003). At the protein level, western blot analysis indicates that the Bβ1 is exclusively expressed in brain tissue and not in the testis, despite the high mRNA expression in that tissue. Closer analysis of specific brain regions has shown high levels of the Bβ1 protein throughout the brain (Strack et. al., 1998).

4.2.1 Transcriptional regulation

The CAG trinucleotide repeat expansion associated with the SCA12 disease is situated just upstream of the transcriptional start site of the Bβ1 specific exon 1.1. A recent study identified the apparent transcriptional regulators for basal expression of the Bβ1 promoter and the effect of the CAG repeat on basal expression (Lin et. al., 2010). Luciferase assays using deletions of the Bβ1 promoter and chromatin immunoprecipitation assays reveal that

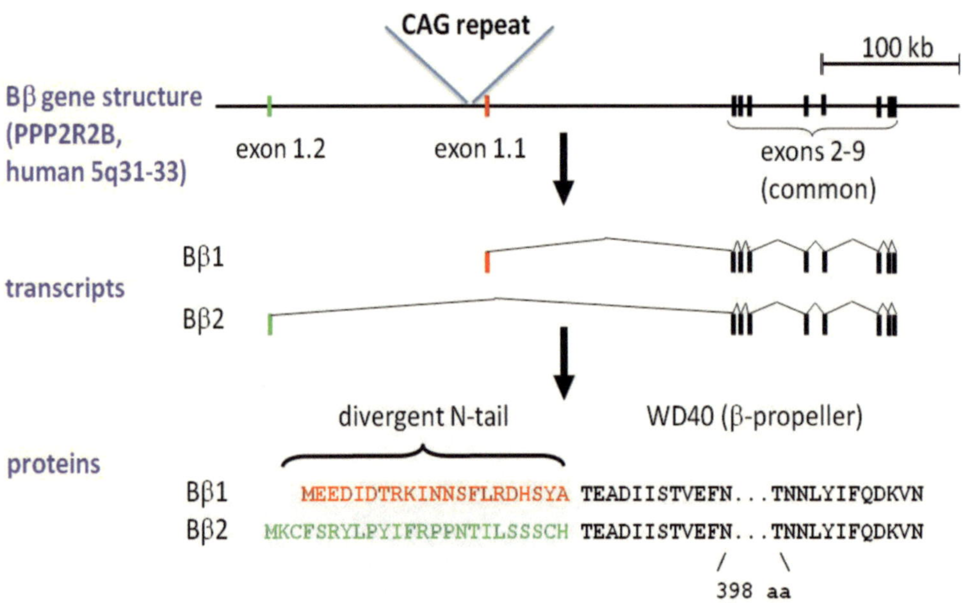

Fig. 3. Schematic representation of PPP2R2B gene structure, splice variant transcripts and proteins. The gene structure shows the CAG repeat expansion location, the Bβ1 (exon 1.1; red) and Bβ2 N-terminal coding sequences (exon 1.2; green). Transcripts and proteins indicate the Bβ1 (red) and Bβ2 (green) splice variant specific transcripts and encoded proteins. Modified from Dagda et. al. (2003).

CREB1, SP1 and TRAP4 bind to and regulate the Bβ1 promoter. Higher luciferase activity is seen in neuronal cell lines and correlates well with the known Bβ1 neuronal expression. Interestingly, increasing the size of the CAG repeat in the Bβ1 promoter increased the promoter activity two-fold. The increased activity is specific to the expansion of the CAG and not a result of changing the spacing of promoter since no change is seen in an AT expansion control (Lin et. al., 2010). A normal length CAG repeat does appear to be important for basal promoter activity since decreasing the number of CAG repeats reduced the promoter activity (Chen et. al., 2009). Independent studies conducted in Japan and Taiwan found that patients suffering from Alzheimer's disease had an increased likelihood of having a reduced number of CAG trinucleotide repeats compared to healthy control subjects (Chen et. al., 2009; Kimura et. al., 2011). Overall, these studies have identified important aspects of the PPP2R2B transcriptional regulation and help to discriminate between the role of the CAG repeat in providing basal transcriptional activation and the pathological effects of increasing or decreasing the trinucleotide repeat number.

A recently identified Japanese autosomal dominant cerebellar ataxia raises more uncertainty about the role of PPP2R2B gene in SCA12. The disease locus for this new ataxia included the PPP2R2B gene but contained no CAG expansion (Sato et. al., 2010). Additionally, all exons and intron/exon borders were sequenced for the entire PPP2R2B gene, including the both first exons (1.1 and 1.2), and no mutations were discovered. Several neuronally expressed genes are within the identified locus and may contain the genetic insult resulting in the ataxia (Sato et al 2010). This does raise the possibility that some of the effects of the CAG expansion in the PPP2R2B gene may be mediated through dysregulation of other nearby genes and not just changes in Bβ gene expression.

4.2.2 PPP2R2B regulation and cancer

Another important form of regulation of Bβ1 occurs in colorectal cancer (CRC) wherein developed cell lines show a decrease or complete absence of Bβ1 expression (Tan et. al., 2010). Furthermore, gene array comparisons of matched patient-derived mucosa controls and CRC tumors indicate a significant decrease in Bβ1 expression in 90% of the tumors. The loss of Bβ1 expression is mediated through hypermethylation of a CpG island that occurs in the Bβ1 promoter. Aberrant methylation of the PPP2R2B gene also appears to be important in breast cancer, as seen in recent reports (Dejeux et. al., 2010; Muggerud et. al., 2010). Finally, an intronic SNP of the PPP2R2B gene, with unknown functional consequence, is correlated with improved prognosis in a breast cancer cohort (Vazquez et. al., 2011). These studies clearly indicate that regulation of the PPP2R2B gene is important in multiple cancers and may provide additional insight into the function of the PPP2R2B gene.

4.3 Protein function

The Bβ1 and Bβ2 splice variants encode proteins that share a common WD40 repeat domain that mediates the recruitment of the A and C subunits of PP2A to make a functional trimeric protein phosphatase. The Bβ1 and Bβ2 proteins differ only in the first 21 and 24 amino acids, respectively, but this leads to a dramatic difference in the protein distribution within the cell.

4.3.1 Bβ1 protein function

Bβ1 has a cytoplasmic distribution and overexpression in cultured primary neurons does not change the morphology, survival or sensitivity to toxic treatments (Figure 4) (Dagda et. al., 2008). Overexpression of Bβ1 in a neuroblastoma cell line does result in increased autophagy (Cheng et. al., 2009). In CRC the loss of Bβ1 following methylation of the CpG island leads to aberrant phosphorylation of several proteins, including the oncogene c-myc. Reexpression of Bβ1 in a colorectal cell line decreases xenograft growth (Tan et. al., 2010). This represents the first described pathway regulated specifically by a Bβ1 containing PP2A trimer. Since some of the proteins regulated by Bβ1 in CRC are also expressed in neuronal tissues, it may be of interest to examine whether the Bβ1-mediated changes in phosphorylation also play a role in SCA12.

4.3.2 Bβ2 protein function

The Bβ2 N-terminus encodes a mitochondrial targeting sequence that results in recruitment of the trimeric PP2A enzyme to the outer mitochondrial membrane (OMM) (Dagda et. al., 2003). In primary hippocampal neurons, PP2A-mediated phosphatase activity at the OMM, through recruitment by Bβ2, results in mitochondrial fragmentation and increased basal death and sensitivity to neurotoxic insults (Figure 4) (Dagda et. al., 2005; Dagda et. al., 2008). Expression of Bβ2 mutants, that either do not target to the OMM or cannot recruit the A and C subunits, prevents the mitochondrial fragmentation and increased neuronal death (Figure 4) (Dagda et. al., 2008). Epitasis experiments indicate that the PP2A/Bβ2-mediated mitochondrial fragmentation precedes and is obligatory to the increased neuronal cell death (Dagda et. al., 2008). An additional study, utilizing neuroblastoma cells, confirmed the increased sensitivity of cells expressing Bβ2 but implicated an increase in autophagy as the culprit in the increased cell death (Cheng et. al., 2009).

Mitochondrial dysfunction is a hallmark of several neurodegenerative diseases, including Alzheimer disease. It can therefore be postulated that the CAG trinucleotide repeat expansion, which is known to increase Bβ1 promoter activity, amplifies both Bβ1 and Bβ2 expression. The Bβ2 upregulation may lead to increased mitochondrial fragmentation and increasing mitochondrial dysfunction in SCA12. Indeed, several other ataxias involve mitochondrial dysfunction. In patients suffering from SCA7, both liver and skeletal muscle biopsies show abnormal mitochondria (Han et. al., 2010). Heterozygous knockout mice for AFG3L2, a mitochondrial-targeted AAA-protease, develop abnormal mitochondria with decreased function and are a model of SCA28 (Maltecca et. al., 2009). Finally, in clinical trials pharmacological treatments with idebenone, an antioxidant thought to counteract mitochondrial dysfunction, have shown some promise in treatment of the genetic neurological disorder Friedreich ataxia (Marmolino, 2011). These examples highlight some of the ataxias associated with mitochondrial dysfunction and exemplify why mitochondrial dysfunction could be an important aspect of SCA12.

4.4 Animal models of SCA12

While characterization of the PPP2R2B gene products has suggested possible pathogenic mechanisms, animal models of SCA12 are urgently needed to test the predictions of the in

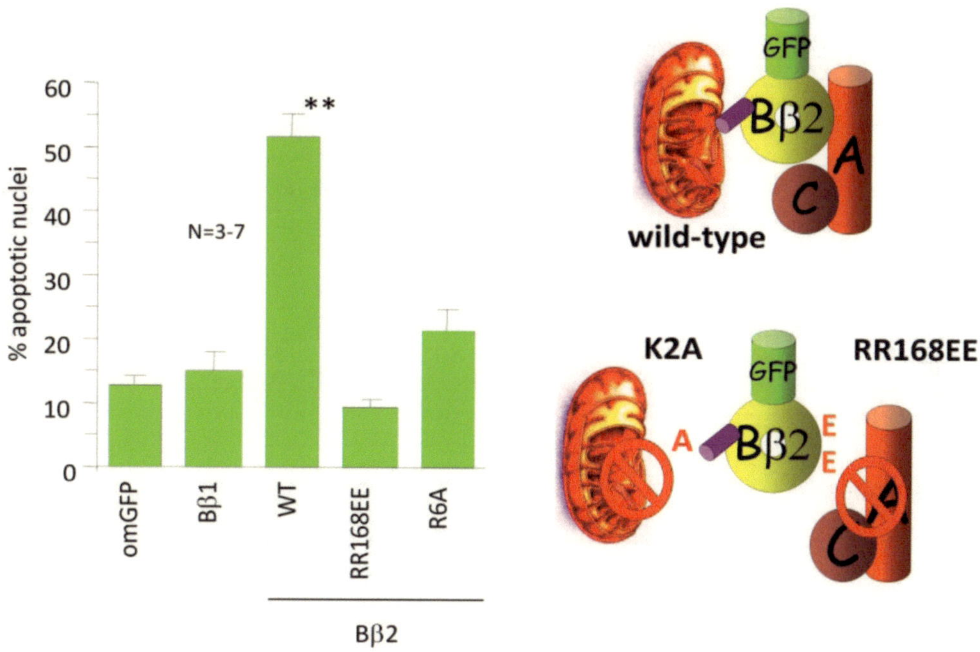

Fig. 4. Mitochondrial targeting of PP2A/Bβ2 is neurotoxic. Hippocampal neurons were transfected with the indicated GFP fusion proteins (om, outer mitochondrial; WT, wild-type) and scored for apoptotic nuclei. Bβ2 mutants that block mitochondrial localization (R6A) or AC dimer recruitment (RR168EE) also block apoptosis induction. Modified from Dagda et. al. (2008).

vitro studies discussed above. A recently developed fly model of SCA12 does display some neuropathies that may be homologous to the human disease (Wang, YC et. al., 2011). In this model, Drosophila overexpresses the human Bβ2 or tws, the fly homolog of Bβ, which results in a dramatic increase in neuronal apoptosis and, for the highest level of tws, a decrease in fly life span. Overexpression of tws results in mitochondrial fragmentation and dysfunction, observed as an increase in reactive oxygen species (ROS) production. Expression of superoxide dismutase 2 or antioxidants treatments reduces ROS production and attenuates the effects of tws overexpression. How the neuropathies and their reversal by pharmacological treatments seen in the fly SCA12 model relate to the human disease remains to be seen.

5. Conclusion

The CAG trinucleotide repeat expansion that occurs in the PPP2R2B gene is now well established as the cause of the autosomal dominant SCA12. This is a rare disease that shows a classical ataxia phenotype. The CAG repeat occurs in the promoter of a neuronally expressed protein, Bβ1, and expansion of the CAG results in increased Bβ1 promoter activity. Aberrant expression of Bβ1 also correlates with several cancers. Expression of another neuronal splice variant of PPP2R2B, Bβ2, increases neuronal death, but its role in SCA12 remains unknown. Despite the identified PPP2R2B gene functions, the underlying molecular basis of the SCA12 disease is not known. Animal models are needed to address the complexity of SCA12 and develop potential therapeutic treatments. The fly model of SCA12 does show mitochondrial dysfunction and recapitulates some neuron specific cell death (Wang, YC et. al., 2011); however, the development of a mammalian model system will likely be required to understand the molecular basis of SCA12 pathogenesis.

6. Acknowledgment

The authors would like to thank Drs. Nicole Worden and Melissa Bose for critically evaluating this manuscript.

7. References

Bahl S, Virdi K, Mittal U, Sachdeva MP, Kalla AK, Holmes SE, O'Hearn E, Margolis RL, Jain S, Srivastava AK& Mukerji M. (2005). Evidence of a common founder for SCA12 in the Indian population. *Annals of Human Genetics*. Vol. 69, No. Pt 5, (September 2005),pp.528-534, ISSN 0003-4800

Brusco A, Cagnoli C, Franco A, Dragone E, Nardacchione A, Grosso E, Mortara P, Mutani R, Migone N& Orsi L. (2002). Analysis of SCA8 and SCA12 loci in 134 Italian ataxic patients negative for SCA1-3, 6 and 7 CAG expansions. *Journal of Neurology*. Vol. 249, No. 7, (Jul 2002), pp.923-929, ISSN 0340-5354

Brussino A, Graziano C, Giobbe D, Ferrone M, Dragone E, Arduino C, Lodi R, Tonon C, Gabellini A, Rinaldi R, Miccoli S, Grosso E, Bellati MC, Orsi L, Migone N& Brusco A. (2010). Spinocerebellar ataxia type 12 identified in two Italian families may mimic sporadic ataxia. *Movement Disorders*. Vol. 25, No. 9, (July 2010),pp.1269-1273, ISSN 1531-8257

Chen CM, Hou YT, Liu JY, Wu YR, Lin CH, Fung HC, Hsu WC, Hsu Y, Lee SH, Hsieh-Li HM, Su MT, Chen ST, Lane HY& Lee-Chen GJ. (2009). PPP2R2B CAG repeat length in the Han Chinese in Taiwan: Association analyses in neurological and psychiatric disorders and potential functional implications. *American Journal of Medical Genetics Part B, Neuropsychiatric genetics*. Vol. 150B, No. 1, (January 2009),pp.124-129, ISSN 1552-485X

Cheng WT, Guo ZX, Lin CA, Lin MY, Tung LC& Fang K. (2009). Oxidative stress promotes autophagic cell death in human neuroblastoma cells with ectopic transfer of mitochondrial PPP2R2B (Bbeta2). *BMC Cell Biology*. Vol. 10, pp.91, ISSN 1471-2121

Cholfin JA, Sobrido MJ, Perlman S, Pulst SM& Geschwind DH. (2001). The SCA12 mutation as a rare cause of spinocerebellar ataxia. *Archives of Neurology*. Vol. 58, No. 11, (Nov 2001), pp.1833-1835, ISSN 0003-9942

Dagda RK, Zaucha JA, Wadzinski BE& Strack S. (2003). A developmentally regulated, neuron-specific splice variant of the variable subunit Bbeta targets protein phosphatase 2A to mitochondria and modulates apoptosis. *Journal of Biological Chemistry*. Vol. 278, No. 27, (July 2003), pp.24976-24985, ISSN 0021-9258

Dagda RK, Barwacz CA, Cribbs JT& Strack S. (2005). Unfolding-resistant translocase targeting: a novel mechanism for outer mitochondrial membrane localization exemplified by the Bbeta2 regulatory subunit of protein phosphatase 2A. *Journal of Biological Chemistry*. Vol. 280, No. 29, (July 2005), pp.27375-27382, ISSN 0021-9258

Dagda RK, Merrill RA, Cribbs JT, Chen Y, Hell JW, Usachev YM& Strack S. (2008). The spinocerebellar ataxia 12 gene product and protein phosphatase 2A regulatory subunit Bbeta2 antagonizes neuronal survival by promoting mitochondrial fission. *Journal of Biological Chemistry*. Vol. 283, No. 52, (December 2008), pp.36241-36248, ISSN 0021-9258

Dejeux E, Ronneberg JA, Solvang H, Bukholm I, Geisler S, Aas T, Gut IG, Borresen-Dale AL, Lonning PE, Kristensen VN& Tost J. (2010). DNA methylation profiling in doxorubicin treated primary locally advanced breast tumours identifies novel genes associated with survival and treatment response. *Molecular Cancer*. Vol. 9, (March 2010), pp.68, ISSN 1476-4598

Fujigasaki H, Verma IC, Camuzat A, Margolis RL, Zander C, Lebre AS, Jamot L, Saxena R, Anand I, Holmes SE, Ross CA, Durr A& Brice A. (2001). SCA12 is a rare locus for autosomal dominant cerebellar ataxia: a study of an Indian family. *Annals of Neurology*. Vol. 49, No. 1, (January 2001), pp.117-121, ISSN 0364-5134

Hallett M. (1991). Classification and treatment of tremor. *Journal of the American Medical Association*. Vol. 266, No. 8, (August 1991), pp.1115-1117, ISSN 0098-7484

Han Y, Deng B, Liu M, Jiang J, Wu S& Guan Y. (2010). Clinical and genetic study of a Chinese family with spinocerebellar ataxia type 7. *Neurology India*. Vol. 58, No. 4, (July-August 2010), pp.622-626, ISSN 0028-3886

Holmes SE, O'Hearn E& Margolis RL. (2003). Why is SCA12 different from other SCAs? *Cytogenetic and Genome Research*. Vol. 100, No. 1-4, pp.189-197, ISSN 1424-859X

Holmes SE, O'Hearn EE, McInnis MG, Gorelick-Feldman DA, Kleiderlein JJ, Callahan C, Kwak NG, Ingersoll-Ashworth RG, Sherr M, Sumner AJ, Sharp AH, Ananth U, Seltzer WK, Boss MA, Vieria-Saecker AM, Epplen JT, Riess O, Ross CA& Margolis RL. (1999). Expansion of a novel CAG trinucleotide repeat in the 5' region of PPP2R2B is associated with SCA12. *Nature Genetics*. Vol. 23, No. 4, (December

Janssens V& Goris J. (2001). Protein phosphatase 2A: a highly regulated family of serine/threonine phosphatases implicated in cell growth and signalling.

Biochemical Journal. Vol. 353, No. Pt 3, (February 2001), pp.417-439, ISSN 0264-6021

Jiang H, Tang B, Xia K, Zhou Y, Xu B, Zhao G, Li H, Shen L, Pan Q& Cai F. (2005-1). Spinocerebellar ataxia type 6 in Mainland China: molecular and clinical features in four families. *Journal of the Neurological Sciences*. Vol. 236, No. 1-2, (September 2005), pp.25-29, ISSN 0022-510X

Jiang H, Tang BS, Xu B, Zhao GH, Shen L, Tang JG, Li QH& Xia K. (2005-2). Frequency analysis of autosomal dominant spinocerebellar ataxias in mainland Chinese patients and clinical and molecular characterization of spinocerebellar ataxia type 6. *Chinese Medical Journal*. Vol. 118, No. 10, (May 2005), pp.837-843, ISSN 0366-6999

Kimura R, Morihara T, Kudo T, Kamino K& Takeda M. (2011). Association between CAG repeat length in the PPP2R2B gene and Alzheimer disease in the Japanese population. *Neuroscience Letters*. Vol. 487, No. 3, (January 2011), pp.354-357, ISSN 1872-7972

Lin CH, Chen CM, Hou YT, Wu YR, Hsieh-Li HM, Su MT& Lee-Chen GJ. (2010). The CAG repeat in SCA12 functions as a cis element to up-regulate PPP2R2B expression. *Human Genetics*. Vol. 128, No. 2, (August 2010), pp.205-212, ISSN 1432-1203

Maltecca F, Magnoni R, Cerri F, Cox GA, Quattrini A& Casari G. (2009). Haploinsufficiency of AFG3L2, the gene responsible for spinocerebellar ataxia type 28, causes mitochondria-mediated Purkinje cell dark degeneration. *The Journal of Neuroscience*. Vol. 29, No. 29, (July 2009), pp.9244-9254, ISSN 1529-2401

Marmolino D. (2011). Friedreich's ataxia: past, present and future. *Brain Research Reviews*. Vol. 67, No. 1-2, (June 2011), pp.311-330, ISSN 1872-6321

Muggerud AA, Ronneberg JA, Warnberg F, Botling J, Busato F, Jovanovic J, Solvang H, Bukholm I, Borresen-Dale AL, Kristensen VN, Sorlie T& Tost J. (2010). Frequent aberrant DNA methylation of ABCB1, FOXC1, PPP2R2B and PTEN in ductal carcinoma in situ and early invasive breast cancer. *Breast Cancer Research*. Vol. 12, No. 1, (January 2010), pp.R3, ISSN 1465-542X

O'Hearn E, Holmes SE, Calvert PC, Ross CA& Margolis RL. (2001). SCA-12: Tremor with cerebellar and cortical atrophy is associated with a CAG repeat expansion. *Neurology*. Vol. 56, No. 3, (February 2001),pp.299-303

Sato K, Yabe I, Fukuda Y, Soma H, Nakahara Y, Tsuji S& Sasaki H. (2010). Mapping of autosomal dominant cerebellar ataxia without the pathogenic PPP2R2B mutation to the locus for spinocerebellar ataxia 12. *Archives of Neurology*. Vol. 67, No. 10, (October 2010), pp.1257-1262, ISSN 1538-3687

Schmidt K, Kins S, Schild A, Nitsch RM, Hemmings BA& Gotz J. (2002). Diversity, developmental regulation and distribution of murine PR55/B subunits of protein phosphatase 2A. *The European Journal of Neuroscience*. Vol. 16, No. 11, (December 2002), pp.2039-2048, ISSN 0953-816X

Schols L, Bauer P, Schmidt T, Schulte T& Riess O. (2004). Autosomal dominant cerebellar ataxias: clinical features, genetics, and pathogenesis. *Lancet Neurology*. Vol. 3, No. 5, (May 2004), pp.291-304, ISSN 1474-4422

Silveira I, Miranda C, Guimaraes L, Moreira MC, Alonso I, Mendonca P, Ferro A, Pinto-Basto J, Coelho J, Ferreirinha F, Poirier J, Parreira E, Vale J, Januario C, Barbot C, Tuna A, Barros J, Koide R, Tsuji S, Holmes SE, Margolis RL, Jardim L, Pandolfo M, Coutinho P& Sequeiros J. (2002). Trinucleotide repeats in 202 families with ataxia: a small expanded (CAG)n allele at the SCA17 locus. *Archives of Neurology*. Vol. 59, No. 4, (Apr 2002), pp.623-629, ISSN 0003-9942

Slupe AM, Merrill RA& Strack S. (2011). Determinants for Substrate Specificity of Protein Phosphatase 2A. *Enzyme Research*. Vol. 2011, pp.398751, ISSN 2090-0414

Srivastava AK, Choudhry S, Gopinath MS, Roy S, Tripathi M, Brahmachari SK& Jain S. (2001). Molecular and clinical correlation in five Indian families with spinocerebellar ataxia 12. *Annals of Neurology*. Vol. 50, No. 6, (December 2001), pp.796-800, ISSN 0364-5134

Strack S, Zaucha JA, Ebner FF, Colbran RJ& Wadzinski BE. (1998). Brain protein phosphatase 2A: developmental regulation and distinct cellular and subcellular localization by B subunits. *The Journal of Comparative Neurology*. Vol. 392, No. 4, (March 1998), pp.515-527, ISSN 0021-9967

Tan J, Lee PL, Li Z, Jiang X, Lim YC, Hooi SC & Yu Q. (2010) B55□-Associated PP2A Complex Controls PDK1-Directed Myc Signaling and Modulates Rapamycin Sensitivity in Colorectal Cancer. *Cancer Cell*. Vol. 18, (November 2010), pp.459-471, ISSN 0028-0836

Teive HA. (2009). Spinocerebellar ataxias. *Arquivos de Neuropsiquiatria*. Vol. 67, No. 4, (December 2009), pp.1133-1142, ISSN 1678-4227

Tsai HF, Liu CS, Leu TM, Wen FC, Lin SJ, Liu CC, Yang DK, Li C& Hsieh M. (2004). Analysis of trinucleotide repeats in different SCA loci in spinocerebellar ataxia patients and in normal population of Taiwan. *Acta Neurologica Scandinavica*. Vol. 109, No. 5, 2004), pp.355-360, ISSN 1600-0404.

Vazquez A, Kulkarni D, Grochola LF, Bond GL, Barnard N, Toppmeyer D, Levine AJ& Hirshfield KM. (2011). A genetic variant in a PP2A regulatory subunit encoded by the PPP2R2B gene associates with altered breast cancer risk and recurrence. *International Journal of Cancer*. Vol. 128, No. 10, (May 2011), pp.2335-2343, ISSN 1097-0215

van de Warrenburg BPC, Sinke RJ, Verschuuren,ÄìBemelmans CC, Scheffer H, Brunt ER, Ippel PF, Maat-Kievit JA, Dooijes D, Notermans NC, Lindhout D, Knoers NVAM& Kremer HPH. (2002). Spinocerebellar ataxias in the Netherlands. *Neurology*. Vol. 58, No. 5, (March 12, 2002), pp.702-708

Wang J, Shen L, Lei L, Xu Q, Zhou J, Liu Y, Guan W, Pan Q, Xia K, Tang B& Jiang H. (2011). Spinocerebellar ataxias in mainland China: an updated genetic analysis among a large cohort of familial and sporadic cases. *Zhong Nan Da Xue Xue Bao Yi Xue Ban*. Vol. 36, No. 6, (June 2011), pp.482-489, ISSN 1672-7347

Wang YC, Lee CM, Lee LC, Tung LC, Hsieh-Li HM, Lee-Chen GJ& Su MT. (2011). Mitochondrial Dysfunction and Oxidative Stress Contribute to the Pathogenesis of Spinocerebellar Ataxia Type 12 (SCA12). *Journal of Biological Chemistry*. Vol. 286, No. 24, (June 2011), pp.21742-21754, ISSN 1083-351X

Worth PF & Wood NW. (2001). Spinocerebellar ataxia type 12 is rare in the United Kingdom. *Neurology*. Vol. 56, No. 3, (Feb 13 2001),pp.419-420, ISSN 0028-3878

8

Autosomal Recessive Spastic Ataxia of Charlevoix-Saguenay (ARSACS): Clinical, Radiological and Epidemiological Aspects

Haruo Shimazaki[1] and Yoshihisa Takiyama[2]
[1]*Division of Neurology, Department of Internal Medicine, Jichi Medical University, Tochigi*
[2]*Department of Neurology, Interdisciplinary Graduate School of Medicine and Engineering, University of Yamanashi, Chuo-City, Yamanashi, Japan*

1. Introduction

Autosomal recessive spastic ataxia of Charlevoix-Saguenay (ARSACS) (OMIM #270550) was originally found among inhabitants of the Charlevoix-Saguenay region of Quebec (Bouchard et al., 1978). ARSACS patients in Quebec show uniform phenotypes characterized by early-onset spastic ataxia, peripheral neuropathy, retinal hypermyelination, hand or foot deformities, and normal mentality. In 2000, the *SACS* gene, which is responsible for ARSACS, was identified in Quebec patients (Engert et al., 2000). Since then, ARSACS has been reported worldwide, especially in the Mediterranean area (El Euch-Fayache et al., 2003; Criscuolo et al., 2004; Grieco et al., 2004; Richter et al., 2004) and Japan (Ogawa et al., 2004; Takiyama, 2006). More *SACS* gene mutations were also identified in other areas (Takiyama, 2007; Ouyang et al., 2008; Vermeer et al., 2008; Gerwig et al., 2010). Meanwhile, ARSACS in non-Quebec patients, especially in Japanese ones, showed marked clinical heterogeneity, i.e., there were patients without spasticity (Shimazaki et al., 2005; Hara et al., 2007; Shimazaki et al., 2007), without retinal hypermyelination (Hara et al., 2007), and with decreased mentality (Shimazaki et al., 2005; Yamamoto et al., 2005; Shimazaki et al., 2007; Hara et al., 2005). The clinical spectrum of the sacsinpathies will expand with the identification of more SACS gene mutations (Gomez, 2004).

We herein review the epidemiology, genetics, clinical phenotypes, radiological and pathological findings in ARSACS cases carrying mutations of the *SACS* gene.

2. Epidemiology

2.1 Quebec

ARSACS is the most common of all inherited spastic ataxias, 320 affected patients having been identified in Quebec (Bouchard et al., 1998). In Quebec, most of the patients' families originate from the Charlevoix and Saguenay-Lac-St. Jean (SLSJ) regions. These regions have a population of about 300,000 inhabitants today that share a limited number of French ancestors who settled first in the Charlevoix region back in the seventeenth and early eighteenth centuries. ARSACS affects 1/1519 individuals in Charlevoix and 1/1952 in the Saguenay-Lac-St. Jean region, where the carrier frequency was estimated to be 1/22 for the 1941-1985 period (De Braekeleer et al., 1993).

2.2 Non-Quebec

SACS gene identification has enabled us to find ARSACS patients worldwide outside Quebec: Tunisia (El Euch-Fayache et al., 2003) in 2003, Italy (Criscuolo et al., 2004; Grieco et al., 2004)in 2004, Japan (Ogawa et al., 2004) in 2004, and Turkey (Richter et al., 2004) in 2004. More cases were then reported in Spain (Criscuolo et al., 2005), France (Anheim et al., 2008), Belgium (Ouyang et al., 2008), the Netherlands (Vermeer et al., 2008), Germany (Gerwig et al., 2010), Maritime Canada (Guernsey et al., 2010), and Morocco and eastern Europe (Baets et al., 2010). In eastern France, ARSACS was identified in two index patients among 102 autosomal recessive cerebellar ataxia (ARCA) ones (Anheim et al., 2008), meanwhile among 43 Dutch ARCA patients, 16 with mutations in the *SACS* gene were identified (Vermeer et al., 2008). In Japan, 17 Japanese ARSACS families have been discovered on SACS gene analysis so far (Ogawa et al., 2004; Hara et al., 2005; Shimazaki et al., 2005; Yamamoto et al., 2005; Ouyang et al., 2006; Yamamoto et al., 2006; Okawa et al., 2006; Hara et al., 2007; Takado et al., 2007; Shimazaki et al., 2007; Kamada et al., 2008; Tsugawa et al., 2009; Haga et al., 2011; Miyatake et al., 2011; Komure et al., 2006). ARSACS might be the second most frequent ARCA next to ataxia with oculomotor apraxia 1 (AOA1) in Japan. Figure 1 shows the geographical distribution and numbers of ARSACS families with *SACS* gene mutations in Japan. We could not find apparent regional accumulation of ARSACS families in Japan. Table 1 lists the previously identified SACS gene mutations that we could confirm in the 17 Japanese ARSACS families. The mutations were unique ones for each family except for one missense mutation (W3248R) found in two unrelated families.

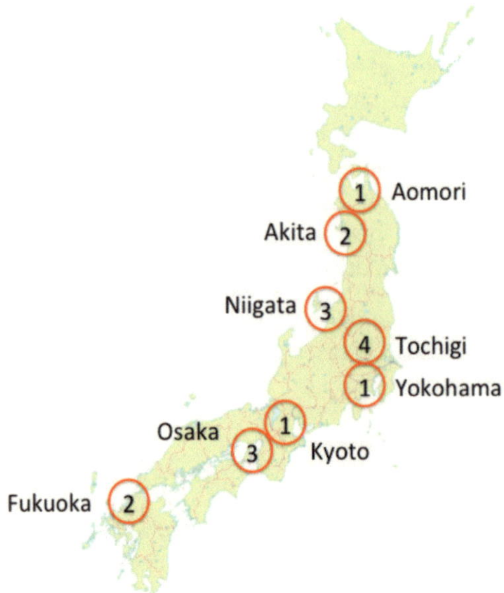
1 Aomori
Akita 2
Niigata 3
4 Tochigi
1 Yokohama
Osaka
1
3
Kyoto
Fukuoka 2

Fig. 1. Regional distribution of ARSACS families in Japan.

ARSACS families show a nationwide distribution in Japan. The numbers in circles are the numbers of families identified in the regions.

Amino acid substitutions	Exon	family	references
W3248R	10	2	Ogawa, 2004, Takiyama, 2006
K2931fsX2952	10	1	Hara, 2005
F1054S	10	1	Shimazaki, 2005
G1734fsX1736	10	1	Yamamoto, 2005
S2058fsX2076	10		
V1231del	10	1	Komure, 2006
P3559L	10		
Q1345X	10	1	Okawa, 2006
R4325X	10	1	Yamamoto, 2006
C395fsX407	8	1	Ouyang, 2006
D687fsX713	8		
R2119X	10	1	Hara, 2007
L308F	8	1	Takado, 2007
D1996fsX1999	10	1	Shimazaki, 2007
N161fsX175	7	1	Kamada, 2008
L802P	10		
G1257X	10	1	Tsugawa, 2009
R3788fsX3820	10		
Y138X	6	1	Haga, 2011
K1755fsX1775	10		
R3636X	10	1	(unpublished)
S4007F	10	1	Miyatake, 2011

Table 1. Previously identified *SACS* gene mutations in Japanese patients.

3. Genetics

3.1 Gene structure and pathological mutations

The *SACS* gene was originally reported to consist of a single gigantic exon spanning 12,794bp encoding an 11,487bp open reading frame (ORF), which represents the largest exon and the largest ORF within an exon found in any vertebrate (Engert et al., 2000). Recently, eight new exons located upstream of the gigantic one were found (Ouyang et al., 2006). More recently, one more upstream non-coding exon was found (Genbank NG_012342, 13-

MAR-2011). The *SACS* gene comprises ten exons with a 13,737 bp ORF encoding 4579 amino acids (Figure 2A).

The *SACS* gene is predicted to encode a 520-kDa multidomain protein, sacsin. The region near the C-terminus exhibits sequence similarity to the J-domain (DnaJ motif) of heat shock protein (HSP) 40 proteins (Parfitt et al., 2009), and the higher eukaryote and prokaryote nucleotide-binding (HEPN) domain (Grynberg, Erlandsen, and Godzik, 2003) (Figure 2B). A ubiquitin-like domain was identified at the N-terminus of sacsin (Parfitt et al., 2009)(Figure 2B). A sacsin repeating region (SRR) is present in triplicate at the N-terminus of sacsin (Anderson, Siller, and Barral, 2010). A xeroderma pigmentosum complementation group C-binding (XPCB) domain (Kamionka and Feigon, 2004) upstream of the DnaJ domain is also predicted.

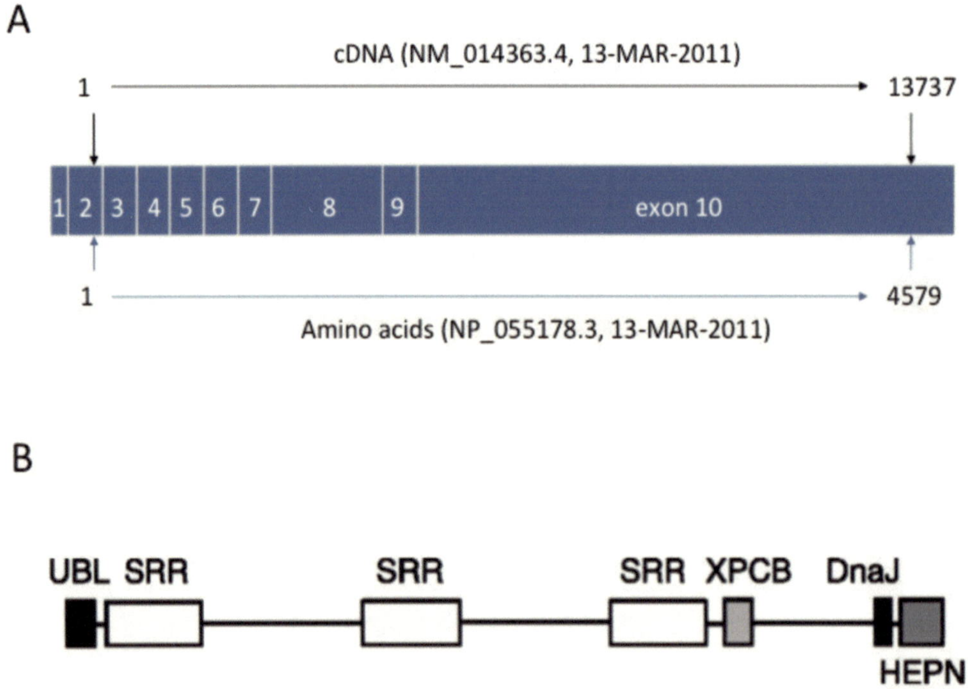

Fig. 2. Primary structure of the *SACS* gene (A) and domain organization of the sacsin protein (B). UBL: ubiquitin-like domain; SRR: sacsin repeating region; XPCB: XPC-binding domain; DnaJ: DnaJ motif (adopted from (Kozlov et al., 2011)).

Seventy-four mutations have been reported as pathological ones in the *SACS* gene (Baets et al., 2010). After publication of that report, we verified the table and found seven additional mutations in exons 6 and 10 of the *SACS* gene in Japanese patients (Table 1) (Komure et al., 2006; Tsugawa et al., 2009; Haga et al., 2011; Miyatake et al., 2011). As far as we know, at least 81 mutations have been found worldwide to date. Most of the mutations are predicted to generate truncated sacsin proteins, and are located in the largest exon, 10. Seventeen mutations were found in exons 4, 6, 7, 8 and 9. On copy number variation (CNV) analysis, an intragenic *SACS* deletion of exons 3-5 was identified (Baets et al., 2010). Two types of large deletions of the whole *SACS* gene and adjacent genes have been reported (Breckpot et al., 2008; Terracciano et al., 2009; McMillan et al., 2009).

3.2 Normal sacsin function

Sacsin is highly expressed in neurons, especially in cerebral corticospinal neurons and cerebellar Purkinje cells (Parfitt et al., 2009). The subcellular localization of sacsin in a cultured neuroblastoma-derived cell line was predominantly cytoplasmic and overlapped with that of mitochondrial protein heat shock protein (HSP) 60 (Parfitt et al., 2009). Because sacsin contains a functional J-domain (DnaJ motif), it has been proposed to act as a co-chaperone of the HSP70 chaperone system (Parfitt et al., 2009). The N-terminal segment of sacsin containing the ubiquitin-like (UbL) domain and the first sacsin repeating region (SRR) exhibits molecular chaperone activity and ATP-hydrolyzing activity (Anderson, Siller, and Barral, 2010, 2011). The UbL domain can interact with the 20 S proteasomal subunit (Parfitt et al., 2009). The HSP70 chaperone machinery is an important component of the cellular response to aggregation prone mutant proteins, and the UbL domain protein is a part of the quality control machinery that regulates protein aggregation. Overall, the main function of sacsin, like other molecular chaperones, is probably to prevent protein misfolding and aggregation. Sacsin prevents polyglutamine-expanded ataxin-1 toxicity (Parfitt et al., 2009). The XPCB domain interacts with ataxin-3, which is involved in spinocerebellar ataxia type 3 (Kamionka and Feigon, 2004). HEPN may stabilize nucleotide binding in complexes formed with the DnaJ domain (Grynberg, Erlandsen, and Godzik, 2003). Recently, the structure and function of the HEPN domain were determined, it being shown that it dimerizes and has a high affinity binding site for GTP, but it does not have GTPase activity (Kozlov et al., 2011).

3.3 Pathogenesis of ARSACS

Although the molecular mechanism underlying ARSACS remains unclear, the autosomal recessive transmission and truncating nature of most *SACS* mutations suggest the loss of sacsin function might cause development of this disease. Several functional alterations of sacsin proteins have been reported. An aspartate to tyrosine mutation (D168Y), located in the first SSR domain, abrogates its ATP-hydrolyzing activity (Anderson, Siller, and Barral, 2010). An asparagine to aspartate mutation (N4549D) in the HEPN domain of the sacsin protein disrupts dimerization and correct protein folding (Kozlov et al., 2011). Premature termination of other mutations and loss of the HEPN domain might lead to ARSACS disease.

4. Clinical phenotypes

4.1 Original Quebec phenotype

ARSACS is clinically characterized by early-onset spastic ataxia, axonal and demyelinating neuropathy, and hypermyelination of retinal nerve fibers (Bouchard et al., 1978; Bouchard, 1991). Unsteadiness of gait is usually the initial symptom. None of the patients ever walk normally, but walking is not delayed in most cases (rarely beyond 18 months of age) (Bouchard et al., 1978; Bouchard, 1991). The disease progression becomes most obvious in the late teens or early twenties, and the mean age for patients becoming wheelchair-bound is 41 years in Quebec patients (Bouchard, 1991). Concerning Quebec patients, ataxia, dysarthria, nystagmus, Babinski sign, hyperreflexia, spasticity, and retinal striations are noted in all of them. Distal amyotrophy of the feet is present in all patients after 20 years old (Bouchard, 1991), and pes cavus is noted in most Quebec patients. With these clinical features, ARSACS is clinically homogeneous in Quebec patients. Bouchard described progressive signs and early non-progressive ones of ARSACS in a review of this disease (Bouchard, 1991). The progressive signs are mostly spastic ataxia of the four limbs, slurred and dysrhythmic speech, discrete to severe distal amyotrophy, and absent ankle jerks after 25 years of age. The early non-progressive signs are increased deep tendon reflexes, a bilateral abnormal plantar response, marked saccadic alteration of smooth pursuit, and prominent myelinated fibers radiating from the disc on the retina.

4.2 Non-Quebec atypical phenotypes

The mean ages at onset are 5.4 and 4.5 years old in Japanese and Tunisian patients, respectively (Takiyama, 2007), while the ages at onset range from one to 1.5 years old in Quebec ones (Bouchard, 1991). Thus, the age at onset in these non-Quebec patients seems to be later than that in Quebec patients. According to a recent report from Belgium, the disease onset was over 20 years in five patients and as late as 40 years in one patient (Baets et al., 2010).

Although ataxia is noted in all non-Quebec ARSACS patients, one report stated that the cerebellar features were very mild in two patients (Baets et al., 2010). Other core clinical features of ARSACS, i.e., dysarthria, nystagmus, distal amyotrophy, Babinski sign, hyperreflexia, and pes cavus, are noted in most non-Quebec patients, which are similar to in Quebec patients.

Non-Quebec patients, however, show some atypical features in comparison with Quebec ones. First, although spasticity is a core clinical feature of ARSACS, we found that two patients in a Japanese family with ARSACS lacked spasticity in the legs and showed areflexia or hyporeflexia (Shimazaki et al., 2005). In Quebec and Tunisian patients, spasticity becomes progressively worse during the disease course and is prevalent in older patients, and tendon reflexes remain preserved throughout the disease, except for ankle jerks (Bouchard et al., 1978; El Euch-Fayache et al., 2003). Since we did not observe the two above patients in their childhood, we were not able to determine whether or not their spasticity had decreased during the disease course or had been absent from the onset (Shimazaki et al., 2005). The cases without spasticity, this depended on the fact that the neuromuscular manifestations were severe enough to diminish muscle tone and masked spasticity, and the planter responses were extensor, demonstrating that pyramidal tract sign was present. Recently, however, we observed another ARSACS patient whose spasticity had disappeared, probably due to the progressive peripheral nerve degeneration in the disease course of 29 years (Shimazaki et al., 2007). Thus, we should recognize that there is a rare ARSACS phenotype without spasticity, and the SACS gene should be analyzed even in cases of early-onset cerebellar ataxia without spasticity. After that, several reports on spasticity-lacking ARSACS patients were published (Hara et al., 2007; Baets et al., 2010; Miyatake et al., 2011).

Second, intellectual impairment is sometimes found in non-Quebec patients. The verbal IQ was 58, 88, 100, and 66 (mean: 78.00) in the four Japanese patients we examined (Takiyama, 2006). Similarly, mental retardation and dementia have been found in Italy (Criscuolo et al., 2004), Japan (Hara et al., 2005), and Turkey (Richter et al., 2004). Meanwhile, the verbal IQ (mean: 92.67) of Quebec patients is considered to be within normal limits, and a number of ARSACS patients have completed the secondary and university levels of education (Bouchard, 1991). Thus, intellectual impairment seems to be variable in ARSACS. Since the mode of inheritance of ARSACS is autosomal recessive, genes other than *SACS* might influence the intellectual impairment.

Defects in conjugate pursuit ocular movements, decreased or absent vibration sense in the toes, hand deformities, and urinary or fecal incontinence are rather frequently noted in Quebec (Bouchard, 1991) and non-Quebec patients (El Euch-Fayache et al., 2003; Takiyama, 2006). Cardiovascular evaluation revealed mitral valve prolapse in a majority of Quebec patients examined (Bouchard, 1991).

Very recently, the disease initially presented with symptoms mainly orienting toward peripheral neuropathy in several patients, and there was one patient who did not exhibit any clinical or electrophysiologic signs of peripheral neuropathy (Baets et al., 2010).

4.3 Ophthalmologic findings

Although increased visibility of myelinated retinal nerve fibers is a hallmark of ARSACS in Quebec patients (Bouchard, 1991), there have been a considerable number of non-Quebec patients without this characteristic sign for ARSACS (El Euch-Fayache et al., 2003; Grieco et al., 2004; Criscuolo et al., 2004; Richter et al., 2004; Hara et al., 2005; Yamamoto et al., 2005; Ouyang et al., 2006; Okawa et al., 2006; Yamamoto et al., 2006; Hara et al., 2007; Baets et al., 2010). Thus, retinal hypermyelination is a variable feature in non-Quebec patients. It is, however, very useful for suspecting a diagnosis of ARSACS, especially in an unusual phenotype without spasticity (Shimazaki et al., 2005). In a case without retinal hypermyelination, ARSACS resembles conditions referred to as early onset cerebellar ataxia with retained tendon reflexes (EOCA) (Chio et al., 1993), Friedreich ataxia with retained reflexes (De Castro et al., 1999), and several clinical descriptions of hereditary spastic paraplegia such as SPG7 (Wilkinson et al., 2004), SPG21 (Simpson et al., 2003), SPG27 (Meijer et al., 2004), and SPG30 (Klebe et al., 2006).

Recently, Desserre et al. have reported that the retinal nerve fiber layer was thickened, as shown using optical coherence tomography (OCT), and that the retina did not show hypermyelinated areas on funduscopy (Desserre et al., 2011). Likewise, Vingolo et al. reported that four patients with ARSACS showed myelinated fibers on funduscopy, and also increased thickness of the retina on OCT, which is a finding not characteristic of persistent myelination of the retina (Vingolo et al., 2011). It is possible that persistent myelination of the retina, a general common finding, was present in those patients without bearing relation to the disease.

5. Neuroradiology

5.1 Brain MRI findings

Some reports have mentioned that characteristic MRI findings in ARSACS are superior cerebellar vermian atrophy and cervical spinal cord atrophy (Bouchard et al., 1998; Takiyama, 2007). Recently, MRI of five patients in Quebec revealed linear hypointensity in T2- and Fluid-Attenuated Inversion Recovery (FLAIR) images of the pons (Martin et al., 2007). Thereafter, the same findings have been reported in only one patient in each of the Netherlands (Van Damme et al., 2009), France (Anheim et al., 2010), and Italy (Terracciano et al., 2010).

We recruited six ARSACS patients with *SACS* mutations in four Japanese families. Brain MRI was performed in all six patients. Brain MRI in the six patients showed superior cerebellar vermian atrophy. In addition, not only pontine linear hypointensity but also middle cerebellar peduncle hypointensity was observed in T2-weighted and FLAIR images (Shimazaki et al., in press) (Table 2). These areas showed isointensity in T1-weighted images. Figure 3 shows representative brain MRI findings in patients 3 (A) and 2 (B). In patient 3, T2*-weighted images were obtained showing no abnormal findings in the pons and middle cerebellar peduncles (Figure 3, A-1).

We found the characteristic MRI findings in the six Japanese ARSACS patients, who all exhibited linear hypointensity in the pons, and a hypointense area in the middle cerebellar peduncles in T2-weighted and FLAIR images (Shimazaki et al., in press). A middle cerebellar peduncle hypointense area has not previously been reported in ARSACS patients, although pontine linear hypointensity was originally reported in five Quebec patients (Martin et al., 2007). Furthermore, as far as we know, hypointensity in these portions has not been described as a MRI finding in spinocerebellar ataxias and hereditary spastic paraplegias.

We thought these hypointense areas were close to the location of the pontocerebellar fibers. We could find low intensity in the middle cerebellar peduncle (MCP) because the pontocerebellar fiber runs from the middle pons to the cerebellum through the MCP. We can detect low MCP intensity in an Italian case (Terracciano et al., 2010). We think an abnormal MCP signal is not specific for Japanese patients.

The hypointensity in the pons and middle cerebellar peduncle might be specific findings for ARSACS cases even in non-Quebec ones with clinical heterogeneity (Shimazaki et al., 2012). Thus, pontine and middle cerebellar peduncle T2 hypointensity detectable on MRI should prompt us to perform *SACS* gene analysis even in such atypical early-onset cerebellar ataxia cases.

5.2 Spinal MRI findings

In Quebec cases, the cervical cord is small and flat (Bouchard, 1991). In our cases, upper cervical cord and medulla oblongata atrophy was not observed in three of the six patients for whom cervical MRI was performed (Shimazaki et al., 2012). Upper cervical atrophy is not a constant feature of ARSACS. In thirteen Belgium cases, cervical spinal cord atrophy was observed on MRI in only one case (Baets et al., 2010).

Case	1	2	3	4	5	6
Age at exam, gender	47, F	43, M	46, M	37, M	33, M	57, F
Age at onset	6	6	3	8	7	3
Cerebellar ataxia	++	+	++	+	++	++
Hyperreflexia	+	+	+	-	-	-
Leg spasticity	+	+	+	-	-	-
Babinski sign	+	+	+	+	+	+
Retinal myelinated fibers	+	+	+	+	+	+
Peripheral neuropathy	+	+	+	+	+	+
Mental impairment	NE	+(WAIS-R)	+(WAIS-R)	NE	+(WAIS-R)	+(MMSE)
Amino acid substitutions	W3248R	W3248R	W3248R	F1054S	F1054S	D1996fsX1999
Superior cerebellar vermian atrophy	+	+	+	+	+	+
Pontine linear hypointensity (T2)	+	+	+	+	+	+
MCP hypointensity (T2)	+	+	+	+	+	+
Medulla oblongata atrophy	-	-	+	+	+	-
Upper cervical cord atrophy	-	-	+	+	+	-
Superior cerebellar CBF decrease	+-	NE	+-	+	+	+

Table 2. Clinical, genetic and MRI findings in the ARSACS patients. NE: not examined; MCP: Middle cerebellar peduncle; CBF: cerebral blood flow in SPECT.

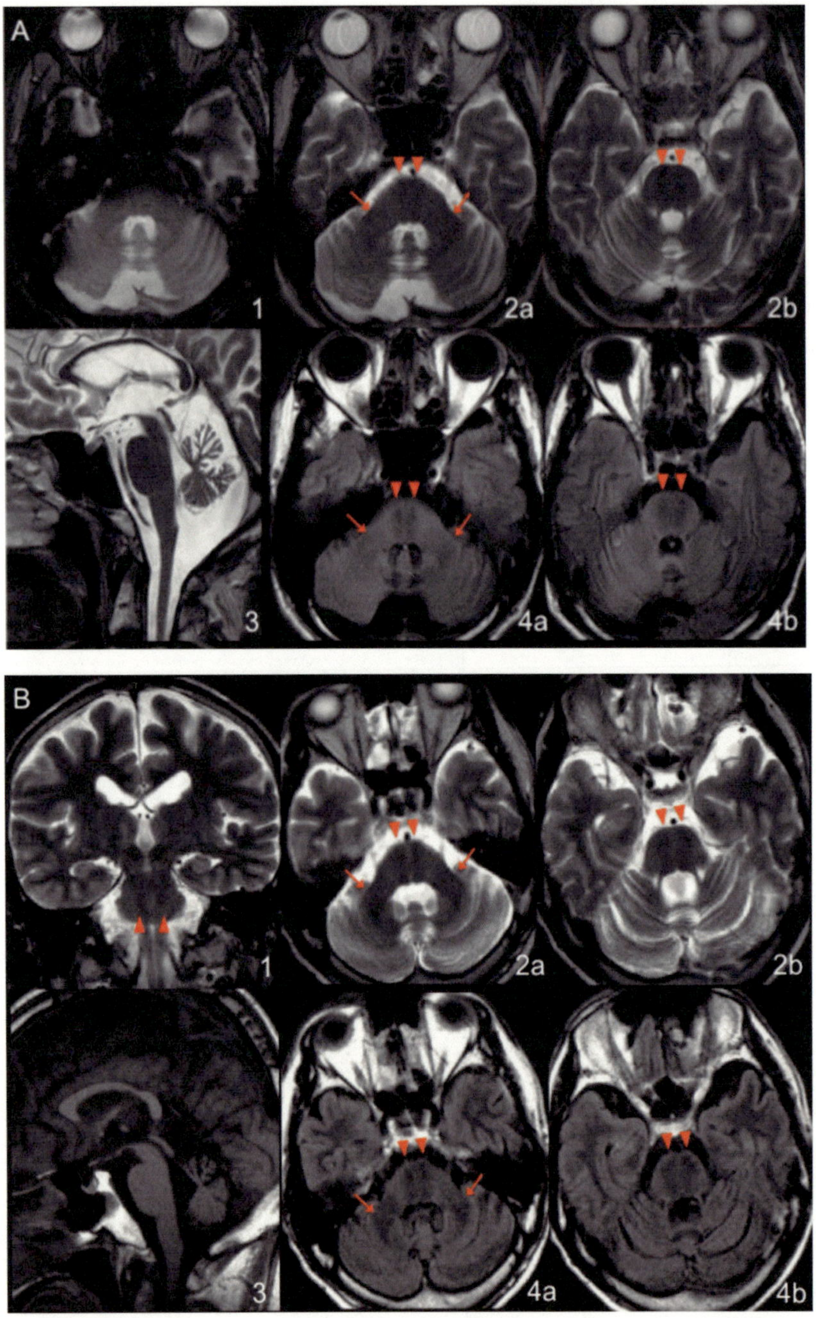

Fig. 3. Representative brain MRI findings in two ARSACS patients. T2-weighted and FLAIR images of patient 3 (A-2a, 2b, 4a, and 4b) and patient 2 (B-1, 2a, 2b, 4a, and 4b) showed hypointensity in the pons (arrowheads) and bilateral middle cerebellar peduncles (arrows). Sagittal sections (A-3 and B-3) revealed superior cerebellar vermian atrophy in all patients. A T2* image of patient 3 (A-1) disclosed no remarkable low intensity in the pontine tegmentum or cerebellar peduncles (Shimazaki et al., 2012).

5.3 SPECT findings

Single photon emission computed tomography (SPECT) of the brain with three-dimensional stereotactic surface projection (3D-SSP) analysis for five cases showed decreased blood flow in the upper cerebellar vermis in three cases (Shimazaki et al., 2007; Shimazaki, Nakano, and Takiyama, 2008) (Figure 4). Meanwhile, early onset cerebellar ataxia with retained tendon reflexes (EOCA) and Friedreich's ataxia often show a reduction in the parietotemporal cortex blood flow as well as cerebellar hypoperfusion (De Michele et al., 1998), this being a different feature from in ARSACS.

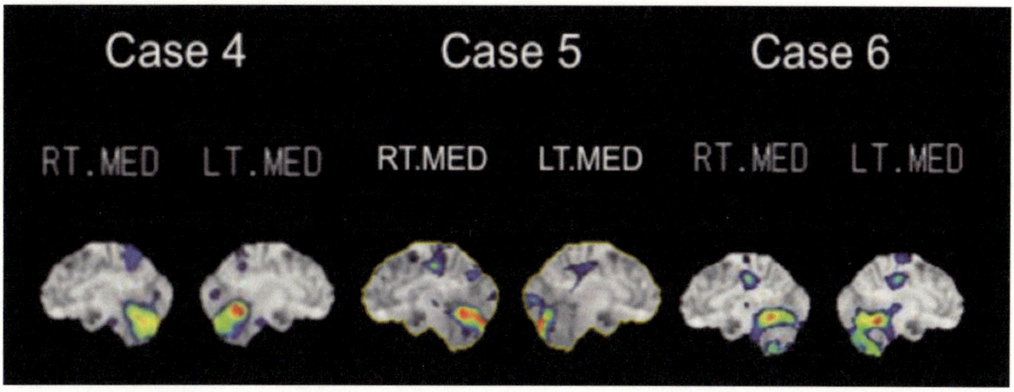

Fig. 4. ^{123}I-IMP SPECT with three-dimensional stereotactic surface projection (3D-SSP) analyses of cases 4, 5, and 6.

The results showed decreased blood flow in the superior cerebellar vermis and cerebellar hemisphere.

6. Neuropathology

6.1 Postmortem autopsy and comparison with the characteristic brain MRI findings

The pathological findings in ARSACS patients have only been reported in a 21-year-old man (Bouchard, 1991) and a 59-year-old man (Richter et al., 1996). The former report of a young man described no findings regarding pontocerebellar fibers, but mentioned a small corticospinal tract and normal pontine nuclei in the pons (Bouchard, 1991). A T2* image of patient 3 disclosed no remarkable low intensity in the pontine tegmentum or cerebellar peduncles. These findings suggest that T2 hypointensity in the pons and cerebellar peduncles is not reflected by iron deposition in these portions. However, a second autopsy on the 59-year-old man revealed the presence of swollen thalamic and cerebellar cortical neurons (Bouchard et al., 1998). Most of these neurons had dense, lipofuscin-like granules within their lysosomes, and the authors suggested that ARSACS may be a lysosomal storage disease (Richter et al., 1996). In neuronal ceroid lipofuscinosis, MRI can often reveal hypointensity of the thalamus and putamen in T2-weighted images, which may reflect the storage of lipofuscin and the increase in the viscosity in these neurons (Autti, Joensuu, and Aberg, 2007). Therefore, the linear hypointensity of the pons that was found among ARSACS patients can also be explained by possible storage of lipofuscin-like materials. Further pathological study is needed to disclose the origin of the T2 hypointensity.

6.2 Nerve and muscle biopsy

Sural nerve biopsy revealed severe axonal degeneration and loss of large myelinated fibers (Peyronnard, Charron, and Barbeau, 1979; Bouchard, 1991; El Euch-Fayache et al., 2003; Takiyama, 2006). These findings in Quebec and non-Quebec patients are consistent with an axonal neuropathy associated with demyelinating features.

Muscle biopsy disclosed typical and obvious neurogenic atrophy, i.e., grouped atrophy in the studied patients (Bouchard, 1991; El Euch-Fayache et al., 2003).

7. Neurophysiology

7.1 Peripheral nerve conduction studies

The peripheral nerve conduction study in Quebec patients revealed an axonal neuropathy with absent sensory action potentials and low motor conduction velocity (Peyronnard, Charron, and Barbeau, 1979; Bouchard, 1991). We have presented the peripheral nerve conduction data for cases 4 and 5 (Shimazaki et al., 2005). In each patient, the motor nerve conduction velocity was mildly reduced in the ulnar and median nerves, and moderately in the posterior tibial nerves. Each compound muscle action potential (CMAP) was markedly decreased. In case 5 (patient 1 of (Shimazaki et al., 2005)), a CMAP was not evoked in the common peroneal nerves. No sensory nerve action potential was evoked in any of the extremities. These data indicate not only a severe to moderate axonal neuropathy but dysmyelinating neuropathy complicated by secondary axonal degeneration as in Quebec and Tunisian patients (Peyronnard, Charron, and Barbeau, 1979; El Euch-Fayache et al., 2003).

7.2 Motor and sensory evoked potentials

Central pathway conduction studies including ones on somatosensory evoked potentials, brainstem auditory evoked potentials, and pattern reversal visual evoked potentials were performed in 67 Quebec patients (De Lean, Mathieu, and Bouchard, 1989). The findings that showed marked delays revealed widespread processes of demyelination in the primary sensory neurons as well as in the central nervous system (Bouchard, 1991). The central sensory and motor pathways were markedly impaired that could be attributed to myelinopathies, and there were high incidences of asymptomatic auditory and visual pathway involvement (Bouchard, 1991).

Electronystagmography showed horizontal gaze nystagmus in all Quebec patients with marked impairment of smooth ocular pursuit and optokinetic nystagmus, and defective fixation suppression of caloric nystagmus (Dionne et al., 1979). Recently, both the masseter and blink reflexes were found to be abnormal in two ARSACS patients (Garcia et al., 2008), whereas the masseter reflex was preserved but a bilateral delay of the late response of the blink reflex was observed in Friedreich' ataxia patients.

8. Therapy and management

Spasticity, the main feature of ARSACS during childhood, is rather mild in most patients. In the teens, however, the spasticity increases in the lower limbs and patients often present a spastic gait with evolving pes cavus (Bouchard et al., 2007). Physical therapy and use of oral medications such as baclofen to control spasticity in the early phase of the disease may prevent tendon shortening and joint contractures. When spasticity becomes significant, intrathecal baclofen may be considered. The most effective surgical procedures were triple arthrodesis with percutaneous lengthening of the Achilles tendon, and adductor and psoas tenotomies combined with neurectomy of the obturator nerve for perineal hygiene in a retrospective study of 26 patients who received surgical orthopaedic treatment (Bouchard and Langlois, 1999).

9. Acknowledgements

This work was supported by Grants-in Aid from the Research Committee for Ataxic Diseases (Y.T. and H.S.), the Ministry of Health, Labour and Welfare of Japan · This work was also supported by Grants-in-Aid from the Research Committee of CNS Degenerative Diseases (Y.T.), and the Ministry of Health, Labor and Welfare of Japan, and supported by a Grant-in-Aid for Scientific Research (C) (23591253 to H.S.) from The Ministry of Education, Culture, Sports, Science and Technology in Japan.

10. References

Anderson, J. F., E. Siller, and J. M. Barral. (2010). The sacsin repeating region (SRR): a novel Hsp90-related supra-domain associated with neuro-degeneration. *J Mol Biol*, Vol.400, No.4, (Jul 2010), pp. 665-674, ISSN 1089-8638

Anderson, J. F., E. Siller, and J. M. Barral. (2011). The Neurodegenerative- Disease-Related Protein Sacsin Is a Molecular Chaperone. *J Mol Biol*, (Jun 2011), [Epub ahead of print], ISSN 1089-8638

Anheim, M., D. Chaigne, M. Fleury, F. M. Santorelli, J. De Seze, A. Durr, A. Brice, M. Koenig, and C. Tranchant. (2008). [Autosomal recessive spastic ataxia of Charlevoix-Saguenay: study of a family and review of the literature]. *Rev Neurol (Paris)*, Vol.164, No.4, (Apr 2008), pp. 363-368, ISSN 0035-3787

Anheim, M., M. Fleury, B. Monga, V. Laugel, D. Chaigne, G. Rodier, E. Ginglinger, C. Boulay, S. Courtois, N. Drouot, M. Fritsch, J. P. Delaunoy, D. Stoppa-Lyonnet, C. Tranchant, and M. Koenig. (2010). Epidemiological, clinical, paraclinical and molecular study of a cohort of 102 patients affected with autosomal recessive progressive cerebellar ataxia from Alsace, Eastern France: implications for clinical management. *Neurogenetics*, Vol.11, No.1, (Feb 2010), pp. 1-12, ISSN 1364-6753

Autti, T., R. Joensuu, and L. Aberg. (2007). Decreased T2 signal in the thalami may be a sign of lysosomal storage disease. *Neuroradiology*, Vol.49, No.7, (Jul 2007), pp. 571-578, ISSN 0028-3940

Baets, J., T. Deconinck, K. Smets, D. Goossens, P. Van den Bergh, K. Dahan, E. Schmedding, P. Santens, V. M. Rasic, P. Van Damme, W. Robberecht, L. De Meirleir, B. Michielsens, J. Del-Favero, A. Jordanova, and P. De Jonghe. (2010). Mutations in SACS cause atypical and late-onset forms of ARSACS. *Neurology*, Vol.75, No.13, (Sep 2010), pp. 1181-1188, ISSN 0028-3878

Bouchard, J. P. (1991). Ressesive spastic ataxia of Charlevoix-Saguenay. In *Hereditary Neuropathies and Spinocerebellar Atrophies. Handbook of Clinical Neurology*, edited by J. M. B. V. de Jong, pp. 451-459, Elsevier , ISBN 0-444-81279-2 , Amsterdam.

Bouchard, J. P., A. Barbeau, R. Bouchard, and R. W. Bouchard. (1978). Autosomal recessive spastic ataxia of Charlevoix-Saguenay. *Can J Neurol Sci*, Vol.5, No.1, (Feb 1978), pp. 61-69, ISSN 0317-1671

Bouchard, J. P., B. Brais, N. Dupre, and G. A. Rouleau. (2007). Hereditary ataxias and spastic parapareses in northeastern Canada. In *Spinocerebellar Degenerations: The Ataxias and Spastic Paraplegias, Blue Books of Neurology*, edited by A. Brice and S. M. Pulst, pp. 222-243, Elsevier, ISBN 0-7506-7503-9, Amsterdam.

Bouchard, J. P., A. Richter, J. Mathieu, D. Brunet, T. J. Hudson, K. Morgan, and S. B. Melancon. (1998). Autosomal recessive spastic ataxia of Charlevoix-Saguenay. *Neuromuscul Disord*, Vol.8, No.7, (Oct 1998), pp. 474-479, ISSN 0960-8966

Bouchard, M., and G. Langlois. (1999). Orthopedic management in autosomal recessive spastic ataxia of Charlevoix-Saguenay. *Can J Surg*, Vol.42, No.6, (Dec 1999), pp. 440-444, ISSN 0008-428X

Breckpot, J., Y. Takiyama, B. Thienpont, S. Van Vooren, J. R. Vermeesch, E. Ortibus, and K. Devriendt. (2008). A novel genomic disorder: a deletion of the SACS gene leading to spastic ataxia of Charlevoix-Saguenay. *Eur J Hum Genet*, Vol.16, No.9, (Sep 2008), pp. 1050-1054, ISSN 1018-4813

Chio, A., L. Orsi, P. Mortara, and D. Schiffer. (1993). Early onset cerebellar ataxia with retained tendon reflexes: prevalence and gene frequency in an Italian population. *Clin Genet*, Vol.43, No.4, (Apr 1993), pp. 207-211, ISSN 0009-9163

Criscuolo, C., S. Banfi, M. Orio, P. Gasparini, A. Monticelli, V. Scarano, F. M. Santorelli, A. Perretti, L. Santoro, G. De Michele, and A. Filla. (2004). A novel mutation in SACS gene in a family from southern Italy. *Neurology*, Vol.62, No.1, (Jan 2004), pp. 100-102, ISSN 0028-3878

Criscuolo, C., F. Sacca, G. De Michele, P. Mancini, O. Combarros, J. Infante, A. Garcia, S. Banfi, A. Filla, and J. Berciano. (2005). Novel mutation of SACS gene in a Spanish family with autosomal recessive spastic ataxia. *Mov Disord*, Vol.20, No.10, (Oct 2005), pp. 1358-1361, ISSN 0885-3185

De Braekeleer, M., F. Giasson, J. Mathieu, M. Roy, J. P. Bouchard, and K. Morgan. (1993). Genetic epidemiology of autosomal recessive spastic ataxia of Charlevoix-Saguenay in northeastern Quebec. *Genet Epidemiol*, Vol.10, No.1, (1993), pp. 17-25, ISSN 0741-0395

De Castro, M., A. Cruz-Martinez, J. J. Vilchez, T. Sevilla, M. Pineda, J. Berciano, and F. Palau. (1999). Early onset cerebellar ataxia and preservation of tendon reflexes: clinical phenotypes associated with GAA trinucleotide repeat expanded and non-expanded genotypes. *J Peripher Nerv Syst*, Vol.4, No.1, (1999), pp. 58-62, ISSN 1085-9489

De Lean, J., J. Mathieu, and J. P. Bouchard. (1989). Central pathway conduction in recessive ataxia of Charlevoix-Saguenay. *Can J Neurol Sci*, Vol.16, (1989), pp. 272, ISSN 0317-1671

De Michele, G., P. P. Mainenti, A. Soricelli, F. Di Salle, E. Salvatore, M. R. Longobardi, A. Postiglione, M. Salvatore, and A. Filla. (1998). Cerebral blood flow in spinocerebellar degenerations: a single photon emission tomography study in 28 patients. *J Neurol*, Vol.245, No.9, (Sep 1998), pp. 603-608, ISSN 0340-5354

Desserre, J., D. Devos, B. G. Sautiere, P. Debruyne, F. M. Santorelli, I. Vuillaume, and S. Defoort-Dhellemmes. (2011). Thickening of Peripapillar Retinal Fibers for the

Diagnosis of Autosomal Recessive Spastic Ataxia of Charlevoix-Saguenay. *Cerebellum*, (May 2011), [Epub ahead of print], ISSN 1473-4230

Dionne, J., G. Wright, H. Barber, R. Bouchard, and J. P. Bouchard. (1979). Oculomotor and vestibular findings in autosomal recessive spastic ataxia of Charlevoix-Saguenay. *Can J Neurol Sci*, Vol.6, No.2, (May 1979), pp. 177-184, ISSN 0317-1671

El Euch-Fayache, G., I. Lalani, R. Amouri, I. Turki, K. Ouahchi, W. Y. Hung, S. Belal, T. Siddique, and F. Hentati. (2003). Phenotypic features and genetic findings in sacsin-related autosomal recessive ataxia in Tunisia. *Arch Neurol*, Vol.60, No.7, (Jul 2003), pp. 982-988, ISSN 0003-9942

Engert, J. C., P. Berube, J. Mercier, C. Dore, P. Lepage, B. Ge, J. P. Bouchard, J. Mathieu, S. B. Melancon, M. Schalling, E. S. Lander, K. Morgan, T. J. Hudson, and A. Richter. (2000). ARSACS, a spastic ataxia common in northeastern Quebec, is caused by mutations in a new gene encoding an 11.5-kb ORF. *Nat Genet*, Vol.24, No.2, (Feb 2000), pp. 120-125, ISSN 1061-4036

Garcia, A., C. Criscuolo, G. de Michele, and J. Berciano. (2008). Neurophysiological study in a Spanish family with recessive spastic ataxia of Charlevoix-Saguenay. *Muscle Nerve*, Vol.37, No.1, (Jan 2008), pp. 107-110, ISSN 0148-639X

Gerwig, M., S. Kruger, F. R. Kreuz, S. Kreis, E. R. Gizewski, and D. Timmann. (2010). Characteristic MRI and funduscopic findings help diagnose ARSACS outside Quebec. *Neurology*, Vol.75, No.23, (Dec 2010), p. 2133, ISSN 1526-632X

Gomez, C. M. (2004). ARSACS goes global. *Neurology*, Vol.62, No.1, (Jan 2004), pp. 10-11, ISSN 0028-3878

Grieco, G. S., A. Malandrini, G. Comanducci, V. Leuzzi, M. Valoppi, A. Tessa, S. Palmeri, L. Benedetti, A. Pierallini, S. Gambelli, A. Federico, F. Pierelli, E. Bertini, C. Casali, and F. M. Santorelli. (2004). Novel SACS mutations in autosomal recessive spastic ataxia of Charlevoix-Saguenay type. *Neurology*, Vol.62, No.1, (Jan 2004), pp. 103-106, ISSN 0028-3878

Grynberg, M., H. Erlandsen, and A. Godzik. (2003). HEPN: a common domain in bacterial drug resistance and human neurodegenerative proteins. *Trends Biochem Sci*, Vol.28, No.5, (May 2003), pp. 224-226, ISSN 0968-0004

Guernsey, D. L., M. P. Dube, H. Jiang, G. Asselin, S. Blowers, S. Evans, M. Ferguson, C. Macgillivray, M. Matsuoka, M. Nightingale, A. Rideout, M. Delatycki, A. Orr, M. Ludman, J. Dooley, C. Riddell, and M. E. Samuels. (2010). Novel mutations in the sacsin gene in ataxia patients from Maritime Canada. *J Neurol Sci*, Vol.288, No.1-2, (Jan 2010), pp. 79-87, ISSN 1878-5883

Haga, R., Y. Miki, Y. Funamizu, T. Kon, C. Suzuki, T. Ueno, H. Nishijima, A. Arai, M. Tomiyama, H. Shimazaki, Y. Takiyama, and M. Baba. (2011). Novel compound heterozygous mutations of the SACS gene in autosomal recessive spastic ataxia of Charlevoix-Saguenay. *Clin Neurol Neurosurg*, (Dec 30 2011), [Epub ahead of print] , ISSN 1872-6968

Hara, K., O. Onodera, M. Endo, H. Kondo, H. Shiota, K. Miki, N. Tanimoto, T. Kimura, and M. Nishizawa. (2005). Sacsin-related autosomal recessive ataxia without prominent retinal myelinated fibers in Japan. *Mov Disord*, Vol.20, No.3, (Mar 2005), pp. 380-382, ISSN 0885-3185

Hara, K., J. Shimbo, H. Nozaki, K. Kikugawa, O. Onodera, and M. Nishizawa. (2007). Sacsin-related ataxia with neither retinal hypermyelination nor spasticity. *Mov Disord*, Vol.22, No.9, (Jul 2007), pp. 1362-1363, ISSN 0885-3185

Kamada, S., S. Okawa, T. Imota, M. Sugawara, and I. Toyoshima. (2008). Autosomal recessive spastic ataxia of Charlevoix-Saguenay (ARSACS): novel compound heterozygous mutations in the SACS gene. *J Neurol*, Vol.255, No.6, (Jun 2008), pp. 803-806, ISSN 0340-5354

Kamionka, M., and J. Feigon. (2004). Structure of the XPC binding domain of hHR23A reveals hydrophobic patches for protein interaction. *Protein Sci*, Vol.13, No.9, (Sep 2004), pp. 2370-2377, ISSN 0961-8368

Klebe, S., H. Azzedine, A. Durr, P. Bastien, N. Bouslam, N. Elleuch, S. Forlani, C. Charon, M. Koenig, J. Melki, A. Brice, and G. Stevanin. (2006). Autosomal recessive spastic paraplegia (SPG30) with mild ataxia and sensory neuropathy maps to chromosome 2q37.3. *Brain*, Vol.129, No.Pt 6, (Jun 2006), pp. 1456-1462, ISSN 1460-2156

Komure, O., E. Murase, T. Saida, M. Nakamura, T. Sano, M. Sanada, and K. Ozawa. (2006). An ARSACS family with compound heterozygous SACS gene mutations. *Rinsho Shinkeigaku*, Vol.46, No.12, (Dec 2006), pp. 1018, ISSN 0009-918X

Kozlov, G., A. Y. Denisov, M. Girard, M. J. Dicaire, J. Hamlin, P. S. McPherson, B. Brais, and K. Gehring. (2011). Structural Basis of Defects in the Sacsin HEPN Domain Responsible for Autosomal Recessive Spastic Ataxia of Charlevoix-Saguenay (ARSACS). *J Biol Chem*, Vol.286, No.23, (Jun 2011), pp. 20407-20412, ISSN 1083-351X

Martin, M. H., J. P. Bouchard, M. Sylvain, O. St-Onge, and S. Truchon. (2007). Autosomal recessive spastic ataxia of Charlevoix-Saguenay: a report of MR imaging in 5 patients. *Am J Neuroradiol*, Vol.28, No.8, (Sep 2007), pp. 1606-1608, ISSN 0195-6108

McMillan, H. J., M. T. Carter, P. J. Jacob, E. E. Laffan, M. D. O'Connor, and K. M. Boycott. (2009). Homozygous contiguous gene deletion of 13q12 causing LGMD2C and ARSACS in the same patient. *Muscle Nerve*, Vol.39, No.3, (Mar 2009), pp. 396-399, ISSN 0148-639X

Meijer, I. A., P. Cossette, J. Roussel, M. Benard, S. Toupin, and G. A. Rouleau. (2004). A novel locus for pure recessive hereditary spastic paraplegia maps to 10q22.1-10q24.1. *Ann Neurol*, Vol.56, No.4, (Oct 2004), pp. 579-582, ISSN 0364-5134

Miyatake, S., H. Tanabe, K. Yatabe, M. Suzuki, K. Ogata, H. Doi, N. Miyake, M. Kawai, and N. Matsumoto. (2011). Identification of a novel homozygous SACS gene mutation in ARSACS. *Rinsho Shinkeigaku*, Vol.51, No.12, (Dec 2011), (in press), ISSN 0009-918X

Ogawa, T., Y. Takiyama, K. Sakoe, K. Mori, M. Namekawa, H. Shimazaki, I. Nakano, and M. Nishizawa. (2004). Identification of a SACS gene missense mutation in ARSACS. *Neurology*, Vol.62, No.1, (Jan 2004), pp. 107-109, ISSN 0028-3878

Okawa, S., M. Sugawara, S. Watanabe, T. Imota, and I. Toyoshima. (2006). A novel sacsin mutation in a Japanese woman showing clinical uniformity of autosomal recessive spastic ataxia of Charlevoix-Saguenay. *J Neurol Neurosurg Psychiatry*, Vol.77, No.2, (Feb 2006), pp. 280-282, ISSN 0022-3050

Ouyang, Y., K. Segers, O. Bouquiaux, F. C. Wang, N. Janin, C. Andris, H. Shimazaki, K. Sakoe, I. Nakano, and Y. Takiyama. (2008). Novel SACS mutation in a Belgian family with sacsin-related ataxia. *J Neurol Sci*, Vol.264, No.1-2, (Jan 2008), pp. 73-76, ISSN 0022-510X

Ouyang, Y., Y. Takiyama, K. Sakoe, H. Shimazaki, T. Ogawa, S. Nagano, Y. Yamamoto, and I. Nakano. (2006). Sacsin-related ataxia (ARSACS): expanding the genotype upstream from the gigantic exon. *Neurology*, Vol.66, No.7, (Apr 2006), pp. 1103-1104, ISSN 1526-632X

Parfitt, D. A., G. J. Michael, E. G. Vermeulen, N. V. Prodromou, T. R. Webb, J. M. Gallo, M. E. Cheetham, W. S. Nicoll, G. L. Blatch, and J. P. Chapple. (2009). The ataxia protein sacsin is a functional co-chaperone that protects against polyglutamine-expanded ataxin-1. *Hum Mol Genet*, Vol.18, No.9, (May 2009), pp. 1556-1565, ISSN 1460-2083

Peyronnard, J. M., L. Charron, and A. Barbeau. (1979). The neuropathy of Charlevoix-Saguenay ataxia: an electrophysiological and pathological study. *Can J Neurol Sci*, Vol.6, No.2, (May 1979), pp. 199-203, ISSN 0317-1671

Richter, A. M., R. K. Ozgul, V. C. Poisson, and H. Topaloglu. (2004). Private SACS mutations in autosomal recessive spastic ataxia of Charlevoix-Saguenay (ARSACS) families from Turkey. *Neurogenetics*, Vol.5, No.3, (Sep 2004), pp. 165-170, ISSN 1364-6745

Richter, A., K. Morgan, J. P. Bouchard, J. Mathieu, J. Lamarche, J. Rioux, et al. (1996). ARSACS: possibly a lysosomal storage disease? *Am J Hum Genet*, Vol.59, (1996), pp. A379, ISSN 0002-9297

Shimazaki, H., I. Nakano, and Y. Takiyama. (2008). Brain MRI and SPECT findings in ARSACS. *Rinsho Shinkeigaku*, Vol.48, No.12, (Dec 2008), p. 1208, ISSN 0009-918X

Shimazaki, H., K. Sakoe, K. Niijima, I. Nakano, and Y. Takiyama. (2007). An unusual case of a spasticity-lacking phenotype with a novel SACS mutation. *J Neurol Sci*, Vol.255, No.1-2, (Apr 2007), pp. 87-89, ISSN 0022-510X

Shimazaki, H., Y. Takiyama, J. Honda, K. Sakoe, M. Namekawa, J. Tsugawa, Y. Tsuboi, C. Suzuki, M. Baba, and I. Nakano. (2012). Middle Cerebellar Peduncles and Pontine T2 Hypo-intensities in ARSACS. *J Neuroimaging*, (Jan 23 2012), [Epub ahead of print], ISSN 1552-6569

Shimazaki, H., Y. Takiyama, K. Sakoe, Y. Ando, and I. Nakano. (2005). A phenotype without spasticity in sacsin-related ataxia. *Neurology*, Vol.64, No.12, (Jun 2005), pp. 2129-2131, ISSN 0028-3878

Simpson, M. A., H. Cross, C. Proukakis, A. Pryde, R. Hershberger, A. Chatonnet, M. A. Patton, and A. H. Crosby. (2003). Maspardin is mutated in mast syndrome, a complicated form of hereditary spastic paraplegia associated with dementia. *Am J Hum Genet*, Vol.73, No.5, (Nov 2003), pp. 1147-1156, ISSN 0002-9297

Takado, Y., K. Hara, T. Shimohata, S. Tokiguchi, O. Onodera, and M. Nishizawa. (2007). New mutation in the non-gigantic exon of SACS in Japanese siblings. *Mov Disord*, Vol.22, No.5, (Apr 2007), pp. 748-749, ISSN 0885-3185

Takiyama, Y. (2006). Autosomal recessive spastic ataxia of Charlevoix-Saguenay. *Neuropathology*, Vol.26, No.4, (Aug 2006), pp. 368-375, ISSN 0919-6544

Takiyama, Y. (2007). Sacsinopathies: sacsin-related ataxia. *Cerebellum*, Vol.6, No.4, (Feb 2007), pp. 353-359, ISSN 1473-4222

Terracciano, A., C. Casali, G. S. Grieco, D. Orteschi, S. Di Giandomenico, L. Seminara, R. Di Fabio, R. Carrozzo, A. Simonati, G. Stevanin, M. Zollino, and F. M. Santorelli. (2009). An inherited large-scale rearrangement in SACS associated with spastic ataxia and hearing loss. *Neurogenetics*, Vol.10, No.2, (Apr 2009), pp. 151-155, ISSN 1364-6753

Terracciano, A., N. C. Foulds, A. Ditchfield, D. J. Bunyan, J. A. Crolla, S. Huang, F. M. Santorelli, and S. R. Hammans. (2010). Pseudodominant inheritance of spastic ataxia of Charlevoix-Saguenay. *Neurology*, Vol.74, No.14, (Apr 2010), pp. 1152-1154, ISSN 1526-632X

Tsugawa, J., Y. Tsuboi, Y. Naitou, S. Ohma, H. Shimazaki, Y. Takiyama, and M. Yamada. (2009). Novel compound heterozygous mutations in a family with sacsin-related ataxia. *Mov Disord*, Vol.24, No.S1, (Jun 2009), p. S1, ISSN 1531-8257

Van Damme, P., P. Demaerel, W. Spileers, and W. Robberecht. (2009). Autosomal recessive spastic ataxia of Charlevoix-Saguenay. *Neurology*, Vol.72, No.20, (May 2009), p. 1790, ISSN 1526-632X

Vermeer, S., R. P. Meijer, B. J. Pijl, J. Timmermans, J. R. Cruysberg, M. M. Bos, H. J. Schelhaas, B. P. van de Warrenburg, N. V. Knoers, H. Scheffer, and B. Kremer. (2008). ARSACS in the Dutch population: a frequent cause of early-onset cerebellar ataxia. *Neurogenetics*, Vol.9, No.3, (Jul 2008), pp. 207-214, ISSN 1364-6745

Vingolo, E. M., R. Di Fabio, S. Salvatore, G. Grieco, E. Bertini, V. Leuzzi, C. Nesti, A. Filla, A. Tessa, F. Pierelli, F. M. Santorelli, and C. Casali. (2011). Myelinated retinal fibers in autosomal recessive spastic ataxia of Charlevoix-Saguenay. *Eur J Neurol*, (Jan 2011), [Epub ahead of print], ISSN 1468-1331

Wilkinson, P. A., A. H. Crosby, C. Turner, L. J. Bradley, L. Ginsberg, N. W. Wood, A. H. Schapira, and T. T. Warner. (2004). A clinical, genetic and biochemical study of SPG7 mutations in hereditary spastic paraplegia. *Brain*, Vol.127, Pt 5, (May 2004), pp. 973-980, ISSN 0006-8950

Yamamoto, Y., K. Hiraoka, M. Araki, S. Nagano, H. Shimazaki, Y. Takiyama, and S. Sakoda. (2005). Novel compound heterozygous mutations in sacsin-related ataxia. *J Neurol Sci*, Vol.239, No.1, (Dec 2005), pp. 101-104, ISSN 0022-510X

Yamamoto, Y., M. Nakamori, K. Konaka, S. Nagano, H. Shimazaki, Y. Takiyama, and S. Sakoda. (2006). Sacsin-related ataxia caused by the novel nonsense mutation Arg4325X. *J Neurol*, Vol.253, No.10, (Oct 2006), pp. 1372-1373, ISSN 0340-5354

9

Neurochemistry and Neuropharmacology of the Cerebellar Ataxias

José Gazulla[1], Cristina Andrea Hermoso-Contreras[2] and María Tintoré[3]
[1]*Department of Neurology, Hospital Universitario Miguel Servet, Zaragoza,*
[2]*School of Medicine, University of Zaragoza, Zaragoza,*
[3]*Nucleic Acid Chemistry Group, Chemistry and Molecular Pharmacology Programme, Institute for Research in Biomedicine of Barcelona, Barcelona,*
Spain

1. Introduction

The aim of this work has been to review the neurochemical alterations described in the cerebellar ataxias, and to enumerate the attempts made at their pharmacological treatment. As will be shown, little use has been made of the neurochemical information available, and the therapeutic trials have been far from successful.

The predominant (though not exclusive) reference to degenerative ataxias is due to the fact that the specificity of the affected cell populations should allow anticipation of more or less specific neurochemical alterations. This information could be used to look for therapeutic strategies, given the absence of curative treatments for the majority of ataxic disorders. This review covers only the pharmacologic attempts performed to treat ataxic symptoms, and is not exhaustive in terms of nosology, genetics or congenital errors of metabolism. The neurochemical basis of some non-degenerative ataxias that demonstrate favourable responses to pharmacological treatment are also reviewed. An outline of the physiological neurotransmission in the cerebellum opens this chapter (Table 1).

2. Neurotransmission in the cerebellum

The cerebellum is made up of four pairs of nuclei located in the deep white matter that covers the fourth ventricle, and is surrounded by a superficial layer of grey matter. The cerebellar cortex has a very uniform cellular structure and great cell density.

In the cortex of the cerebellum, there are several types of inhibitory interneurons that utilize γ-aminobutyric acid (GABA) as neurotransmitter. These are Golgi cells (that coexpress GABA with glycine), stellate cells, basket cells and Lugaro cells.

Purkinje cells are also GABAergic; they are the only ones whose axons exit the cortex of the cerebellum, projecting towards the cerebellar and vestibular nuclei. They use taurine as an osmotic regulator.

The excitatory amino acid glutamate is used in the cerebellar cortex by granule cells and unipolar brush cells. The axons of the granule cells constitute the parallel fibres of the molecular layer.

Most of the afferent fibres of the cerebellum are excitatory and use glutamate as main neurotransmitter. The climbing fibres that leave the contralateral inferior olive and synapse with the Purkinje cell dendrites are mostly glutamatergic, in addition to using aspartate and homocysteic acid. The mossy fibres are more numerous and originate in a number of areas, such as the pontine nuclei, reticular formation, spinal cord, deep cerebellar nuclei (as collaterals to the nuclear axons) and unipolar brush cells. They reach the dendrites of the granule cells in the so called glomerular structures. The great majority of mossy fibres use glutamate; a small proportion, acetylcholine (afferents from the vestibular nuclei and others from the cerebellar nuclei) and peptides such as enkephalins, cholecystokinin, corticotrophin, or calcitonin gene related peptide (CGRP). Part of the climbing and mossy fibres which originate in precerebellar structures, emit a collateral ramification that reaches the deep cerebellar nuclei on their trajectory toward the cortex. The efferent nuclear fibres are excitatory, with the exception of those destined for the inferior olives, which have an inhibitory function.

In addition to the mossy and climbing fibres, there is a group of beaded fibres that use monoamines as neurotransmitters, and reach the three layers of the cerebellar cortex.

Glutamate	Mossy fibers Climbing fibers Granule cells Parallel fibers Unipolar brush cells
GABA	Golgi cells Stellate cells Basket cells Lugaro cells Purkinje cells
Glycine	Golgi cells (coexpressed with GABA)
Noradrenaline	Origin in locus ceruleus
Serotonin	Origin in reticular formation
Acetylcholine	Origin in vestibular nuclei
Histamine	Origin in hipothalamus

Table 1. Neurotransmitters in the cerebellum (references 1-7).

A contingent of noradrenergic fibres stems from the locus ceruleus, and there seems to be a group of dopaminergic afferents of indeterminate origin. Serotonergic fibres originate at the paramedian and lateral reticular nuclei, the periolivary reticular formation and the lateral tegmental region; it has not been possible to demonstrate connections between the raphe nuclei and the cerebellar cortex. Some histaminergic fibres reach the cerebellar cortex from the hypothalamus.

Nitric oxide (NO) is a non-synaptic neurotransmitter present in the cerebellar cortex, mostly generated in the soma and parallel fibres of the granule cells. This substance spreads through the cell membranes and acts on glial cells and some neurons, stimulating the synthesis of cyclic guanosine-monophosphate. Basket and unipolar brush cells also synthesise NO, although not so Purkinje cells (1-7).

In conclusion, neurotransmission in the cerebellum implicates the amino acids glutamate and GABA, which establish an equilibrium between excitatory and inhibitory phenomena (Table 1).

Figures of the anatomy of the cerebellum and its connections, and of the neurochemical organization of the cerebellar cortex may be found the works of Colin et al (5), and Ottersen et al (1).

3. Neurochemistry and pharmacological therapy of the cerebellar ataxias

The abundance of neurotransmitters in the cerebellum complicates the task of determining which among them are implicated in disease pathogenesis. In addition, neurochemical data about many diseases is fragmentary. This section reviews the available neurochemical information (Table 2) and attempts at pharmacological treatment (Table 3) of the following conditions:

1. Cortical cerebellar atrophies
2. Atrophies of the cerebellar cortex and afferent fibres from the brainstem (olivopontocerebellar atrophies, OPCA).
3. Spinocerebellar atrophies.
4. Degenerations of the dentate nucleus and efferent tracts of the cerebellum.
5. Episodic ataxias.

4. Cortical cerebellar atrophies

The cortical cerebellar atrophy (CCA) of idiopathic etiology constitutes a relatively straightforward neurochemical model: the loss of Purkinje cells in the cerebellar vermis (8) causes a selective decrease of the concentration of GABA in the dentate nuclei (9) and cerebrospinal fluid (CSF) (10-13), with no reduction in that of glutamate (9), homovanillic acid (HVA), 5-hydroxiindolacetic acid (5-HIAA), or the noradrenergic metabolite 3-methoxy-4-hydroxyphenylglycol (MHPG) (14). Reduced consumption of glucose in the cerebellum has been determined by positron emission tomography (PET) (15). This condition presents as a late-onset, pure cerebellar syndrome (8). Autosomal dominant spinocerebellar ataxias (SCA) that exhibit a progressive and isolated cerebellar syndrome include SCA 5, 6, 11, 15, 22, 26 and 30.

Cortical cerebellar atrophy	Decreased content of GABA in the dentate nuclei and CSF.
Oivopontocerebellar atrophy	Decreased levels of GABA and glutamate in the cerebellar cortex, and of GABA in the dentate nuclei. Decreased concentration of dopamine and HVA in putamen, caudate and nucleus accumbens. CSF: decreased levels of GABA and glutamate
Friedreich's ataxia	Decreased glutamate concentration in the grey substance and dorsal columns in the lumbar spinal cord. Low glutamate and GABA concentrations in the cerebellar cortex.
Machado-Joseph disease	Decreased HVA in CSF.
Dentatorubral-pallidoluysian atrophy	Decreased GABA and substance P in globus pallidus and substantia nigra, and of choline-acetyltransferase in putamen and caudate nucleus. Reduced GABA in CSF.
Episodic ataxia type 6	Defective glutamate uptake

Table 2. Neurochemistry of the cerebellar ataxias.

Cortical cerebellar atrophy	Anticholinesterase drugs: physostigmine (13,53) Serotonergic drugs: L-5-hydroxytryptophan (38-41), buspirone (43-47), tandospirone (48) Serotonergic antagonists: ondansetron (49) Peptides: TRH (51,52) GABAergic drugs: gabapentin (25), pregabalin (31) NMDA agonists: D-cicloserine (54) Carbonic anhidrase inhibitors: acetazolamide (55,56) Piracetam (32,33)
Oivopontocerebellar atrophy	Anticholinesterase drugs: physostigmine (53,94) Serotonergic drugs: L-5-hydroxytryptophan (40,91), buspirone (46) Dopaminergic drugs: amantadine (89) Peptides: TRH (52) Cholinergic drugs: lecithin (95), L-acetylcarnitine (99) GABAergic drugs: vigabatrin (90), gabapentin (103), zolpidem (101) Glucocorticoid drugs: betamethasone (105) Glutamatergic drugs: ramified amino acids (100) Riluzole (102)
Friedreich's ataxia	Cholinergic drugs: L-acetylcarnitine (99) Serotonergic drugs: L-5-hydroxytryptophan (40,91) Tandospirone (48) Dopaminergic drugs: amantadine (89,115) GABAergic drugs: vigabatrin (116) Peptides: TRH (52) Iron chelators: deferiprone (133) Antioxidant agents: idebenone (118-121,123, 126,127) Erythropoietin (131, 132)
Machado-Joseph disease	Tetrahydrobiopterin (140) Trimethoprim-sulfametoxazole (141,145) Serotonergic drugs: buspirone (92), fluoxetin (120), tandospirone (147, 48) Antiepileptic drugs: lamotrigine (146) Antiarrhythmic drugs: mexiletine (148) Riluzole (102)
Episodic ataxia type 1 Episodic ataxia type 2 Episodic ataxia type 3 Episodic ataxia type 4 Episodic ataxia type 5	Acetazolamide, phenytoin (156) Acetazolamide (161) Acetazolamide (164) Dimenhydrinate (166) Acetazolamide (169)

Table 3. Pharmacological therapy of the cerebellar ataxias. Boliographic references are in brackets.

A deficiency of GABA in the cerebellum may lead to cerebellar ataxia, as suggested by abnormal GABAergic neurotransmission in the presence of antibodies directed against the enzyme glutamic decarboxylase (GAD) (16), and the coexistence of ataxia with the aforementioned antibodies (17-19). Anti-GAD antibodies are present in juvenile neuronal ceroid-lipofuscinosis, a disorder that may associate ataxia (20), and a selective vulnerability of GABAergic neurons has been found in other lysosomal disorders (21). Besides, an amelioration of ataxia was achieved with the use of GABAergic drugs in a case of adult GM2 gangliosidosis (22), and administration of gabapentin improved motor coordination in potassium/sodium hyperpolarization-activated cyclic nucleotide-gated channel 1 (HCN1) knockout mice, which exhibit a decreased content of GABA in the cerebellum (23).

The pharmacological trials in CCA are reviewed in the following section.

An open-label trial of gabapentin reported a substantial clinical improvement, and statistically significant differences in the scores of some items selected from the International Cerebellar Ataxia Rating Scale (ICARS) (24). Ten patients were initially given a single dose of 400 mg of gabapentin, followed by doses between 900 and 1600 mg per day during four weeks. Every patient experienced an improvement in ataxia, and in three, gait became normal (25). Gabapentin interacts with the $\alpha 2$-δ subunit of the P/Q type voltage-dependent calcium channels (VDCC) (26), stimulates GABAergic neurotransmission by presynaptic mechanisms (27) and increases the concentration of GABA in the brain of healthy adults (28). More recently, gabapentin treatment decreased ICARS scores by more than 10% in 11 patients with SCA 6 (caused by an abnormal expansion in *CACNA1A*, 19p13, that encodes the α1A subunit of the P/Q-type VDCC), indicating that the drug could be beneficial in this disease (29).

Pregabalin, a molecule closely related to gabapentin, improved the scores in the Scale for the Assessment and Rating of Ataxia (SARA) (30) in a single blind, placebo controlled trial that included two patients with CCA (31).

A patient with cortical cerebellar ataxia was administered piracetam in a single-blind trial. Piracetam (a derivative of GABA that binds to H^3-glutamate sites) improved tandem gait and gait ataxia in a dose of 60 g per day, and the authors concluded that this drug might have an anti-ataxic effect when used in high doses (32). Subsequently, 60 g per day of piracetam was given to a group of two patients with hereditary CCA, and six with other hereditary ataxias (excluding Friedreich ataxia, FRDA), in an open-label trial. The reduction obtained in the mean total score of ICARS (from 39.4±17, to 30.9±14.9), and in that of the posture and gait item, reached statistical significance (33).

Chan-Palay et al induced ataxia in animals through thiamine deprivation, and found a loss of serotonergic fibres in the nervous system (34). As a consequence, the authors suggested that a deficiency of serotonin might constitute the neurochemical basis for ataxia in humans (35). Anyway, neither a deficiency of serotonin nor atrophy of structures that could cause serotonergic denervation have been demonstrated in humans with CCA. The modulating effect of serotonin on GABAergic neurotransmission could explain some of the results reported below (36,37).

In two studies on the serotonergic precursor L-5-hydroxytryptophan, improved stance and speech were obtained in patients with degenerative and secondary ataxias, CCA among them (38,39). However, in a double-blind placebo crossover study of 13 patients with CCA, seven with OPCA, and 19 with FRDA, no improvement in ataxia was observed (40), although the inclusion of different diseases in the mentioned trials prevented a clear assessment of the effect of L-5-hydroxytryptophan on CCA. In addition, this drug was administered to six patients with CCA in an open-label study, without finding changes in the amplitude of voluntary movement or in the latency of electromyographic activity in antagonist muscles, showing that L-5-hydroxytryptophan was not an effective therapeutic agent for CCA (41).

The drug buspirone stimulates the serotonergic 5-HT1A receptor. It is currently used as an anxiolytic (42), so this effect must be ruled out in its assessment as a treatment for CCA (43-47). Trouillas et al studied the effect of buspirone on CCA in an open-label (42) and in two placebo-controlled studies (44,45). They defined their results as "a progressive modulation, rather than a radical transformation of ataxic symptoms" (43,45), referring to the limited and delayed improvement achieved. Lou et al (46) used buspirone in an open-label study in 14 patients with CCA and six with OPCA; the drug was administered in accordance with the severity of the ataxia. The authors found that buspirone was effective in cases of mild or moderate ataxia, though they did not individualize its effect on any of the two disorders. Andrade-Filho et al (47) noted improvement in 11 patients with CCA, with the addition of buspirone to other anti-ataxic and antiepileptic drugs. However, the methodology employed in this work did not make clear the aetiology of the ataxias, nor did it measure accurately the effectiveness of the drug.

The serotonergic agonist tandospirone was given during four weeks to 5 patients with SCA 6, 5 with SCA 1, 6 with SCA 2, 14 with Machado Joseph disease (MJD), and 9 with multisystem atrophy. This was an open-label, non blinded trial, and obtained reductions in the ICARS scores of the SCA 6 (p 0.043) and MJD (p 0.005) subgroups that reached statistical significance. It must be remarked, however, that the two tables in this article mentioned different values for the pre-treatment mean ICARS score of the cerebellar-multisystem atrophy subgroup, that the discussion incorporated results not specified in the corresponding section, and that the value of probability ($p<0.0001$) for the reduction of ICARS scores after treatment with tandospirone for the entire group, was out of proportion with the results of p for every subgroup of patients (48).

A double-blind, placebo controlled study of the serotonergic antagonist ondansetron showed worsening of the knee-heel manoeuvre in 15 patients with CCA (49).

Thyrotropin-releasing hormone (TRH) increases noradrenaline turnover, facilitates cholinergic transmission, and adjusts GABAergic neurotransmission (50). Although its intravenous administration had no effect on one patient with familial CCA (51), a study of patients with CCA, OPCA and FRDA showed an amelioration of postural instability (52). Obviously, the risk of hyperthyroidism prevents the prolonged use of this potentially beneficial agent.

The use of the anti-cholinesterase drug physostigmine in two double-blind, placebo controlled studies in patients with CCA, obtained no improvement in ataxia. The authors of both articles concluded that physostigmine was not effective in the treatment of this disease (13,53).

The amino-acid D-cycloserine, a partial agonist of the N-metil-D-aspartate (NMDA) glutamate receptor, was used in a placebo controlled trial in two patients with CCA, two with SCA 6 (53), 10 patients with multisystem atrophy and one with degenerative spinocerebellar ataxia. Mild improvements were found in some items of ICARS, and it was suggested that activation of NMDA receptors could lead to symptomatic improvement in spinocerebellar ataxia (54).

Finally, the use of acetazolamide in three patients with SCA 6 was found to have no effect on ataxia (55). Nevertheless, an open-label study of 9 patients with SCA 6 treated with 500 mg per day of acetazolamide, achieved a statistically significant improvement in ICARS scores and in the results of posturographic analysis (56).

Some forms of CCA have a non-degenerative etiology. Chronic abuse of ethanol may cause loss of neurons with GABA-A receptors, especially in the Purkinje cell layer, and vermian atrophy. Abstention from alcohol has been proposed to halt progression of ataxia (57).

Cerebellar paraneoplastic degeneration is a remote consequence of cancer. It is characterised histologically by loss of Purkinje cells and the presence of perivascular and leptomeningeal inflammatory infiltrates (58). An autoimmune cause is invoked by the presence of antibodies directed against epitopes common to the tumour and: 1) Purkinje cells (Yo, Tr) (59,60), 2) Hu and Ri nuclear proteins (60), 3) Tr dendritic protein (61), 4) P/Q-type VDCC (62,63), and 5) mGluR1 type glutamate metabotropic receptors (64). The latter are capable of altering both the acute and plastic response of Purkinje cells, causing cerebellar dysfunction (64). Antineoplastic treatment is recommended, or immunotherapy in its defect (60).

5. Olivopontocerebellar atrophies

The olivopontocerebellar atrophies comprise a heterogeneous group of disorders (degenerative diseases, prionopathies, hereditary errors of metabolism and mitochondrial encephalopathies) whose histological substrate is: 1) loss of neurons in the inferior olive and ventral portion of the pons; 2) loss of mossy and climbing fibres, and 3) atrophy of the cerebellar cortex (65). There is depletion of Purkinje and granule cells in the cerebellar cortex, especially in the hemispheres (8). This expresses clinically a global cerebellar syndrome, accompanied by additional neurological signs. It may be sporadic or familial; familial cases are associated with a greater frequency of medullar signs (with the exception of spasticity), dystonia and oculomotor abnormalities (65). Autosomal dominant spinocerebellar ataxias in which OPCA constitutes the pathological or radiological substrate are SCA 1, 2, 7, 12 and 13 (66).

A fourth part of sporadic OPCA cases develop multisystem atrophy (which associates parkinsonism and autonomic failure) (66,67). Analysis of pathological material has shown immunoreactive inclusions to alpha-synuclein in oligodendrocytes (68) and neurons (69) in this disease. However, this is not the case with SCA1 or SCA2 (disorders caused by expansion of CAG triplets in 6p22.3 and 12q24.13), in which olivopontocerebellar atrophy constitutes the pathological basis (66). The frequency of associated lesions (locus coeruleus, red nucleus, substantia nigra, dentate, hypoglossal and dorsal motor nuclei, nucleus ambiguus, etc) with those described, blurs the nosological limits of OPCA (70).

Neurochemical studies in OPCA have demonstrated an important decrease of GABA content in the dentate nuclei (9,71,72) and cerebellar cortex (71).

The content of glutamate in the cerebellum varied between an important reduction and normality, in different sources (9,71,72). Kanazawa et al established correlation in brains with OPCA, between: 1) the content of glutamate in the anterior vermis, and the density of granule cells; 2) the concentration of glutamate in the posterior vermis and the cerebellar hemispheres, and the cellular density of the inferior olive; 3) the content of GABA in the dentate nuclei, and the density of Purkinje cells (9).

In an autoradiographic receptor study, Albin and Gilman found a statistically significant reduction in the density of GABA, benzodiazepine (BZD) and glutamate receptors in the cerebellar cortex of OPCA brains, compatible with loss of granule and Purkinje cells (73). A PET study found diminished flumazenil binding in the brainstem and cerebellum, confirming the deficiency of GABA observed in OPCA (74).

A study of a patient with sporadic OPCA found IgM antibodies directed against the glutamate receptor subunit GluR2. Antibodies were demonstrated on Purkinje cells, basal portion of the pons and inferior olive, by immunohistochemical methods. The antibodies were shown to be able to depolarise neurons *in vitro*, a fact that pointed to excitotoxicity of autoimmune origin in the genesis of the disease (75).

A low activity of the enzyme glutamate dehydrogenase was previously considered a biochemical hallmark of OPCA (76), although later studies demonstrated a lack of specificity of this metabolic alteration (77,78).

PET studies have shown decreases in dopamine and HVA levels in the striatum in familial (79) and sporadic (80) OPCA. The density of dopamine D2 receptors was normal in the putamen and caudate nuclei in one parkinsonian patient who exhibited OPCA at autopsy, demonstrating the possibility of presynaptic parkinsonism in this disease (81).

A reduced acetylcholinesterase activity and a low density of muscarinic receptors in the cerebellar cortex were found in familial OPCA, suggesting that cholinergic denervation was a major neurochemical anomaly in this variant (82,83). Nevertheless, choline-acetyltransferase activity in mossy fibres (1,3) was greater in familial OPCA than in control cases (82), disproving the previously mentioned proposal.

In CSF, in addition to a low content of GABA (9-11), a low glutamate level was found in sporadic OPCA (11), as well as low levels of HVA, thiamine and MHPG in hereditary OPCA (84-86), with those of tryptophan and 5-HIAA in normal ranges (85).

In addition, a decrease in the levels of pontine and cerebellar N-acetylaspartate (reflecting neuronal loss), was found by high field proton magnetic resonance spectroscopy (^{1}H MRS) in patients with SCA 2 and cerebellar multisystem atrophy. An increase in myoinositol, that points to involvement of glial cells, was also found in multisystem atrophy (87).

To summarise, deficiencies of GABA, glutamate, dopamine and possibly noradrenaline, are present in the nervous system of OPCA patients, although no deficiencies of serotonin or acetylcholine have been documented (79,85).

In an ataxia-telangiectasia (AT) brain with cerebellar, inferior olive and dentate nuclei atrophy, the contents of GABA and glutamate in the cerebellar cortex, and of GABA in the dentate nuclei, were lower than those in controls (88). These neurochemical findings were similar to those in hereditary OPCA (71), and demonstrate that the neurochemical abnormalities of the ataxias are independent of the underlying condition.

The neurochemical complexity of OPCA makes successful pharmacological therapy difficult. As outlined below, a large number of clinical trials have been done, in an attempt to find a remedy.

A double-blind placebo controlled study using amantadine hydrochloride in 30 patients with OPCA without akinesia, obtained improvements in simple and movement reaction times in response to visual and auditory stimuli, that reached statistical significance. The beneficial results were attributed, either to a dopaminergic effect of the drug, or to blockade of NMDA receptors, an effect similar to that exercised by memantine (89).

In a group of 14 patients (one with sporadic OPCA, four with familial OPCA and nine with FRDA), a double-blind comparative trial of vigabatrin (an irreversible inhibitor of GABA-transaminase) with placebo, yielded no apparent benefit (90).

A previously mentioned trial (40) did not find improvement in ataxia with L5-hydroxytryptophan in a group that included seven patients with OPCA. This conclusion was shared by Currier et al, using the same drug in a group that included three patients with OPCA (91).

A group of 20 patients (5 with SCA 2, 2 with SCA 3, 4 with FRDA, and the remaining with other degenerative ataxias) was given buspirone at doses of 60 mg per day, in a double-blind, placebo-controlled, cross-over trial; buspirone was not superior to placebo in the amelioration of ataxia (92). The potential effects of oestrogen on neuroprotection, and of buspirone on ataxia, were combined in an open-label study with 18 OPCA patients. The participants were allocated either to buspirone, 15 mg/day, or to buspirone and oestrogen, 0.625 mg/day. No statistically significant differences were found in ICARS scores, compared with baseline, in any group, although a trend of improvement in gait speed and knee-tibia test was observed in the first one, suggesting that oestrogen was not beneficial in cerebellar dysfunction (93). The work of Lou et al, using buspirone in seven patients with OPCA and 14 with CCA, has been detailed earlier (46).

In another previously mentioned study, the administration of physostigmine to 10 patients with OPCA and nine with CCA gave no apparent benefit (53), although this drug was found to have a favourable effect when used in a heterogeneous group that included three cases of OPCA (94).

The administration of the cholinergic precursor lecithin to 11 patients with OPCA induced a clinical worsening coincident with elevated plasma choline levels (95). Results obtained with choline chloride (96) and physostigmine, led Harding (97) and Manyam (13) to conclude that cholinergic drugs were not effective to treat cerebellar ataxias, probably because no deficit in cholinergic neurotransmission has been confirmed in these diseases (50). In spite of this, a double-blind, placebo controlled analysis of the cholinomimetic agent L-acetylcarnitine obtained a mild improvement in the coordination items of ICARS, in a group of 14 patients with sporadic and hereditary OPCA (98), and in another group of 11 patients with FRDA (99).

Based on the hypothesis that stimulation of glutamate metabolism could favour its neurotransmission in the cerebellum, and so prevent excitotoxic damage, Mori et al gave branched amino-acids to a group of 16 patients (five with sporadic OPCA, and 11 with SCA6 and SCA7) in a double-blind crossover study. They used doses of 1.5g, 3g, 6g and placebo (100). Starting with an ICARS score average of 42.44 ± 16.60, reductions of 2.92 ± 3.35 were obtained with a 1.5g dose, and of 4.31 ± 4.57 with a 3g dose. These modest results were nevertheless statistically significant, though the effect on patients with OPCA could not be individualized.

The favourable effect of TRH in a group of patients with several types of ataxia (including 12 with OPCA) has been referred to already (52).

In four out of five patients with SCA 2, an improvement of ataxia and intention tremor was observed after administration of zolpidem in single doses of 10 mg. In one patient, a SPECT scan verified normalization of a previously diminished Tc^{99}exametazime binding. The drug's beneficial effect was attributed to reversion of a phenomenon of diaschisis (101).

In a randomized, double-blind, placebo-controlled trial, 40 patients (4 with SCA 2, 6 with multisystem atrophy, 8 with FRDA, and others with degenerative and acquired ataxias) were assigned to riluzole (100 mg/day) or placebo, during 8 weeks. The number of patients with a 5-point drop in ICARS compared to baseline (primary endpoint of the study) was significantly higher in the riluzole group after 4 and 8 weeks of treatment, with a mean change of – 7.05 [± 4.96] points in the total score, versus 0.16 [± 2.65] with placebo (102).

Gabapentin was found to improve gait in a patient with sporadic OPCA, and dysarthria and oscillopsia in another (103). Duhigg described an unexpected regression of ataxia in a patient with OPCA that received 30 mg/day of propranolol (104).

Finally, inhaled betamethasone led to improvement in the ataxia of a patient with infantile AT (105), whilst pregabalin in combination with tiagabine ameliorated ataxia in a patient with adult-onset AT (106).

6. Spinocerebellar atrophies

The most frequent and severe spinocerebellar atrophy is Friedreich's ataxia. FRDA has autosomal recessive inheritance, and an early onset. It is associated with scoliosis, pes cavus, cardiomyopathy, dysarthria, deep tendon areflexia, loss of vibration sense and extensor plantar responses (107). The lesions are located mainly in the spinal cord, where macroscopic atrophy, loss of fibres in the dorsal columns, dorsal and ventral spinocerebellar bundles, and direct and crossed corticospinal tracts, are present. Neuronal loss is found in the gracilis and cuneatus nuclei, Clarke's dorsal nuclei and in the dorsal root ganglia. The dorsal roots are atrophic, and there is depletion of myelinated fibres in the sensory nerves. Neuronal depopulation and loss of iron in the dentate nuclei, as well as atrophy of the superior cerebellar peduncles are also found, while the cerebellar cortex is preserved (8,97,108). Hypertrophic changes are present in the heart, with increased connective tissue and loss of cardiomyocytes (108).

The genetic anomaly in FRDA is an abnormal expansion of a GAA triplet in the first intron of the *FXN* gene on chromosome 9q13, that inhibits the transcription of the mitochondrial protein frataxin. Its deficiency interferes with the synthesis of iron-sulphur complexes, and with iron transport. These cause an accumulation of reactive iron in the mitochondria, interfere with oxidative phosphorylation and allow the formation of toxic oxygen radicals (109).

Neurochemical studies in FRDA have demonstrated low concentrations of glutamate and glycine in the grey matter of the lumbar cord and of glutamate in the dorsal columns, which reflect the loss of corticospinal and sensory glutamatergic fibres (110,111). There was also a reduction in the concentrations of glutamate and GABA in the vermis and the cerebellar hemispheres (112).

HVA and 5-HIIA CSF levels were reduced in patients with FRDA (85); this was not the case with CSF levels of GABA and homocarnosine (113), nor with the density of BZD receptors in the brain (114).

Pharmacological therapy has only achieved partially favourable results in FRDA. As previously mentioned, the results of trials with L-hydroxytryptophan (40,94), physostigmine (53), TRH (52), vigabatrin (91), riluzole (102) and buspirone (92), in groups that included patients with several types of ataxia, did not permit individualization of the effect of these drugs on FRDA.

Botez et al did not find improvement in ataxia when treating a group of 27 patients with FRDA with amantadine hydrochloride (90). The same result was reported by Filla et al, in a double-blind cross-over trial using amantadine hydrochloride in 12 patients with FRDA (115). No benefit was obtained, either, in an open-label assay of vigabatrin in nine patients with FRDA (116).

Idebenone (a government-supported drug for treatment of FRDA in Canada, among other countries) is a synthetic analogue of coenzyme Q10 with powerful antioxidant properties, whose effectiveness on the ataxia and cardiomyopthy of FRDA is currently being investigated.

A positive effect of idebenone on the cardiomyopathy of FRDA reported in a preliminary trial (117) was confirmed in a randomized placebo-controlled trial with 29 patients, in which a reduction of the thickness of the interventricular septum and posterior wall of the left ventricle, that reached statistical significance, was evidenced by echocardiography (118). Another study found that six (among eight) patients with FRDA exhibited an important reduction of cardiac hypertrophy (119), although no improvement in ataxia was noticed in any of these trials.

In a study with an examination period that ranged from 6 to 84 months, Ribat et al observed that ataxia and cardiac ejection fraction deteriorated in 88 patients with FRDA while receiving 5 mg/kg per day of idebenone (in spite of finding decreased cardiac hypertrophy by echocardiography), as well as in 16 non-treated patients (120). An increase in interventricular septum and left posterior wall thickness was observed in patients without previous myocardiopathy, who received 5 mg/kg per day of idebenone. The authors concluded that idebenone did not prevent the development of myocardiopathy, although no worsening was found in patients with known cardiac disease (121).

The phase 3 Idebenone Effects on Neurological ICARS Assessments (IONIA) study randomized 70 ambulatory FRDA patients aged 8 to 18, with ICARS scores between 10 and 54, to placebo and idebenone at doses of 10-20, and 30-54 mg/kg per day. No improvement in left ventricular hypertrophy or cardiac function could be demonstrated over a six month period (122).

Artuch et al (123) reported a statistically significant amelioration in cerebellar function, compared with baseline evaluation, in paediatric patients with FRDA receiving idebenone.

Recently, emphasis has been placed on the use of high doses of idebenone in an effort to improve ataxia in FRDA (124,125); accordingly, a randomized, double-blind, placebo-controlled phase 2 six-month trial (National Institutes of Health Collaboration with Santhera in Ataxia [NICOSIA]) of this drug at doses of 5, 15 and 45 mg/kg per day, was performed on 48 ambulatory FRDA patients aged between 8 and 18, with ICARS scores between 10 and 54. Increasing doses of idebenone were associated with reductions in ICARS scores in a dose-dependent manner, even though overall statistically significant differences were not obtained; thus concluding that high doses of idebenone might be necessary to attain beneficial effects on neurological function (126).

In contrast, the "neurological" arm of the IONIA trial achieved a minimal mean reduction in ICARS scores, which did not reach statistical significance when compared to placebo (127).

The drug mitoquinone (an antioxidant derived from idebenone), which is active in the mitochondrion though not so in the cytosol, is expected to be an effective therapeutic agent in FRDA (128)

A double-blind study of 5-hydroxytryptophan and placebo in 19 patients with FRDA (129), and of an open-label study of amantadine in 16 (130), only gave slightly positive results. A similar benefit was obtained in a previously mentioned study that used L-acetylcarnitine in 11 patients with FRDA (100).

It was demonstrated recently that human recombinant erythropoietin (rhuEPO) increased frataxin in lymphocytes from patients with FRDA, in vitro; this effect was independent from the EPO receptor (131). Thus, a persistent and significant increase in frataxin levels was found in peripheral blood lymphocytes of seven (among 10) patients with FRDA who received 5.000 units of rhuEPO subcutaneously, three times a week during 8 weeks; reductions in the urinary oxidative stress marker 8-hydroxi-2′-deoxyguanosine excretion, and in SARA scores, were also found (132). The same favourable results (that reached statistical significance) were replicated in a study involving 8 patients with FRDA, who received 2.000 units of rhuEPO three times a week during six months; unfortunately, the design of the trial could not rule out a placebo effect of the drug (133).

More specific therapeutic approaches for FRDA are under investigation, such as the histone deacetylase inhibitors, which impair abnormal DNA transcription in FRDA; peroxisome proliferator-activated receptor gamma agonists, that enhance cell antioxidant activity and frataxin levels; deferiprone (a mitochondrion-specific iron chelator) reduced iron content in the dentate nuclei (as measured by MRI), and improved neuropathy and gait ataxia in the youngest patients among 9 adolescents with FRDA (134); gene-based strategies, as the use of viral vectors that express frataxin, which corrected sensitivity to oxidative stress in FRDA fibroblasts (128,135); and finally, pluripotent stem cells induced from FRDA fibroblasts were able to differentiate into neurons and cardiomyocytes (136).

An isolated deficiency of vitamin E, caused by mutations in the gene that encodes the alpha-tocopherol transfer protein in 8q13, can present with an identical phenotype to FRDA. The neurological manifestations stabilise or may partially revert with administration of vitamin E (137).

7. Degenerations of the dentate nucleus and efferent tracts of the cerebellum

This section deals about about Machado-Joseph disease and dentatorubral-pallidoluysian atrophy (DRPLA).

MJD, also designated SCA3, is caused by an unstable expansion of a CAG triplet in the *ataxin 3* gene in14q32.1, and exhibits dominant transmission (138). The lesions are found in the dentate nuclei and superior cerebellar peduncles, and respect the cerebellar cortex, striatum, inferior olive and corticospinal tracts. The pontine nuclei are sometimes affected. The dorsal columns, spinocerebellar tracts and Clarke's dorsal nuclei degenerate in the spinal cord (110). Associated lesions may be present in the anterior horns, oculomotor and subthalamic nuclei, substantia nigra, medial longitudinal fascicle, and peripheral nerves. Among the manifestations of MJD, ataxia is related to lesions in the dentate or pontine nuclei; oculomotor disorders, to those in the brainstem; and parkinsonism, to those in the substantia nigra. The frequent spasticity cannot be explained by the aforementioned findings (138).

Neurochemical abnormalities in MJD consist of a reduced CSF concentration of HVA, even in cases without apparent parkinsonism (85,139). Concentrations of 5-HIAA and MHPG were reduced in CSF in one patient with MJD (136), although these changes were not found in every instance (85,139).

Attempts at pharmacological therapy in MJD are outlined below.

Based on the finding that trimethoprim increased the concentration of tetrahydrobiopterin (THB) in CSF in MJD, Sakai et al administered 1 mg/kg of THB and placebo to five patients for 10 day periods, in a crossover scheme. They reported a statistically significant improvement in the performance of some timed tests of motor function, though deglutition and tendon hypereflexia were not modified (140).

A double-blind, placebo-controlled, crossover trial of trimethoprim-sulfamethoxazole (TS) in 20 patients with SCA3, employed: 1) a clinical scale of ataxia and other non-cerebellar symptoms; 2) posturographic analysis; 3) the Schoppe motor performance test; and 4) achromatic and colour discrimination visual sensitivity tests. After six months of TS administration, none of the patients showed improvement in any of the enumerated tests. No differences were noted in sub-group analysis according to age, sex, duration of illness, phenotype, age at onset, or number of CAG triplets (141). These categorical results contrast with the more favourable outcomes obtained in a study that included eight patients with MJD (142), and with three other reports of individual patients (143-145) that received TS. The reason for the differing results could lie in the absence of molecular diagnosis in the latter studies, or in other methodological differences (141).

An open-label study on the use of the antidepressant drug fluoxetine involved doses of 20 mg per day given to 13 patients with MJD. In spite of a statistically significant improvement according to the Montgomery-Asberg depression rating scale, the EDSS and UPDRS scales showed no differences in motor function. The study concluded that serotonergic stimulation was not effective in the treatment of MJD (146).

Buspirone, at a dose of 60 mg per day, did not improve ataxia in a group of 20 patients that included 4 with SCA 3 (92).

Another open-label study used 10 to 30 mg per day doses of tandospirone. Seven out of 10 patients with MJD had their ICARS scores slightly improved, with additional mitigation of symptoms potentially caused by 5-HT1 receptor dysfunction (insomnia, anorexia, depression and cold lower extremities). The authors concluded that MJD manifested symptoms derived from these receptors, and recommended further tests with tandospirone in this disease (147). An open-label trial of tandospirone in 39 patients (14 with MJD among them) has already been commented on (48).

The antiarrhythmic drug mexiletine was shown to alleviate muscle cramps in MJD, without improving ataxia (148).

Liu et al gave 50 mg/day of lamotrigine to six patients with MJD, and observed improvement in one leg stance and tandem gait. They proposed that this beneficial effect could be due to enhanced expression of ataxin 3, induced by the drug (149).

Dentatorubral-pallidoluysian atrophy is a dominantly transmitted illness caused by an abnormal expansion of a CAG triplet in the atrophyn gene, in 12p13.31, that codifies polyglutamine sequences of abnormal length that exert a toxic action (as in other diseases caused by expansion of CAG triplets) (150). An important neuronal loss in the dentate and red nuclei is found. Less intense degeneration of the subthalamic nuclei and external part of the globus pallidus is also present, while the cerebellar cortex is preserved. Some studies have described spinal cord lesions identical to FRDA in DRPLA, in addition to those described (151); demyelinization in the superior cerebellar peduncles and efferent tracts of the pallidum has been noted, as well. These lesions may be asymmetric (152). Polyglutamine nuclear inclusions have been found in neurons and oligodendrocytes (153).

The clinical manifestations of DRPLA are heterogeneous. Cerebellar ataxia and dementia are considered cardinal signs, accompanied by progressive myoclonic epilepsy in cases with onset before the age of 20, or choreoathetosis and psychiatric symptoms when onset occurs later. It has been determined that there is an inverse correlation between the number of CAG triplets and age at onset of the disease. The differential diagnosis includes Huntington's disease due to the possible association of chorea and dementia (150).

The neurochemical alterations in DRPLA are centred on a reduction of GABA and substance P in the globus pallidus and substantia nigra, and reduced choline-acetyltransferase activity in the caudate and putamen, in spite of preservation of the small striatal neurons; this result points to cell hypofunction as its cause (154). In CSF, the concentration of GABA was found to be very low in five cases of DRPLA, whilst levels of HVA and 5-HIAA were normal (151).

Recently, an accumulation of 8-hydroxi-2'-deoxyguanosine and 8-hydroxyguanosine, and a reduction of immunoreactivity to Cu/Zn superoxide dismutase, were found in the lentiform and dentate nuclei of DRPLA brains, suggesting the possibility that oxidative stress might play a part in the genesis of this disease (155).

No clinical assay dedicated to the treatment of ataxia caused by DRPLA has been performed to date.

8. Episodic ataxias

Episodic ataxias are transmitted by autosomal dominant inheritance, and are amenable to drug treatment.

Episodic ataxia type 1 (EA1), also known as episodic ataxia with myokymia, has its onset in infancy or early adolescence, and associates interictal myokymia in the face and limbs (identified by electromyography) with brief episodes of unsteadiness, tremor and dysarthria. The attacks are brought about by voluntary movement or startle, and may occur many times every day. They can be prevented with acetazolamide or phenytoin. EA1 is caused by mutations in the *KCNA1* gene in 12p13, which encodes the voltage- dependent potassium channel KCNA1, widely expressed in the cerebellum and peripheral nerve (156-159). It has been demonstrated that the mutated channels increase cellular excitability, and prevent physiological repolarization (160).

Episodic ataxia type 2 (EA2) is caused by mutations in *CACNA1A*, that give rise to truncated α1A subunits (161). Electrophysiological characterisation of the abnormal proteins has demonstrated reduced channel conductance, causing an abnormally low calcium ingress, with the consequent cell damage (162,163).

EA2 appears in infancy and is associated with crises of ataxia, vertigo and nausea that last hours or days and are precipitated by emotional stress, fatigue or ingestion of coffee or ethanol. Interictal nystagmus, permanent ataxia and atrophy of the cerebellar vermis may coexist. Diagnosis may be difficult, as EA2 may be confused with anxiety or paroxysmal vertigo. The ataxic episodes respond to prophylaxis with acetazolamide (156,161).

Episodic ataxia type 3 (EA3) appears between the age of one year, and forty. It is associated with ataxia, vertigo and tinnitus, frequently headache, diplopia and blurred vision; interictal myokymia is also present. It may be distinguished from EA1 by the presence of vertigo and tinnitus, and from EA2 by the absence of interictal nystagmus and the short duration of the attacks, which are prevented by acetazolamide (164). The responsible gene is located in 1q42 (165).

Episodic ataxia type 4 (EA4), or vestibulocerebellar ataxia, was described by Farmer and Mustian in 1963 and is characterised by vertigo, diplopia, and mild or moderate ataxia that lasts from a few minutes to several weeks. It appears at an average age of 23 years (166). Defects have been found in smooth ocular pursuit and suppression of the vestibulo-ocular reflex, in addition to gaze-evoked nystagmus (167). Some patients develop progressive ataxia (166). EA4 responds to prophylaxis with dimenhydrinate (166) and is genetically distinct from SCA1, 2, 3, 4, 5, EA1, EA2 and DRPLA (168).

Episodic ataxia type 5 (EA5) is caused by a point mutation in *CACNB4* (2q22-q23), that causes a change of one amino-acid (C104F) in the β4 subunit of the VDCC. It was described in patients with French-Canadian ancestry, and its clinical symptoms (ataxia and vertigo) and duration are similar to EA2; there is interictal nystagmus and it responds to prophylaxis with acetazolamide. The main difference is a later age of onset (169).

Episodic ataxia type-6 (EA6) was described in a ten year-old child that exhibited transitory episodes of ataxia and dysarthria in addition to epilepsy, migraine and alternating hemiplegia. A heterozygote mutation was identified in *SLC1A3* (5p13), the gene that encodes the excitatory amino-acid transporter 1 (EAAT1, GLAST1), pointing to abnormal reuptake of synaptic glutamate as the causing factor of the neurological syndrome (170).

9. Conclusions

As may be deduced from the exposed data, pharmacological trials of cerebellar ataxias have been flawed by a number of factors, like the recruitment of very scarce numbers of patients, the predominance of clinical assays which include patients with more than one disease, the lack of an ataxia rating scale of generalized use and that of quantitative means of measuring ataxic symptoms, the absence of standard doses of the drugs under investigation, and probably the most important, the usual lack of application of the available pathophysiological data to the trials performed to date.

The basic neurochemical anomaly in idiopathic CCA consists in a lowering of the cerebellar content of GABA. In OPCA, deficits of glutamate, dopamine, and probably, noradrenaline, are present as well. Glutamate is essentially the deficient neurotransmitter in FRDA. A deficiency of serotonin has not been demonstrated conclusively in degenerative ataxias. The neurotransmitter abnormalities of MJD and DRPLA have not been well defined yet. Thus, it seems obvious that the neurochemical complexity of these disorders is one of the reasons for the lack of effective treatments.

Some tests have shown that the drugs gabapentin, pregabalin and tiagabine are effective in ataxias that associate a predominant deficiency of GABA in the cerebellum, like CCA and OPCA. Presumably, the more selective the deficit of GABA, the more effective the GABAergic substitution.

Agents capable of restoring the physiological action of glutamate (associated with neuroprotective molecules to prevent excitotoxic phenomena) could be useful in disorders like OPCA and FRDA. Conversely, the usefulness of the peptide TRH is conditioned by the risk of hyperthyroidism. Idebenone and other agents used to treat FRDA have to prove their effectiveness on ataxia, in a definite manner. The lack of effectiveness of physostigmine and choline chloride discards them as therapeutic agents for CCA and OPCA. The use of serotonergic agents in the cerebellar ataxias must be considered controversial at least, due to insufficient neurochemical evidence, and that of riluzole should be investigated in depth, as it could benefit patients with multisystem atrophy.

Given the severity of many of the ataxias considered in this work, treatable causes, such as vitamin E deficiency, should be ruled out when faced with phenotypes similar to FRDA. In a similar way, therapeutic trials with acetazolamide should be undertaken in cases with uncertain diagnoses, with the aim of recognising ataxias that respond to this drug.

Research aimed at identifying effective drugs to treat the cerebellar ataxias should, ideally, look for agents able to neutralize the causes of these diseases. However, as this is not possible in most cases, neurochemical evidence might provide useful clues in the search for therapeutic remedies (171,172). The study of animal and experimental models of disease, the use of precise methods for the measurement of ataxia (clinical semi-quantitative scales, quantitative movement analysis, etc) and the recruitment of homogenous study populations (22), are all highly recommended. In this way, the currently exiguous therapeutic panorama of the cerebellar ataxias could be amplified until etiological remedies are found.

10. References

[1] Ottersen OP, Walberg F. Neurotransmitters in the cerebellum. In: Manto MU, Pandolfo M, editors. The cerebellum and its disorders. Cambridge: Cambridge University Press, 2002: 38-48.

[2] Mugnaini E. GABAergic inhibition in the cerebellar system. In: Martin DL, Olsen RW, editors. GABA in the Nervous System: the view at fifty years. Philadelphia: Lippincott, Williams & Wilkins, 2000: 383-407.

[3] Ottersen OP. Neurotransmitters in the cerebellum. Rev Neurol (Paris) 1993; 149: 629-636.

[4] Kwong WH, Chan WY, Lee KKH, Fan M, Yew DT. Neurotransmitters, neuropeptides and calcium binding proteins in developing human cerebellum: a review. J Histochem 2000; 32: 521-534.

[5] Colin F, Ris L, Godaux E. Neuroanatomy of the cerebellum. In: Manto MU, Pandolfo M, editors. The cerebellum and its disorders. Cambridge: Cambridge University Press, 2002: 6-27.

[6] Bastian AJ, Thach WT. Structure and function of the cerebellum. In: Manto MU, Pandolfo M, editors. The cerebellum and its disorders. Cambridge: Cambridge University Press, 2002: 49-66.

[7] Trouillas P. Bases théoriques et propositions pour une neuropharmacologie de l´ataxie cérébelleuse. Rev Neurol (Paris) 1993; 149: 637-646.

[8] Oppenheimer DR. Diseases of the basal ganglia, cerebellum and motor neurons. In: Adams JH, Corsellis JAN, Duchen LW, editors. Greenfield´s Neuropathology. Londres: Edward Arnold, 1982: 699-747.

[9] Kanazawa I, Kwak S, Sasaki H, Mizusawa H, Muramoto O, Yoshizawa K, et al. Studies on neurotransmitter markers and neuronal cell density in the cerebellar system in olivopontocerebellar atrophy and cortical cerebellar atrophy. J Neurol Sci 1985; 71: 193-208.

[10] Ogawa N, Kuroda H, Ota Z, Yamamoto M, Otsuki S. Cerebrospinal fluid gamma-aminobutiric acid variations in cerebellar ataxia. Lancet 1982; 2:215.

[11] Kuroda H, Ogawa N, Yamawaki Y, Nukina I, Ofuji T, Yamamoto M, et al. Cerebrospinal fluid GABA levels in various neurological and psychiatric diseases. J Neurol Neurosurg Psychiatry 1982; 45: 257-260.

[12] Tohgi H, Abe T, Hashiguchi K, Takahashi S, Nozaki Y, Kikuchi T. A significant reduction of putative transmitter amino acids in cerebrospinal fluid of patients with Parkinson´s disease and spinocerebellar degeneraton. Neurosci Letter 1991; 126: 155-158.

[13] Manyam BV, Giacobini E, Ferraro TN, Hare TA. Cerebrospinal fluid as a reflector of central cholinergic and amino acid neurotransmitter activity in cerebellar ataxia. Arch Neurol 1990; 47: 1194-1199.

[14] Aldo WF, van de Warrenburg BPC, Munneke M, van Geel WJA, Bloem BR, et al. CSF analysis differentiates multiple-system atrophy from idiopathic late-onset cerebellar ataxia. Neurology 2006; 67: 474-479.

[15] Otsuka M, Ichiya Y, Kubawara Y, Hosokawa S, Akashi Y, Yoshida T, et al. Striatal 18F-Dopa uptake and brain glucose metabolism by PET in patients with syndrome of progressive ataxia. J Neurol Sci 1994; 124: 198-203.

[16] Ishida K, Mitoma H, Song S, Uchihara T, Inaba K, Eguchi S, et al. Selective suppression of cerebellar GABAergic transmission by an autoantibody to glutamic acid decarboxylase. Ann Neurol 1999; 46: 263-267.

[17] Saiz A, Arpa J, Sagasta A, Casamitjana R, Zarranz JJ, Tolosa E, et al. Autoantibodies to glutamic acid decarboxylase in three patients with cerebellar ataxia, late-onset diabetes mellitus, and polyendocrine autoimmunity. Neurology 1997; 49: 1026-1030.

[18] Honnorat J, Saiz A, Giometto B, Vincent A, Brieva L, de Andrés C, et al. Cerebellar ataxia with anti-glutamic acid decarboxylase antibodies. Arch Neurol 2001; 58: 225-230.

[19] Vulliemoz S, Vanini G, Truffert A, Chizzolini C, Seeck M. Epilepsy and cerebellar ataxia associated anti-glutamic acid decarboxylase antibodies. J Neurol Neurosurg Psychiatry 2007 ; 78 : 187-189.

[20] Chattopadhyay S, Kriscenski-Perry E, Wenger DA, Pearce DA. An autoantibody to GAD65 in sera of patients with juvenile neuronal ceroid lipofuscinosis. Neurology 2002; 59: 1816-1817.

[21] Walkley SU, Baker HJ, Rattazzi MC, Haskins ME, Wu JY. Neuroaxonal dystrophy in neuronal storage disorders: evidence for major GABAergic neuron involvement. J Neurol Sci 1991; 104: 1-8.

[22] Gazulla J, Benavente I. Gangliosidosis GM2 del adulto: mejoría de la ataxia con fármacos GABAérgicos. Neurología 2002; 17: 157-161.

[23] Massella A, Gusciglio M, D'Intimo G, Sivilia S, Ferraro L, Calzá L, et al. Gabapentin treatment improves motor coordination in a mouse model of progressive ataxia. Brain Res 2009; 1301: 135-142.

[24] Trouillas P, Takayanagi T, Currier RD, Subramony SH, Wessel K, Bryer A, et al. International Cooperative Ataxia Rating Scale for pharmacological assessment of the cerebellar syndrome. J Neurol Sci 1997; 145: 205-211.

[25] Gazulla J, Errea JM, Benavente I, Tordesillas C. Treatment of ataxia in cortical cerebellar atrophy with the GABAergic drug gabapentin. A preliminary study. Eur Neurol 2004; 52: 7-11.

[26] Greenberg DA. Calcium channels in neurological disease. Ann Neurol 1997; 42: 275-282.

[27] Moshé SL. Mechanisms of action of anticonvulsant agents. Neurology 2000; 55 (Suppl 1): S32-S40.

[28] Kuzniecky R, Ho S, Pan J, Martin R, Gilliam F, Faught E, et al. Modulation of cerebral GABA by topiramate, lamotrigine, and gabapentin in healthy adults. Neurology 2002; 58: 368-372.

[29] Nakamura K, Yoshida K, Miyakazi D, Morita H, Ikeda S. Spinocerebellar ataxia type 6 (SCA 6): clinical pilot trial with gabapentin. J Neurol Sci 2009; 278: 107-111.

[30] Schmitz-Hübsch T, du Montcel ST, Baliko L, Berciano J, Boesch S, Depondt C, et al. Scale for the assessment and rating of ataxia: development of a new clinical scale. Neurology 2006; 66: 1717-1720.

[31] Gazulla J, Benavente I. Single-blind, placebo-controlled pilot study of pregabalin for ataxia in cortical cerebellar atrophy. Acta Neurol Scand. 2007; 116: 235-8.

[32] Vural M, Ozekmekci S, Apaydin H, Altinel A. High-dose piracetam is effective on cerebellar ataxia in patient with cerebellar cortical atrophy. Mov Disord 2003; 18: 457-459.

[33] Ince Gunal D, Agan K, Afsar N, Borucu D, Us O. The effect of piracetam on ataxia: clinical observations in a group of autosomal dominant cerebellar ataxia patients. J Clin Pharm Ther. 2008; 33: 175-8.

[34] Chan-Palay V, Plaitakis A, Nicklas W, Berl S. Autoradiographic demonstration of loss of labeled indoleamine axons in chronic diet-induced thiamine deficiency. Brain Res 1977; 138: 380-384.
[35] Trouillas P. The cerebellar serotonergic system and its possible involvement in cerebellar ataxia. Can J Neurol Sci 1993; 20 (S3): S78-S82.
[36] Lee MA, Strahlendorf JC, Strahlendorf HK. Modulatory action of serotonin on glutamate-induced excitation of cerebellar Purkinje cells. Brain Res 1986; 361: 107-113.
[37] Strahlendorf JC, Lee MA, Strahlendorf HK. Serotonin modulates muscimol- and baclofen-elicited inhibition of cerebellar Purkinje cells. Eur J Pharmacol 1991; 201: 239-242.
[38] Trouillas P, Garde A, Robert JM, Renaud B, Adeleine P, Bard J, et al. Régression du syndrome cérébelleux sous administration a long terme de 5-HTP ou de l´association 5-HTP-bensérazide. 26 observations quantifiées et traitées par ordinateur. Rev Neurol (Paris) 1982; 138: 415-435.
[39] Trouillas P, Brudon F, Adeleine P. Improvement of cerebellar ataxia with levorotatory form of 5-hydroxytryptophan. Arch Neurol 1988; 45: 1217-1222.
[40] Wessel K, Hermsdörfer J, Deger K, Herzog T, Huss GP, Kömpf D, et al. Double-blind crossover study of hydroxytryptophan in patients with degenerative cerebellar diseases. Arch Neurol 1995; 52: 451-455.
[41] Manto M, Hildebrand J, Godaux E, Roland H, Blum S, Jacquy J, et al. Analysis of FRDAst movements in cerebellar cortical atrophy: Failure of L-hydroxytryptophan to improve cerebellar ataxia. Arch Neurol 1997; 54: 1192-1194.
[42] Hurlé MA, Monti J, Flórez J. Fármacos ansiolíticos y sedantes. Farmacología de los trastornos del sueño. In: Flórez J, Armijo JA, Mediavilla A, editors. Farmacología humana. Barcelona: Elsevier Masson SA, 2008: 543-566.
[43] Trouillas P, Xie J, Getenet JC, Adeleine P, Nighoghossian N, Honnorat J, et al. Effet de la buspirone, un agoniste sérotoninergique 5-HT1A sur l´ataxie cérébelleuse: un étude pilote. Rev Neurol (Paris) 1995; 151: 708-713.
[44] Trouillas P, Xie J, Adeleine P. Treatment of cerebellar ataxia with buspirone: a double-blind study. Lancet 1996; 348: 759.
[45] Trouillas P, Xie J, Adeleine P, Michel D, Vighetto A, Honnorat J, et al. Buspirone, a 5-hydroxytryptamine1A agonist, is active in cerebellar ataxia. Results of a double-blind drug placebo study in patients with cerebellar cortical atrophy. Arch Neurol 1997; 54: 749-752.
[46] Lou JS, Goldfarb L, McShane L, Gatev P, Hallett M. Use of buspirone for treatment of cerebellar ataxia. An open-label study. Arch Neurol 1995; 52: 982-988.
[47] Andrade-Filho AS, Passos-Almeida J, Andrade-Souza VM, Sena-Pereira LR. Clorhidrato de buspirona en el tratamiento de la ataxia cerebelosa. Rev Neurol (Barcelona) 2002; 35: 301-305.
[48] Takei A, Hamada S, Homma S, Hamada K, Tashiro K, Hamada T. Difference in the effects of tandospirone on ataxia in various types of spinocerebellar degeneration: an open-label study. Cerebellum 2010; 9: 567-570.
[49] Bier JC, Dethy S, Hildebrand J, Jacquy J, Manto M, Martin JJ, et al. Efectos del preparado oral de ondansetrón sobre la disfunción cerebelosa. Un estudio multicéntrico doble ciego. J Neurol Ed Esp 2003; 1: 90-94.
[50] Berciano J, Pascual J. Farmacoterapia de los síndromes espinocerebelosos. Neurología 1990; 5: 200-204.

[51] Gracia Naya M, Pina Latorre MA. Ensayo terapéutico en una familia con atrofia cerebelosa tardía. Neurología 1991; 6: 188-189.
[52] Sobue I, Yamamoto H, Konayaga M, Lida M, Takayanegi T. Effect of thyrotropin-releasing hormone on ataxia of spinocerebellar degeneration. Lancet 1980; 1; 418-419.
[53] Wessel K, Langenberger K, Nitschke MF, Kompf D. Double-blind crossover study with physostigmine in patients with degenerative cerebellar diseases. Arch Neurol 1997; 54: 397-400.
[54] Ogawa M, Shigeto H, Yamamoto T, Oya Y, Wada K, Nishikawa T, et al. D-cycloserine for the treatment of ataxia in spinocerebellar degeneration. J Neurol Sci 2003; 210: 53-56.
[55] Jen JC, Yue Q, Karrim J, Nelson SF, Baloh RW. Spinocerebellar ataxia type 6 with positional vertigo and acetazolamide responsive episodic ataxia. J Neurol Neurosurg Psychiatry 1998; 65: 565-568.
[56] Yabe I, Sasaki H, Yamashita I, Takei A, Tashiro K. Clinical trial of acetazolamide in SCA 6, with assessment using the Ataxia Rating Scale and body stabilometry. Acta Neurol Scand 2001; 104: 44-47.
[57] Manto MU, Jacquy J. Alcohol toxicity in the cerebellum: clinical aspects. In: Manto MU, Pandolfo M, editors. The cerebellum and its disorders. Cambridge: Cambridge University Press, 2002: 336-341.
[58] Henson RA, Urich H. Cancer and the nervous system. London: Blackwell Scientific, 1982: 346-367.
[59] Furneaux HM, Rosenblum MK, Dalmau J, Wong E, Woodruff P, Graus F, et al. Selective expression of Purkinje-cell antigens in tumor tissue from patients with paraneoplastic cerebellar degeneration. N Engl J Med 1990; 322: 1844-1851.
[60] Hildebrand J, Balériaux D. Cerebellar disorders in cancer. In: Manto MU, Pandolfo M, editors. The cerebellum and its disorders. Cambridge: Cambridge University Press, 2002: 265-287.
[61] Bernal F, Shams´ili S, Rojas I, Sánchez-Valle R, Saiz A, Dalmau J, et al. Anti-Tr antibodies as markers of paraneoplastic cerebellar degeneration and Hodgkin´s disease. Neurology 2003; 60: 230-234.
[62] Graus F, Lang B, Pozo-Rosich P, Saiz A, Casamitjana R, Vincent A. P/Q type calcium-channel antibodies in paraneoplastic cerebellar degeneration with lung cancer. Neurology 2002; 59: 764-766.
[63] Fukuda T, Motomura M, Nakao Y, Shiraisi H, Yoshimura T, Iwanaga K, et al. Reduction of P/Q-type calcium channels in the postmortem cerebellum of paraneoplastic cerebellar degeneration with Lambert-Eaton myasthenic syndrome. Ann Neurol 2003; 53: 21-28.
[64] Coesmans M, Sillevis Smitt PA, Linden DJ, Shigemoto R, Hirano T, Yamakawa Y, et al. Mechanisms underlying cerebellar motor deficits due to mGluR1-autoantibodies. Ann Neurol 2003; 53: 325-336.
[65] Berciano J. Olivopontocerebellar atrophy. A review of 117 cases. J Neurol Sci 1982; 53: 253-272.
[66] Berciano J, Boesch S, Pérez-Ramos JM, Wenning GK. Olivopontocerebellar atrophy: toward a better nosological definition. Mov Disord 2006; 10: 1607-1613.
[67] Gilman S, Little R, Johanns J, Heumann M, Kluin KJ, Junck L, et al. Evolution of sporadic olivopontocerebellar atrophy into multiple system atrophy. Neurology 2000; 55: 527-532.

[68] Berciano J. Multiple system atrophy and idiopathic late-onset cerebellar ataxia. In: Manto MU, Pandolfo M, editors. The cerebellum and its disorders. Cambridge: Cambridge University Press, 2002: 178-197.
[69] Tu P, Galvin JE, Baba M, Giasson B, Tomita T, Leight S, et al. Glial cytoplasmatic inclusions in white matter oligodendrocytes of multiple system atrophy brains contain insoluble α-sinuclein. Ann Neurol 1998; 44: 415-422.
[70] Berciano J. La nosología de la atrofia olivopontocerebelosa. Revisión crítica. Arch Neurobiol 1981; 44: 163-181.
[71] Perry TL, Kish SJ, Hansen S, Currier RD. Neurotransmitter amino acids in dominantly inherited cerebellar disorders. Neurology 1981; 31: 237-242.
[72] Kish SJ, Perry TL, Hornykiewicz O. Benzodiazepine receptor binding in cerebellar cortex: observations in olivopontocerebellar atrophy. J Neurochem 1984; 42: 466-469.
[73] Albin RL, Gilman S. Autoradiographic localization of inhibitory and excitatory amino acid neurotransmitter receptors in human normal and olivopontocerebellar atrophy cerebellar cortex. Brain Res 1990; 522: 37-45.
[74] Gilman S, Koeppe RA, Junck L, Kluin KJ, Lohman M, St Laurent RT. Benzodiazepine receptor binding in cerebellar degenerations studied with positron emission tomography. Ann Neurol 1995; 38: 176-185.
[75] Gahring LC, Rogers SW, Twyman RE. Autoantibodies to glutamate receptor subunit GluR2 in nonFRDAmilial olivopontocerebellar degeneration. Neurology 1997; 48: 494-500.
[76] Duvoisin RC, Chokroverty S, Lepore F, Nicklas W. Glutamate dehydrogenase deficiency in patients with olivopontocerebellar atrophy. Neurology 1983; 33: 1322-1326.
[77] Duvoisin RC, Nicklas W, Ritchie V, Sage S, Chokroverty S. Low leukocyte glutamate dehydrogenase activity does not correlate with any particular type of multiple system atrophy. J Neurol Neurosurg Psychiatry 1988; 51: 1508-1511.
[78] Grossman A, Rosenberg RN, Warmoth L. Glutamate and malate dehydrogenase activities in Joseph disease and olivopontocerebellar atrophy. Neurology 1987; 37: 106-111.
[79] Kish SJ, Robitaille Y, El-Awar M, Clark B, Schut L, Ball MJ, et al. Striatal monoamine neurotransmitters and metabolites in dominantly inherited olivopontocerebellar atrophy. Neurology 1992; 42: 1573-1577.
[80] Rinne JO, Burn DJ, Mathias CJ, Quinn NP, Marsden CD, Brooks DJ. Positron emission tomography studies on the dopaminergic system and striatal opioid binding in the olivopontocerebellar atrophy variant of multiple system atrophy. Ann Neurol 1995; 37: 568-573.
[81] Pascual J, Pazos A, del Olmo E, Figols J, Leno C, Berciano J. Presynaptic parkinsonism in olivopontocerebellar atrophy: clinical, pathological, and neurochemical evidence. Ann Neurol 1991; 30: 425-428.
[82] Kish SJ, Schut L, Simmons J, Gilbert J, Chang LJ, Rebbetoy M. Brain acetylcholinesterase activity is markedly reduced in dominantly-inherited olivopontocerebellar atrophy. J Neurol Neurosurg Psychiatry 1988; 51: 544-548.
[83] Whitehouse PJ, Muramoto O, Troncoso JC, Kanazawa I. Neurotransmitter receptors in olivopontocerebellar atrophy: an autoradiographic study. Neurology 1986; 36: 193-197.

[84] Higgins JJ, Harley-White J, Kopin IJ. Low lumbar CSF concentrations of homovanilic acid in the autosomal dominant ataxias. J Neurol Neurosurg Psychiatry 1995; 58: 760.
[85] Botez MI, Young SN. Biogenic amine metabolites and thiamine in cerebrospinal fluid in heredo-degenerative ataxias. Can J Neurol Sci 2001; 28: 134-140.
[86] Orozco G, Estrada R, Perry TL, Araña J, Fernández R, González-Quevedo A, et al. Dominantly inherited olivopontocerebellar atrophy from Eastern Cuba. Clinical, neuropathological, and biochemical findings. J Neurol Sci 1989; 93: 37-50.
[87] Öz G, Iltis I, Hutter D, Thomas W, Bushara KO, Gomez CM. Distinct neurochemical profiles of spinocerebellar ataxias 1, 2, 6 and cerebellar multiple system atrophy. Cerebellum 2010; DOI 10.1007/s12311-010-0213-6.
[88] Perry TL, Kish SJ, Hinton D, Hansen S, Becker LE, Gelfand EW. Neurochemical abnormalities in a patient with ataxia-telangiectasia. Neurology 1984; 34: 187-191.
[89] Botez MI, Botez-Marquard T, Elie R, Pedraza OL, Goyette K, Lalonde R. Amantadine hydrochloride treatment in heredodegenerative ataxias: a double blind study. J Neurol Neurosurg Psychiatry 1996; 61: 259-264.
[90] Bonnet AM, Esteguy M, Tell G, Schechter PJ, Hardenberg J, Agid Y. A controlled study of oral vigabatrin (γ-vinilGABA) in patients with cerebellar ataxia. Can J Neurol Sci 1986; 13: 331-333.
[91] Currier RD, Collins GM, Subramony SH, Haerer AF. Treatment of hereditary ataxia with the levorotatory form of hydroxytryptophan. Arch Neurol 1995; 52: 440-441.
[92] Assadi M, Campellone JV, Janson CG, Veloski JJ, Schwartzman RJ, Leone P. Treatment of spinocerebellar ataxia with buspirone. J Neurol Sci 2007; 260: 143-146.
[93] Heo JH, Lee ST, Chu K, Kim M. The efficacy of combined estrogen and buspirone treatment in olivopontocerebellar atrophy. J Neurol Sci 2008; 271: 87-90.
[94] Kark RAP, Budelli MAR, Wachsner R. Double-blind, triple-crossover trial of low doses of oral physostigmine in inherited ataxias. Neurology 1981; 31: 188-192.
[95] Finocchiaro G, Di Donato S, Madonna M, Fusi R, Ladinsky H, Consolo S. An approach using lecithin treatment for olivopontocerebellar atrophies. Eur Neurol 1985; 24: 414-421.
[96] Lawrence CM, Millac P, Stout GS, Ward JW. The use of choline chloride in ataxic disorders. J Neurol Neurosurg Psychiatry 1980; 43: 452-454.
[97] Harding AE. The hereditary ataxias and related disorders. Edinburgh, Churchill Livingstone, 1984.
[98] Pourcher E, Barbeau A. Field testing of an ataxia scoring and staging system. Can J Neurol Sci 1980; 7: 339-344.
[99] Sorbi S, Forleo P, FRDAni C, Piacentini S. Double-blind, crossover, placebo-controlled clinical trial with L-acetylcarnitine in patients with degenerative cerebellar ataxia. Clin Neuropharmacol 2000; 23: 114-118.
[100] Mori M, Adachi Y, Mori N, Kurihara S, Kashiwaya Y, Kusumi M, et al. Double-blind crossover study of branched-chain amino acid therapy in patients with spinocerebellar degeneration. J Neurol Sci 2002; 195: 149-152.
[101] Clauss R, Sathekge M, Nel W. Transient improvement of spinocerebellar ataxia witrh zolpidem. N Engl J Med 2004; 351: 511-512.
[102] Ristori G, Romano S, Visconti A, Cannoni S, Spadaro M, Frontali M, et al. Riluzole in cerebellar ataxia. A randomized, double-blind, placebo-controlled trial. Neurology 2010; 74: 839-845.

[103] Gazulla J, Benavente I. Mejoría sintomática de la atrofia olivopontocerebelosa con gabapentina. Rev Neurol 2005; 40: 285-288
[104] Duhigg WJ. Effects of propranolol on ataxic syndromes. Arch Neurol 1985; 42: 15.
[105] Buoni S, Zannolli R, Sorrentino L, Fois A. Betamethasone and improvement of neurological symptoms in ataxia-telangiectasia. Arch Neurol 2006; 63: 1479-1482.
[106] Gazulla J, Benavente I, Sarasa M. Ataxia-telangiectasia del adulto. Observación clínica y terapéutica. Neurología 2006; 21: 447-451.
[107] Harding AE. Friedreich´s ataxia: a clinical and genetic study of 90 families with an analysis of early diagnostic criteria and intrafamilial clustering of clinical features. Brain 1981; 104: 589-620.
[108] Koeppen AH. Neuropathology of the inherited ataxias. In: Manto MU, Pandolfo M, editors. The cerebellum and its disorders. Cambridge: Cambridge University Press, 2002: 387-405.
[109] Pandolfo M. The molecular basis of Friedreich ataxia. Neurología 2000; 59: 325-329.
[110] Butterworth RF, Giguere JF. Glutamic acid in spinal-cord gray matter in Friedreich´s ataxia. N Engl J Med 1982; 307: 897.
[111] Butterworth RF, Giguere JF. Amino acids in autopsied human spinal cord. Selective changes in Friedreich´s ataxia. Neurochem Pathol 1984; 2: 7-17.
[112] Huxtable R, Azari J, Reisine T, Johnson P, Yamamura H, Barbeau A. Regional distribution of amino acids in Friedreich´s ataxia brains. Can J Neurol Sci 1979; 6: 255-258.
[113] Bonnet AM, Tell G, Schechter PJ, Grove J, Saint-Hilaire MH, de Smet Y, et al. Cerebrospinal fluid GABA and homocarnosine concentration in patients with Friedreich´s ataxia, Parkinson´s disease, and Huntington´s chorea. Mov Disord 1987; 2: 117-123.
[114] Chavoix C, Samson Y, Pappata S, Prenant C, Maziere M, Seck A, et al. Positron emission tomography study of brain benzodiazepine receptors in Friedreich´s ataxia. Can J Neurol Sci 1990; 17: 404-409.
[115] Filla A, De Michele G, Orefice G, Santorelli F, Trombetta L, Banfi S, et al. A double-blind cross-over trial of amantadine hydrochloride in Friedreich´s ataxia. Can J Neurol Sci 1993; 20: 52-55.
[116] De Smet Y, Mear JY, Tell G, Schechter PH, Lhermitte F, Agid Y. Effect of gamma-vinyl GABA in Friedreich´s ataxia. Can J Neurol Sci 1982; 9: 171- 173.
[117] Rustin P, von Kleist-Retzow JC, Chantrel-Groussard K, Sidi D, Munnich A, Rotig A. Effect of idebenone on cardiomyopathy in Friedreich´s ataxia: a preliminary study. Lancet 1999; 354: 477-479.
[118] Mariotti C, Solari A, Torta D, Marano L, Florentini C, Di Donato S. Idebenone treatment in Friedreich patients: one-year-long randomized placebo-controlled trial. Neurology 2003; 60: 1676-1679.
[119] Buyse G, Mertens L, Di Salvo G, Matthijs I, Weidemann F, Eyskens B, et al. Idebenone treatment in Friedreich's ataxia: neurological, cardiac, and biochemical monitoring. Neurology 2003; 60: 1679-1681.
[120] Ribat P, Pousset F, Tanguy ML, Rivaud-Pechoux S, Le Ber I, Gasparini F, et al. Neurological, cardiological, and oculomotor progression in 104 patients with Friedreich ataxia during long-term follow-up. Arch Neurol 2007; 64: 558-564.
[121] Rinaldi C, Tucci T, Maione S, Giunta A, De Michele G, Filla A. Low-dose idebenone treatment in Friedreich's ataxia with and without cardiac hypertrophy. J Neurol 2009; 256: 1434-1437.

[122] Lagedrost S, Sutton MSJ, Cohen MS, Satou GM, Kaufman BD, Perlman SL, et al. Idebenone in Friedreich ataxia cardiomyopathy-results from a 6-month phase III study (IONIA). Am Heart J 2011; 161: 639-645.

[123] Artuch R, Aracil A, Mas A, et al. Friedreich's ataxia: Idebenone treatment in early stage patients. Neuropediatrics 2002; 33: 190-193.

[124] Di Prospero NA, Sumner CJ, Penzak SR, Ravina B, Fischbeck KH, Taylor JP. Safety, tolerability and pharmacokinetics of high-dose idebenone in patients with Friedreich ataxia. Arch Neurol 2007; 64: 803-808.

[125] Schulz JB, Di Prospero NA, Fischbeck K. Clinical experience with high-dose idebenone in Friedreich ataxia. J Neurol 2009; 256 (suppl 1): 42-45.

[126] Di Prospero NA, Baker A, Jeffries N, Fischbeck KH. Neurological effects of high-dose idebenone in patients with Friedreich's ataxia: a randomized, placebo-controlled trial. Lancet Neurol 2007; 6: 878-886.

[127] Lynch DR, Perlman SL, Meier T. A phase 3, placebo-controlled trial of idebenone in Friedreich ataxia. Arch Neurol 2010; 67: 941-947.

[128] Mancuso M, Orsucci D, Choub A, Siciliano G. Current and emerging treatment options in the management of Friedreich ataxia. Neuropsychiatr Dis Treat 2010; 6: 491-499.

[129] Trouillas P, Serratrice G, Laplane D, Rascol A, Augustin P, Barroche G, et al. Levorotatory form of 5-hydroxytryptophan in Friedreich´s ataxia. Results of a double-blind drug-placebo cooperative study. Arch Neurol 1995; 52: 456-460.

[130] Peterson PL, Saad J, Nigro MA. The treatment of Friedreich´s ataxia with amantadine hydrochloride. Neurology 1988; 38: 1478-1480.

[131] Sturm B, Helminger M, Steinkellner H, Heidai MM, Goldenberg H, Scheiber-Mojdehkar B. Carbamylated erythropoietin increases frataxin independent from the erythropoietin receptor. Eur J Clin Invest 2010; 40: 561-565.

[132] Boesch S, Sturm B, Hering S, Goldenberg H, Poewe W, Scheiber-Mojdehkar B. Friedreich's ataxia: clinical pilot trial with recombinant human erythropoietin. Ann Neurol 2007; 62: 521-524.

[133] Boesch S, Sturm B, Hering S, Scheiber-Mojdehkar B, Steinkellner H, Goldenberg H, Poewe W. Neurological effects of recombinant human erythropoietin in Friedreich's ataxia: a clinical pilot trial. Mov Disord 2008; 23: 1940-1944.

[134] Boddaert N, Le Quan Sang KH, Rötig A, Leroy-Willig A, Gallet S, Brunelle F, Sidi D, et al. Selective iron chelation in Friedreich ataxia: biologic and clinical implications. Blood. 2007; 110: 401-8.

[135] Tsou AY, Friedman LS, Wilson RB, Lynch DR. Pharmacotherapy for Friedreich ataxia. CNS Drugs 2009; 2009: 213-223.

[136] Liu J, Verma PJ, Evans-Galea MV, Delatycki MB, Michalska A, Leung J, et al. Generation of induced pluripotent stem cell lines from Friedreich ataxia patients. Stem Cell Rev 2010; doi: 10.1007/s12015-010-9210-x.

[137] Hammans SR. The inherited ataxias and the new genetics. J Neurol Neurosurg Psychiatry 1996; 61: 327-332.

[138] Subramony SH, Vig PJS. Spinocerebellar ataxia type 3. In: Manto MU, Pandolfo M, editors. The cerebellum and its disorders. Cambridge: Cambridge University Press, 2002: 428-439.

[139] Kitamura J, Kubuki Y, Tsuruta K, Kurihara T, Matsukara S. A new FRDAmily with Joseph disease in Japan. Homovanillic acid, magnetic resonance, and sleep apnea studies. Arch Neurol 1989; 46: 425-428.

[140] Sakai T, Antoku Y, Matsuishi T, Iwashita H. Tetrahydrobiopterin double-blind crossover trial in Machado-Joseph disease. J Neurol Sci 1996; 136: 71-72.
[141] Schulte T, Mattern R, Berger K, Szymanski S, Klotz P, Kraus PH, et al. Double-blind crossover trial of trimethoprim-sulfamethoxazole in spinocerebellar ataxia type 3/Machado-Joseph disease. Arch Neurol 2001; 58: 1451-1457.
[142] Sakai T, Matsuishi T, Yamada S, Komori H, Iwashita H. Sulfamethoxazole-trimethoprim double-blind, placebo-controlled, crossover trial in Machado-Joseph disease: sulFRDAmethoxazole-trimethoprim increases cerebrospinal fluid level of biopterin. J Neural Transm Gen Sect 1995; 102: 159-172.
[143] Mello KA, Abbott BP. Effect of sulfamethoxazole and trimethoprim on neurologic dysfunction in a patient with Joseph´s disease. Arch Neurol 1988; 45: 210-213.
[144] Sangla S, De Boucker T, Cheron F, Cambier J, Dehen H. Amélioration d´une maladie de Joseph par le sulfaméthoxazole-triméthoprime. Rev Neurol (Paris) 1990; 146: 213-214.
[145] Azulay JP, Blin O, Mestre D, Sangla I, Serratrice G. Contrast sensitivity improvement with sulfamethoxazole and trimethoprim in a patient with Machado-Joseph disease without spasticity. J Neurol Sci 1994; 123: 95-99.
[146] Monte TL, Rieder CRM, Tort AB, Rockennback I, Pereira ML, Silveira I, et al. Use of fluoxetine for treatment of Machado-Joseph disease: an open-label study. Acta Neurol Scand 2003; 107: 207-210.
[147] Takei A, Fukazawa T, Hamada T, Sohma H, Yabe I, Sasaki H, et al. Effects of tandospirone on "5-HTA1 receptor-associated symptoms" in patients with Machado-Joseph disease: an open-label study. Clin Neuropharmacol 2004; 27: 9-13.
[148] Kanai K, Kuwabara S, Arai K, Sung JY, Ogawara K, Hattori T. Muscle cramp in Machado-Joseph disease: altered motor axonal excitability properties and mexiletine treatment. Brain 2003; 126: 965-973.
[149] Liu C-S, Hsu H-M, Cheng W-L, Hsieh M. Clinical and molecular events in patients with Machado-Joseph disease under lamotrigine therapy. Acta Neurol Scand 2005; 111: 385-390.
[150] Tsuji S. Dentatorubral-pallidoluysian atrophy. In: Manto MU, Pandolfo M, editors. The cerebellum and its disorders. Cambridge: Cambridge University Press, 2002: 481-490.
[151] Iizuka R, Hirayama K. Dentato-rubro-pallido-luysian atrophy. In: Vynken PJ, Bruyn GW, Klawans HL, editors. Handbook of Clinical Neurology, volume 5 (49). Amsterdam: Elsevier Science Publishers, 1986: 437-443.
[152] Smith JK. Dentatorubropallidoluysian atrophy. In: Vynken PJ, Bruyn GW, editors. Handbook of Clinical Neurology, volumen 21. Amsterdam: Elsevier North Holland, 1975: 519-534.
[153] Yamada M, Sato T, Tsuji S, Takahashi H. Oligodendrocytic polyglutamine pathology in dentatorubral-pallidoluysian atrophy. Ann Neurol 2002; 52: 670-674.
[154] Kanazawa I, Sasaki H, Muramoto O, Matsushita M, Mizutani Y, Iwabuchi K, et al. Studies on neurotransmitter markers and striatal neuronal cell density in Huntington´s disease and dentatorubropallidoluysian atrophy. J Neurol Sci 1985; 70: 151-165.
[155] Miyata R, Hayashi M, Tanuma N, Shioda K, Fukatsu R, Mizutani S. Oxidative stress in neurodegeneration in dentatorubral-pallidoluysian atrophy. J Neurol Sci 2008; 264: 133-139.

[156] Berciano J, Infante J, Mateo I, Combarros O. Ataxias y paraplejías hereditarias: revisión clínicogenética. Neurología 2002; 17: 40-51.

[157] Adelman JP, Bond CT, Pessia M, Maylie J. Episodic ataxia results from voltage-dependent potassium channels with altered functions. Neuron 1995; 15: 1449-1554.

[158] Rajakulendran S, Schorge S, Kullmann DM, Hanna MG. Episodic ataxia type 1: a neuronal potassium channelopathy. Neurotherapeutics 2007; 4: 258-266.

[159] Tomlinson SE, Tan SV, Kullmann DM, Griggs RC, Burke D, Hanna MG, Bostock H. Nerve excitability studies characterize Kv1.1 fast potassium channel dysfunction in patients with episodic ataxia type 1. Brain 2010; 133: 3530-3540.

[160] Brunt ERP, van Weerden TW. Familial paroxysmal kinesegenic ataxia and continuous myokimia. Brain 1990; 113: 1361-1382.

[161] D'Adamo MC, Imbrici P, Pessia M. Episodic ataxias as ion channel diseases. In: Manto MU, Pandolfo M, editors. The cerebellum and its disorders. Cambridge: Cambridge University Press, 2002: 562-572.

[162] Spacey SD, Hildebrand ME, Materek LA, Bird TD, Snutch TP. Functional implications of a novel EA2 mutation in the P/Q-type calcium channel. Ann Neurol 2004; 56: 213-220.

[163] Cuenca-León E, Banchs I, Serra SA, Latorre P, Fernàndez-Castillo N, Corominas R, et al. Late-onset episodic ataxia type 2 associated with a novel loss-of-function mutation in the CACNA1A gene. J Neurol Sci 2009; 280: 10-14.

[164] Steckley JL, Ebers GC, Cader MZ, McLachlan RS. An autosomal dominant disorder with episodic ataxia, vertigo, and tinnitus. Neurology 2001; 57: 1499-1502.

[165] Cader MZ, Steckley JL, Dyment DA, McLachlan RS. A genome-wide screen and linkage mapping for a large pedigree with episodic ataxia. Neurology 2005; 65: 156-158.

[166] Farmer TW, Mustian VM. Vestibulocerebellar ataxia. A newly defined hereditary syndrome with periodic manifestations. Arch Neurol 1963; 8: 21-30.

[167] Small K, Pollock SC. Ocular motility in North Carolina autosomal dominant ataxia. J Neuroophthalmol 1996; 16: 91-95.

[168] Damji KF, Allingham RR, Pollock SC, Small K, Lewis KE, Stajich JM, et al. Periodic vestibulocerebellar ataxia, an autosomal dominant ataxia with defective smooth pursuit, is genetically distinct from other autosomal dominant ataxias. Arch Neurol 1996; 53: 338-344.

[169] Escayg A, De Waard M, Lee DD, Bichet D, Wolf P, Mayer T, et al. Coding and noncoding variation of the human calcium-channel beta(4)-subunit gene CACNB4 in patients with idiopathic generalized epilepsy and episodic ataxia. Am J Hum Genet 2000; 66: 1531-1539.

[170] Jen JC, Wan J, Palos TP, Howard BD, Baloh R. Mutation in the glutamate transporter EAAT1 causes episodic ataxia, hemiplegia, and seizures. Neurology 2005; 65: 529-534.

[171] Matilla-Dueñas A, Sánchez I, Corral-Juan M, Dávalos A, Alvarez R, Latorre P. Cellular and molecular pathways triggering neurodegeneration in the spinocerebellar ataxias. Cerebellum 2010; 9: 148-166.

[172] Schöls L, Bauer P, Schmidt T, Schulte T, Riess O. Autosomal dominant cerebellar ataxias: clinical features, genetics, and pathogenesis. Lancet Neurol 2004; 3: 291-304.